Hepatobiliary Disorders

Hepatobiliary Disorders

Edited by Gracie Douglas

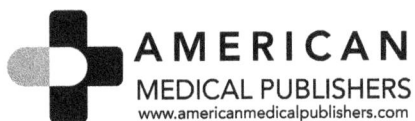

AMERICAN
MEDICAL PUBLISHERS
www.americanmedicalpublishers.com

American Medical Publishers,
41 Flatbush Avenue,
1st Floor, New York,
NY 11217, USA

Visit us on the World Wide Web at:
www.americanmedicalpublishers.com

ISBN: 978-1-63927-193-1

Cataloging-in-Publication Data

    Hepatobiliary disorders / edited by Gracie Douglas.
       p. cm.
    Includes bibliographical references and index.
    ISBN 978-1-63927-193-1
    1. Liver--Diseases. 2. Biliary tract--Diseases. I. Douglas, Gracie.
RC845 .H46 2022
616.362--dc23

Table of Contents

Preface

This book has been an outcome of determined endeavour from a group of educationists in the field. The primary objective was to involve a broad spectrum of professionals from diverse cultural background involved in the field for developing new researches. The book not only targets students but also scholars pursuing higher research for further enhancement of the theoretical and practical applications of the subject.

The study of liver and biliary disorders is undertaken within the field of hepatology. Liver diseases are caused by a variety of factors. Some of these are viral hepatitis and other infectious diseases, inflammatory liver conditions, conditions arising due to high alcohol consumption and toxins, malignant neoplasm of the liver and intrahepatic bile ducts, metabolic diseases and vascular disorders of the liver, etc. Diseases of the gallbladder and biliary tract include malignant neoplasms, cholecystitis, cholelithiasis, biliary dyskinesia, spasm of sphincter of Oddi, etc. The investigation of biliary and liver diseases is done through specialized imaging techniques. Non-invasive non-therapeutic investigations are possible with the aid of endoscopic ultrasound and magnetic resonance cholangiopancreatography. Endoscopic retrograde cholangiopancreatography combines fluoroscopy and endoscopy to diagnose and treat disorders of the biliary or pancreatic ductal systems. It can address inflammatory strictures, leaks acquired from surgery or trauma, and cancer. The anatomy of the biliary tract can be visualized with percutaneous transhepatic cholangiography. This book elucidates the causes, symptoms and pathophysiology of hepatobiliary diseases in a comprehensive manner. It strives to provide a fair idea about the modern practices in the management of hepatobiliary disorders. A number of latest researches have been included to keep the readers up-to-date with the global concepts in these medical conditions.

It was an honour to edit such a profound book and also a challenging task to compile and examine all the relevant data for accuracy and originality. I wish to acknowledge the efforts of the contributors for submitting such brilliant and diverse chapters in the field and for endlessly working for the completion of the book. Last, but not the least; I thank my family for being a constant source of support in all my research endeavours.

Editor

Surgical outcomes of hepatocellular carcinoma with biliary tumor thrombus

Wenhui Qiao[1†], Feng Yu[2†], Lupeng Wu [3], Bin Li [3] and Yanming Zhou[3*]

Abstract

Background: Hepatocellular carcinoma (HCC) with biliary tumor thrombus (BTT) is rare and its impact on postoperative prognosis remains controversial. The aim of this study was to evaluate the published evidence concerning the outcome of surgical resection of HCC with BTT.

Methods: Eligible studies were identified by searching PubMed and reviewed systematically. Comparisons of the clinicopathologic features and surgical outcomes for HCC patients with or without BTT were analyzed using meta-analytical techniques.

Results: Twenty retrospective studies containing 598 patients that met the selection criteria were included for review. The perioperative mortality was 2.1 % (range, 0–10 %), and the median 5-year overall survival (OS) was 24 % (range, 0–48 %) with a recurrence rate of 63.9 % (range, 42–91 %). Pooled analysis of 13 comparative studies showed that HCC patients with BTT had a higher incidence of vascular invasion (odds ratio [OR]: 4.70, 95 % CI: 2.90–7.60; P <0.001), a higher frequency of poor differentiation (OR: 2.07, 95 % CI: 1.23–3.49; P = 0.006), and a shorter 5-year OS rate (OR: 0.31, 95 % CI: 0.21–0.64; P <0.001) than those without BTT.

Conclusions: Although HCC with BTT has more aggressive biological characteristics and is an indicator of poor prognosis, surgical resection can still provide long-term survival for some patients.

Keywords: Hepatocellular carcinoma, Biliary tumor thrombus, Resection, Prognosis

Background

Hepatocellular carcinoma (HCC) is the fifth most common neoplasm in the world and is the third leading cause of cancer-related death worldwide, with more than 500 000 new cases diagnosed each year [1]. Surgical resection remains the mainstay of curative treatment for this disease. Portal vein thrombus is a frequent event in HCC and has important impact on patient survival after surgical resection [2], while biliary tumor thrombus (BTT) is relatively rare with a reported incidence of 0.53–12.9 % in autopsy and surgical specimens [3–9]. In this regard, few reports are available in the literature

addressing the role of surgical resection for this special clinical entity. In addition, the prognostic impact of BTT is controversial [5, 6, 9]. The current study assesses the published literature on surgical resection for HCC with BTT and compares the clinicopathologic features and long-term postoperative outcomes between HCC patients with BTT and those without BTT.

Methods
Systematic search strategy

A comprehensive systematic review of all published literature from 1966 to September 2015 was undertaken using PubMed database. The following Medical Subject Headings terms were used: "hepatocellular carcinoma," "biliary tumor thrombus," "bile duct tumor thrombus," and "bile duct thrombus." Reference lists of all retrieved articles were manually searched to identify further potentially relevant articles. This study was performed

* Correspondence: zhouymsxy@sina.cn
†Equal contributors
3Department of Hepato-Biliary-Pancreato-Vascular Surgery, First affiliated Hospital of Xiamen University, Xiamen, China
Full list of author information is available at the end of the article

according to Preferred Reporting Items for Systematic Reviews and Meta-analyses (PRISMA) guideline guidelines [10].

Inclusion and exclusion criteria

English language studies with a sample size of at least 10 patients that reported long-term survival data following surgical resection for HCC with BTT were included. Animal studies, letters, reviews, abstracts, editorials, expert opinions, duplicates, studies with fewer than 10 patients, studies involving patients who were treated with nonsurgical management or liver transplantation were excluded.

Data extraction and quality assessment

Information on study design, first author, country or region, year of publication, study population characteristics, and outcomes of interest were independently extracted by two authors (Yanming Zhou and Feng Yu). Discrepancies between the two reviewers were resolved by discussion and consensus. Study methodology quality was categorized according to the Evidence-based Medicine Levels of Evidence [11].

Macroscopic BTT was defined when it was present in the common hepatic duct or the first to second branches of the bile duct and microscopic BTT was defined when it was present in the third order or more peripheral branches of the bile duct [12].

The primary outcome measures were 1-, 3- and 5-year overall survival (OS) following surgical resection.

Statistical analysis

Data extracted for BTT group were reported as total and percentage for categorical variables and as median values and range for continuous variables, unless otherwise stated. The results of comparative studies of patients with BTT and without BTT were pooled by the use of Review Manager.software, version 5.1 (The Cochrane Collaboration, Software Update, Oxford). Dichotomous variables were expressed as odds ratio (OR) with a 95 % confidence interval (95 % CI), and continuous variables were expressed as the weighted mean difference (WMD) with a 95 % CI. χ^2 test and I^2 were used to assess heterogeneity between studies. The random-effect model was used if there was significant heterogeneity ($P < 0.1$); otherwise, the fixed-effect model was used. Publication bias was evaluated via funnel plot. Statistical significance was set at $P < 0.05$.

Results

Systematic review

Among 154 potentially relevant papers identified by the initial search, 20 finally met the inclusion criteria in this review and are summarised in Table 1 [3–9, 12–26]. All studies were retrospectively designed, originated from Asia (Japan, $n = 8$ [5, 6, 12, 13, 15, 20, 21, 25]; Mainland China, $n = 7$ [7, 8, 14, 16, 17, 19, 26]; Korea, $n = 2$ [18, 22]; Taiwan, $n = 1$ [9]; India, $n = 1$ [23]; Hong Kong, $n = 1$ [24]) and classified as level-4 evidence. The sample size of each study varied from 13 to 73 patients. Thirteen studies utilised patients without BTT as a control group for comparison [5, 6, 9, 13, 15–17, 19–24].

The included papers described 598 patients who underwent surgical resection for HCC with BTT, including 526 (88 %) patients who had macroscopic BTT and 72 (12 %) patients who had microscopic BTT. Most (80.2 %, 441/550) patients were men. The median or mean age ranged from 47.1 to 60 (median = 54.2) years. Hepatitis B surface antigen (HBsAg) and hepatitis C virus antibody (Anti-HCV) were positive in 60.7 % (324/533) and 14.9 % (50/335) of patients, respectively. Mean or median tumor size ranged from 3.8 to 6.4 (median = 5.4) cm. Cirrhosis, tumor multiplicity, vascular invasion, poor differentiation, intrahepatic metastasis, and tumor capsule absence, occurred in 60.4 % (229/379), 36.8 % (127/345), 67.1 % (306/456), 47.9 % (188/392), 31.6 % (92/291), and 66.7 % (140/210) of patients, respectively.

Table 2 shows the operative intervention and postoperative outcomes. Among 573 patients with available information, hepatectomy with or without tumor thrombectomy was carried out in 423 (73.8 %), followed by hepatectomy combined bile duct resection in 144 (25.1 %), thrombectomy only in 4 (0.7 %), and thrombectomy with hepatic artery ligation and cannulation in 2 (0.35 %). There were 13 perioperative deaths (2.1 %) (range, 0–10 %). The median overall survival was 26.1 months (range, 11.4–47 months). The median 1-, 3- and 5-year OS rates were 72 % (range, 38–93 %), 39 % (range, 11–77 %) and 24 % (range, 0–48 %), respectively. Disease recurrence developed in 64.8 % (310/478) patients.

Meta-analysis

A total of 13 comparative studies including 334 patients with BTT and 6361 without BTT were included for analysis [5, 6, 9, 13, 15–17, 19–24]. Table 3 presents a summary of outcomes. Table 3 presents a summary of the outcomes. There was no significant difference in clinicopathological characteristics between the two groups in terms of sex, age, hepatitis viral status (hepatitis B or C virus), presence of cirrhosis, tumor size and multiplicity, tumor capsule absence, and intrahepatic metastasis, while vascular invasion (OR: 4.70, 95 % CI: 2.90–7.60; P <0.001) and poor differentiation (OR: 2.07, 95 % CI: 1.23–3.49; P = 0.006) were more frequently observed in BTT group than those in non-BTT group.

The 1-, 3- and 5-year OS rates in patients with BTT were significantly lower than those in patients without BTT (OR: 0.48, 95 % CI: 0.31–0.73; P <0.001; OR: 0.45, 95 % CI: 0.29–0.680; P <0.001; OR: 0.31, 95 % CI: 0.21 – 0.64; P < 0.001, respectively) (Figs. 1, 2 and 3).

Table 1 Clinical background of included studies

First author (Year)	No.	M/F	Age (years)[a]	BTT type Ma/Mi	HBsAg n (%)	Anti-HCV n (%)	Cirrhosis n (%)	TS (cm)[a]	MT n (%)	VI n (%)	PD n (%)	IM n (%)	TCA n (%)
Satoh (2000) [5]	17	15/2	58.2	17/0	5 (29.4)	–	–	–	–	11 (64.8)	5 (29.4)	–	–
Shiomi (2001) [6]	17	15/2	58.8	17/0	7 (46.7)	3 (17.6)	6 (35 %)	6.1	12/16 (75)	13 (76)	0 (0)	5 (29)	–
Peng (2004) [7]	15[b]	10/5	49	15/0	13 (86.7)	–	–	5.1	2 (13.3)	5 (33.3)	–	–	–
Qin (2004) [8]	34	28/6	48.5	34/0	34 (100)	–	32 (94.1)	6.4	–	–	–	–	34 (100)
Yeh (2004) [9]	17	14/3	52.3	17/0	–	–	–	3.8	–	12/16 (75)	3/11 (27.2)	5/16 (83.3)	2/11 (18.2)
Esaki (2005) [12]	38	32/6	62	19/19	8 (21.1)	–	10 (26.3)	6.2	19 (50)	27 (71)	11 (28.9)	19 (50)	–
Ikenaga (2009) [13]	15	12/3	66	10/5	4 (27.7)	7 (46.7)	–	5.0	6 (40)	12/14 (85.7)	–	10 (66.7)	2 (13.3)
Luo (2009) [14]	48[c]	–	–	48/0	–	–	–	6.2	–	–	–	–	–
Noda (2011) [15]	22	21/1	58	22/0	15 (68.1)	5 (22.7)	6 (27.2)	>5, n=9	20 (90.9)	13 (59)	18 (81.8)	–	–
Shao (2011) [16]	27	24/3	47.1	24/3	26 (96.7)	0 (0)	18 (66.7)	>5, n=10	–	17 (62.9)	26 (96.3)	5 (18.5)	21 (77.7)
Yu (2011) [17]	20[d]	17/3	50.6	20/0	16 (80)	–	14 (70)	4.5	–	12 (60)	13 (65)	4 (20)	15 (75)
Moon (2013) [18]	73	52/21	54.2	73/0	59 (80.8)	2 (2.8)	62 (84.9)	5.8	11 (15)	53 (72.6)	54 (74)	25 (34.2)	–
Meng (2014) [19]	35	24/11	51.3	28/7	26 (74.3)	0 (0)	25 (65.8)	>5, n=24	15 (42.8)	10 (25.8)	10 (25.8)	–	24 (68.6)
Oba (2014) [20]	13	12/1	61	13/0	4 (30.7)	5 (38.5)	3 (23)	4.4	2 (15.4)	12 (92.3)	–	–	–
Kasai (2015) [21]	44	35/9	64	44/0	8 (18.2)	21 (52.5)	14 (31.8)	5.8	16 (36.4)	31 (70.4)	18 (40.9)	8 (25.8)	–
Kim (2015) [22]	31	21/10	53	0/31	26 (83.9)	1 (3.2)	–	4.8	–	28 (90.3)	1 (3.2)	–	7 (22.5)
Rammohan (2015) [23]	39	28/11	52.1	39/0	7 (17.9)	2 (5.1)	Excluded	5.6	–	–	–	–	–
Wong (2015) [24]	37	29/8	57	37/0	30 (81.1)	–	–	6	15 (29.7)	25 (67.6)	11 (29.7)	–	35 (94.6)
Yamamoto (2015) [25]	19	19/0	67	19/0	7 (36.8)	4 (21)	6 (31.5)	4.3	–	–	–	–	–
Zeng (2015) [26]	37	33/4	50	30/7	29 (78.4)	–	33 (89.2)	4.9	9 (24.3)	25 (67.5)	23 (62.2)	6 (16.2)	–

M male, F female, Ma macroscopic, Mi microscopic, HBsAg hepatitis B surface antigen, anti-HCV hepatitis C virus antibody, ST solitary tumor, TS tumor size, MT multiple tumor, VI vascular invasion, PD poor differentiation, IM intrahepatic metastasis, TCA tumor capsule absence

[a] mean or median

[b] including 1 patients underwent liver transplantation; [c] including 5 patients underwent liver transplantation; [d] including 2 patients underwent liver transplantation

Table 2 Operative intervention and outcomes

References	Hx ± Tb n (%)	Hx + BDR n (%)	Tb only n (%)	Mortality n (%)	Median survival (Months)	Overall survival (%) 1-year 3-years 5-years	Recurrence n (%)
5	12 (70.6)	5 (29.4)	0 (0)	0 (0)	–	58 30 16	10/15 (66.7)
6	12 (70.6)	5 (29.4)	0 (0)	0 (0)	17.6	75 47 28	11 (64.7)
7	7 (50)	4 (28.5)	3 (21.4)	1 (7.1)	14	73 51 21	7 (100)
8	30 (88.2)	1 (2.9)	1 (2.9)	1 (2.9)	–	71 11 –	14/28 (50)
9	–	–	–	1 (5.9)	20.8	60 20 6.7	11/16 (68.7)
12	33 (86.8)	5 (13.2)	0 (0)	0 (0)	31	79 45 33	29 (76.3)
13	12 (80)	3 (20)	0 (0)	0 (0)	11.4	46 23 0	11 (73.3)
14	40 (93)	3 (7)	0 (0)	1 (2.1)	37	93 56 24	10 (21)
15	20 (90.9)	2 (9.1)	0 (0)	0 (0)	–	62 30 30	13/16 (81.2)
16	26 (96.3)	1 (3.7)	0 (0)	1 (3.7)	–	70 26 7.4	25/26 (96.1)
17	12 (66.7)	6 (33.3)	0 (0)	2 (10)	–	73 21 –	7/13 (53.8)
18	42 (57.5)	31 (42.5)	0 (0)	3 (4.1)	–	77 41 32	52/70 (74.3)
19	25 (71.4)	10 (28.6)	0 (0)	0 (0)	19	38 20 11	–
20	7 (53.8)	6 (46.2)	0 (0)	0 (0)	47	92 77 48	6 (46.1)
21	37 (84)	7 (16)	0 (0)	2 (4.5)	23.7	70 38 31	30/41 (73.2)
22	31 (100)	0 (0)	0 (0)	0 (0)	–	90 61 –	20 (64.5)
23	30 (76.9)	9 (23.1)	0 (0)	2 (5.1)	28.6	82 48 10	–
24	9 (24.3)	28 (75.7)	0 (0)	0 (0)	44	69 54 39	23 (62.1)
25	15 (78.9)	4 (21.1)	0 (0)	0 (0)	–	82 39 32	10/15 (66.7)
26	23 (62.2)	14 (37.8)	0 (0)	0 (0)	–	64 24 18	21 (56.8)

Hx hepatectomy, *Tb* thrombectomy, *BDR* bile duct resection

Table 3 Results of meta-analysis comparing hepatocellular carcinoma with or without biliary tumor thrombus

Outcome of interest	No. of studies	No. of patients BTT Non-BTT	OR/WMD	95 % CI	P value	HG P value
Clinicopathological characteristics						
Male	12	317 5806	1.07	0.97, 1.43	0.67	0.69
Age	9	256 3840	0.01	−1.01, 1.02	0.99	0.01
Hepatitis B surface antigen	11	297 5150	1.33	0.99, 1.79	0.06	0.35
Hepatitis C virus antibody	9	243 4274	0.72	0.37, 1.39	0.33	0.03
Cirrhosis	6	158 3569	0.72	0.51, 1.00	0.05	0.11
Tumor size	7	177 4028	−0.89	−2.63, 0.85	0.32	<0.001
Multiple tumor	6	166 3662	1.85	0.76, 4.52	0.18	<0.001
Tumor capsule absence	7	176 2305	1.26	0.63, 2.51	0.62	0.02
Intrahepatic metastases	5	109 1710	1.47	0.93, 2.33	0.10	0.40
Vscular invasion	12	293 5939	4.70	2.90, 7.60	<0.001	0.001
Poor differentiation	8	227 4003	2.07	1.23, 3.49	0.006	0.05
Long-term outcomes						
1-year overall survival	12	280 4739	0.48	0.31, 0.72	<0.001	0.02
3-year overall survival	12	280 4739	0.45	0.29, 0.68	<0.001	0.007
5-year overall survival	10	231 4021	0.31	0.21, 0.64	<0.001	0.02

BTT biliary tumor thrombus, *OR* odds ratio, *WMD* weighted mean difference, *CI* confidence interval, *HG* heterogeneity

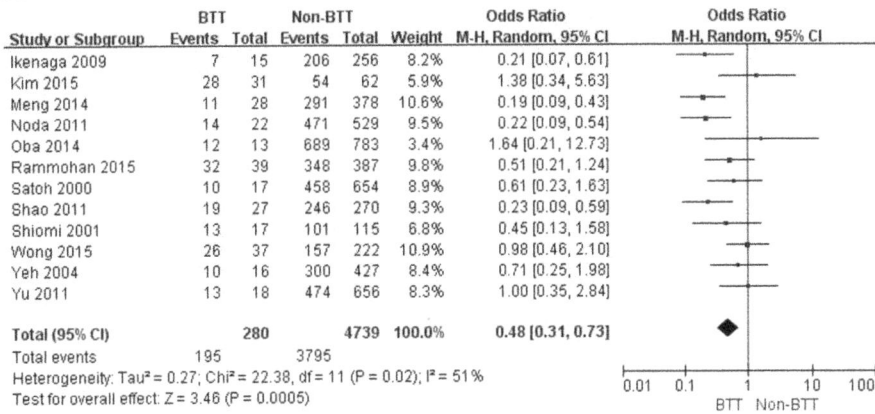

Study or Subgroup	BTT Events	Total	Non-BTT Events	Total	Weight	Odds Ratio M-H, Random, 95% CI
Ikenaga 2009	7	15	206	256	8.2%	0.21 [0.07, 0.61]
Kim 2015	28	31	54	62	5.9%	1.38 [0.34, 5.63]
Meng 2014	11	28	291	378	10.6%	0.19 [0.09, 0.43]
Noda 2011	14	22	471	529	9.5%	0.22 [0.09, 0.54]
Oba 2014	12	13	689	783	3.4%	1.64 [0.21, 12.73]
Rammohan 2015	32	39	348	387	9.8%	0.51 [0.21, 1.24]
Satoh 2000	10	17	458	654	8.9%	0.61 [0.23, 1.63]
Shao 2011	19	27	246	270	9.3%	0.23 [0.09, 0.59]
Shiomi 2001	13	17	101	115	6.8%	0.45 [0.13, 1.58]
Wong 2015	26	37	157	222	10.9%	0.98 [0.46, 2.10]
Yeh 2004	10	16	300	427	8.4%	0.71 [0.25, 1.98]
Yu 2011	13	18	474	656	8.3%	1.00 [0.35, 2.84]
Total (95% CI)		280		4739	100.0%	0.48 [0.31, 0.73]
Total events	195		3795			

Heterogeneity: Tau² = 0.27; Chi² = 22.38, df = 11 (P = 0.02); I² = 51%
Test for overall effect: Z = 3.46 (P = 0.0005)

Fig. 1 Result of the meta-analysis on 1-year overall survival

Discussion

HCC patients with BTT usually respond poorly to nonsurgical treatments, such as transcatheter arterial chemoembolization (TACE), percutaneous transhepatic biliary drainage, and radiation. Oba et al. [20] reported that the 1-, 3-, and 5-year OS rate in their 25 patients was 14 %, 5 % and 0 % after nonsurgical treatment, respectively. Luo et al. [14] reported a 5-year OS rate of 0 % for patients treated with TACE (n = 27) or biliary decompression (n = 40). In this study, patients who received surgical resection had a 5-year OS rate of 24 %, which is far better than the results of the nonsurgical treatments discussed above. So it seems justified to carry out surgical resection for this group of patients.

We found that long-term survival in patients with BTT was significantly shorter than that in patients without BTT. This may be a consequence of the fact that BTT has more aggressive biologically characteristics. As

showed in the current study, the incidence of vascular invasion and poor differentiation, two powerful unfavorable prognostic factors, were more frequently observed in BTT group than those in non-BTT group.

The high incidence of postoperative recurrence limits the potential for surgical cure of HCC. Postoperative recurrence is usually classified as early (≤1 year) and late (>1 year) recurrence. Early recurrence was found to be associated with worse prognosis compared with late recurrence.[27] Ikenaga et al. [13] reported that 53 % of their patients in BTT group developed recurrences in the remnant liver within 3 months after surgery. Qin [8], Noda [15], Shao [16], Zeng [26] and their colleagues reported that more than 50 % of their BTT patients experienced recurrences during the first year after surgery. Shao et al. [16] found that patients with BTT had a higher rate of early recurrence than those without BTT (70.3 % vs. 34.8 %; P < 0.001). In aggregate, these results suggest that patients with BTT had a higher propensity for early recurrence. It is widely accepted that early recurrence is mainly caused by intrahepatic metastasis from the primary tumor via the venous circulation [27].

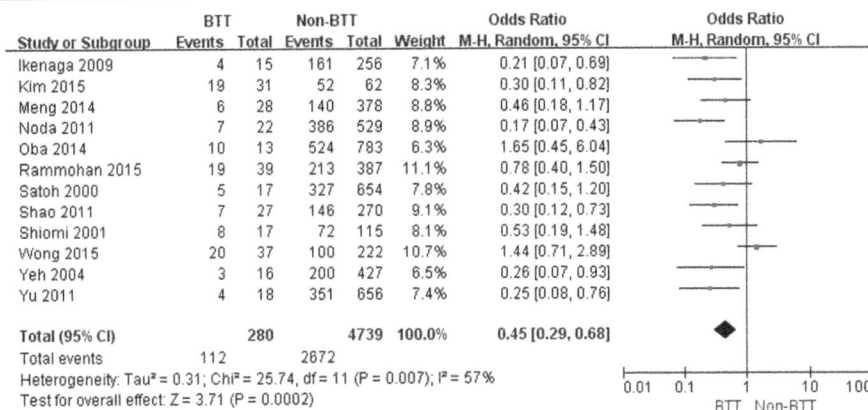

Study or Subgroup	BTT Events	Total	Non-BTT Events	Total	Weight	Odds Ratio M-H, Random, 95% CI
Ikenaga 2009	4	15	161	256	7.1%	0.21 [0.07, 0.69]
Kim 2015	19	31	52	62	8.3%	0.30 [0.11, 0.82]
Meng 2014	6	28	140	378	8.8%	0.46 [0.18, 1.17]
Noda 2011	7	22	386	529	8.9%	0.17 [0.07, 0.43]
Oba 2014	10	13	524	783	6.3%	1.65 [0.45, 6.04]
Rammohan 2015	19	39	213	387	11.1%	0.78 [0.40, 1.50]
Satoh 2000	5	17	327	654	7.8%	0.42 [0.15, 1.20]
Shao 2011	7	27	146	270	9.1%	0.30 [0.12, 0.73]
Shiomi 2001	8	17	72	115	8.1%	0.53 [0.19, 1.48]
Wong 2015	20	37	100	222	10.7%	1.44 [0.71, 2.89]
Yeh 2004	3	16	200	427	6.5%	0.26 [0.07, 0.93]
Yu 2011	4	18	351	656	7.4%	0.25 [0.08, 0.76]
Total (95% CI)		280		4739	100.0%	0.45 [0.29, 0.68]
Total events	112		2672			

Heterogeneity: Tau² = 0.31; Chi² = 25.74, df = 11 (P = 0.007); I² = 57%
Test for overall effect: Z = 3.71 (P = 0.0002)

Fig. 2 Result of the meta-analysis on 3-year overall survival

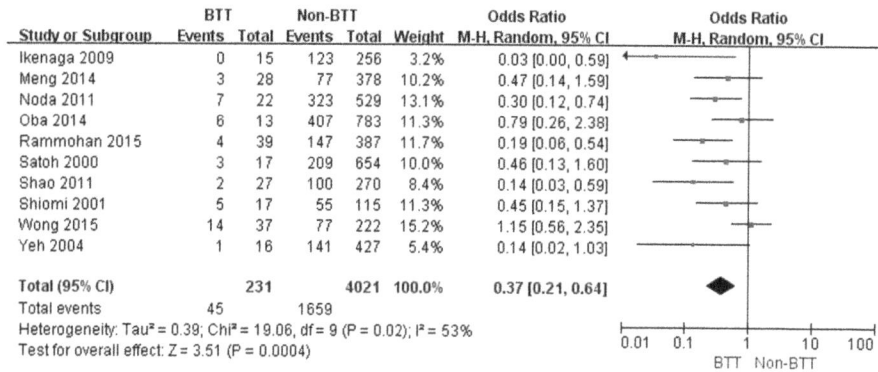

Study or Subgroup	BTT Events	Total	Non-BTT Events	Total	Weight	Odds Ratio M-H, Random, 95% CI
Ikenaga 2009	0	15	123	256	3.2%	0.03 [0.00, 0.59]
Meng 2014	3	28	77	378	10.2%	0.47 [0.14, 1.59]
Noda 2011	7	22	323	529	13.1%	0.30 [0.12, 0.74]
Oba 2014	6	13	407	783	11.3%	0.79 [0.26, 2.38]
Rammohan 2015	4	39	147	387	11.7%	0.19 [0.06, 0.54]
Satoh 2000	3	17	209	654	10.0%	0.46 [0.13, 1.60]
Shao 2011	2	27	100	270	8.4%	0.14 [0.03, 0.59]
Shiomi 2001	5	17	55	115	11.3%	0.45 [0.15, 1.37]
Wong 2015	14	37	77	222	15.2%	1.15 [0.56, 2.35]
Yeh 2004	1	16	141	427	5.4%	0.14 [0.02, 1.03]
Total (95% CI)		**231**		**4021**	**100.0%**	**0.37 [0.21, 0.64]**
Total events	45		1659			

Heterogeneity: Tau² = 0.39; Chi² = 19.06, df = 9 (P = 0.02); I² = 53%
Test for overall effect: Z = 3.51 (P = 0.0004)

Fig. 3 Result of the meta-analysis on 5-year overall survival

As most patients with BTT also had vascular invasion, it is understandable that BTT is likely to recur early after resection. On the other hand, Ikenaga et al. [13] reported two cases of BTT patients without vascular invasion who developed early recurrence in the remnant liver. Similarly, Shao et al. [16] reported nine cases of BTT patients without vascular invasion who experienced early recurrence. These data indicate that dissemination via the bile duct system is another gate of intrahepatic metastasis. In the American Joint Committee on Cancer (AJCC)/International Union Against Cancer (UICC) staging system, information of BTT is not required [28]. In contrast, in the Liver Cancer Study Group of Japan (LCSGJ) staging system, patients with BTT are assigned to the advanced stage and had a less favorable prognosis [29]. Based on the results of the present study, the LCSGJ staging system appears to be more appropriate for HCC lesions than the AJCC/UICC system.

The necessity of bile duct resection for HCC with macroscopic BTT is a subject of debate. Some authors found that BTT rarely invaded the bile duct wall around the hepatic hilus and could be easily removed [5, 6, 15, 25]. Besides, analysis of the OS rate by some studies showed

that bile duct resection did not seem to provide any significant benefit [5, 6, 15], and therefore they suggested that such resection should be avoided unless essential for technical purposes. Whereas other authors advocated routine bile duct resection for HCC patients with BTT, knowing that it may minimize recurrence due to better eradication of the microscopic tumor [24, 26]. As all these studies involved the analysis of only a small number of patients, comparisons of the results between the two groups may be of limited value, and therefore future studies with a larger number of patients are required.

There have been relatively few studies in the literature reporting the practice and outcome of liver transplantation for the treatment of HCC with BTT. Peng et al. [7] reported one patient who died of recurrence at 27 months after liver transplantation. Hwang et al. [30] reported a 5-year OS rate of 50 % in a cohort of 14 patients. Although these authors believed that liver transplantation may be a potential treatment option for HCC with BTT, it is prudent to draw any firm conclusion before more results are obtained from further studies with larger sample sizes.

The present study has several limitations. First, all the included studies were performed in the Asia-Pacific region, which may affect the generalizability. In addition, the retrospective nature of eligible studies is vulnerable to introduce potential bias. For example, there were differences in observation periods, disease stages and surgical methods between the institutions. For this reason, significant heterogeneity was tested in the meta-analytic statistical outcomes. Finally, as only 13 of the 20 included studies were eligible for meta-analysis, the impact of BTT on the prognosis may be underestimated.

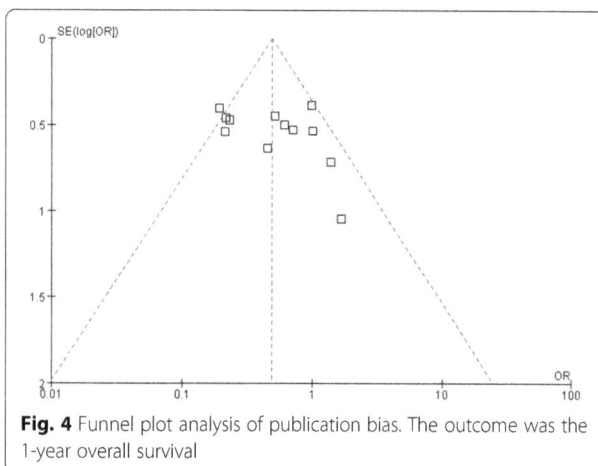

Fig. 4 Funnel plot analysis of publication bias. The outcome was the 1-year overall survival

Conclusions

HCC with BTT has aggressive biological characteristics and is an indicator of poor prognosis. However, surgical resection can still provide long-term survival for some patients. More effective adjuvant therapies need to be developed to improve the outcome. Adoptive immunotherapy [31], antiviral therapy [32, 33], intrahepatic injection of 131I-lipiodol [34], and sorafenib- or peretinoin-based chemotherapy [35, 36] may provide beneficial effects.

Competing interests

The authors declare that they have no competing interests.

Authors' contributions

YZ and FY participated in the design and coordination of the study, carried out the critical appraisal of studies and wrote the manuscript. WQ, LW, and BL developed the literature search, carried out the extraction of data, assisted in the critical appraisal of included studies and assisted in writing up. LW,YZ, and FY carried out the statistical analysis of studies. All authors read and approved the final manuscript.

Acknowledgements

We thank Doctor Yanfang Zhao (Department of Health Statistics, Second Military Medical University, Shanghai, China) for her critical revision of the meta-analysis section.

Author details

[1]Department of General Surgery, First Hospital of Lanzhou University, Lanzhou, China. [2]Department of Hepatobiliary Surgery, No.101 Hospital of CPLA, Wuxi, China. [3]Department of Hepato-Biliary-Pancreato-Vascular Surgery, First affiliated Hospital of Xiamen University, Xiamen, China.

References

1. Llovet JM, Burroughs A, Bruix J. Hepatocellular carcinoma. Lancet. 2003; 362:1907–17.
2. Zhou YM, Yang JM, Li B, Yin ZF, Xu F, Wang B, et al. Risk factors for early recurrence of small hepatocellular carcinoma after curative resection. Hepatobiliary Pancreat Dis Int. 2010;9:33–7.
3. Kojiro M, Kawabata K, Kawano Y, Shirai F, Takemoto N, Nakashima T. Hepatocellular carcinoma presenting as intrabile duct tumor growth: a clinicopathologic study of 24 cases. Cancer. 1982;49:2144–7.
4. Huang JF, Wang LY, Lin ZY, Chen SC, Hsieh MY, Chuang WL, et al. Incidence and clinical outcome of icteric type hepatocellular carcinoma. J Gastroenterol Hepatol. 2002;17:190–5.
5. Satoh S, Ikai I, Honda G, Okabe H, Takeyama O, Yamamoto Y, et al. Clinicopathologic evaluation of hepatocellular carcinoma with bile duct thrombi. Surgery. 2000;128:779–83.
6. Shiomi M, Kamiya J, Nagino M, Uesaka K, Sano T, Hayakawa N, et al. Hepatocellular carcinoma with biliary tumor thrombi: aggressive operative approach after appropriate preoperative management. Surgery. 2001;129:692–8.
7. Peng SY, Wang JW, Liu YB, Cai XJ, Xu B, Deng GL, et al. Hepatocellular carcinoma with bile duct thrombi: analysis of surgical treatment. Hepatogastroenterology. 2004;51:801–4.
8. Qin LX, Ma ZC, Wu ZQ, Fan J, Zhou XD, Sun HC, et al. Diagnosis and surgical treatments of hepatocellular carcinoma with tumor thrombosis in bile duct: experience of 34 patients. World J Gastroenterol. 2004;10:1397–401.
9. Yeh CN, Jan YY, Lee WC, Chen MF. Hepatic resection for hepatocellular carcinoma with obstructive jaundice due to biliary tumor thrombi. World J Surg. 2004;28:471–5.
10. Moher D, Liberati A, Tetzlaff J, Altman DG. Preferred reporting items for systematic reviews and meta-analyses: the PRISMA statement. BMJ. 2009; 339:b2535.
11. CEBM. Oxford Center for Evidence-Based Medicine:. http://www.cebm.net/oxford-centre-evidence-based-medicine-levels-evidence-march-2009/. [accessed 30 July 2015].
12. Esaki M, Shimada K, Sano T, Sakamoto Y, Kosuge T, Ojima H. Surgical results for hepatocellular carcinoma with bile duct invasion: a clinicopathologic comparison between macroscopic and microscopic tumor thrombus. J Surg Oncol. 2005;90:226–32.
13. Ikenaga N, Chijiiwa K, Otani K, Ohuchida J, Uchiyama S, Kondo K. Clinicopathologic characteristics of hepatocellular carcinoma with bile duct invasion. J Gastrointest Surg. 2009;13:492–7.
14. Xiangji L, Weifeng T, Bin Y, Chen L, Xiaoqing J, Baihe Z, et al. Surgery of hepatocellular carcinoma complicated with cancer thrombi in bile duct:

efficacy for criteria for different therapy modalities. Langenbecks Arch Surg. 2009;394:1033–9.
15. Noda T, Nagano H, Tomimaru Y, Murakami M, Wada H, Kobayashi S, et al. Prognosis of hepatocellular carcinoma with biliary tumor thrombi after liver surgery. Surgery. 2011;149:371–7.
16. Shao W, Sui C, Liu Z, Yang J, Zhou Y. Surgical outcome of hepatocellular carcinoma patients with biliary tumor thrombi. World J Surg Oncol. 2011;9:2.
17. Yu XH, Xu LB, Liu C, Zhang R, Wang J. Clinicopathological characteristics of 20 cases of hepatocellular carcinoma with bile duct tumor thrombi. Dig Dis Sci. 2011;56:252–9.
18. Moon DB, Hwang S, Wang HJ, Yun SS, Kim KS, Lee YJ, et al. Surgical outcomes of hepatocellular carcinoma with bile duct tumor thrombus: a Korean multicenter study. World J Surg. 2013;37:443–51.
19. Meng KW, Dong M, Zhang WG, Huang QX. Clinical characteristics and surgical prognosis of hepatocellular carcinoma with bile duct invasion. Gastroenterol Res Pract. 2014;2014:604971.
20. Oba A, Takahashi S, Kato Y, Gotohda N, Kinoshita T, Shibasaki H, et al. Usefulness of resection for hepatocellular carcinoma with macroscopic bile duct tumor thrombus. Anticancer Res. 2014;34:4367–72.
21. Kasai Y, Hatano E, Seo S, Taura K, Yasuchika K, Uemoto S. Hepatocellular carcinoma with bile duct tumor thrombus: surgical outcomes and the prognostic impact of concomitant major vascular invasion. World J Surg. 2015;39:1485–93.
22. Kim JM, Kwon CH, Joh JW, Sinn DH, Park JB, Lee JH, et al. Incidental microscopic bile duct tumor thrombi in hepatocellular carcinoma after curative hepatectomy: a matched study. Medicine (Baltimore). 2015;94:e450.
23. Rammohan A, Sathyanesan J, Rajendran K, Pitchaimuthu A, Perumal SK, Balaraman K, et al. Bile duct thrombi in hepatocellular carcinoma: is aggressive surgery worthwhile? HPB (Oxford). 2015;17:508–13.
24. Wong TC, Cheung TT, Chok KS, Chan AC, Dai WC, Chan SC, et al. Outcomes of hepatectomy for hepatocellular carcinoma with bile duct tumour thrombus. HPB (Oxford). 2015;17:401–8.
25. Yamamoto S, Hasegawa K, Inoue Y, Shindoh J, Aoki T, Sakamoto Y, et al. Bile duct preserving surgery for hepatocellular carcinoma with bile duct tumor thrombus. Ann Surg. 2015;261:e123–5.
26. Zeng H, Xu LB, Wen JM, Zhang R, Zhu MS, Shi XD, et al. Hepatocellular carcinoma with bile duct tumor thrombus: a clinicopathological analysis of factors predictive of recurrence and outcome after surgery. Medicine (Baltimore). 2015;94:e364.
27. Poon RT, Fan ST, Ng IO, Lo CM, Liu CL, Wong J. Different risk factors and prognosis for early and late intrahepatic recurrence after resection of hepatocellular carcinoma. Cancer. 2000;89:500–7.
28. Chun YH, Kim SU, Park JY, do Kim Y, Han KH, Chon CY. Prognostic value of the 7th edition of the AJCC staging system as a clinical staging system in patients with hepatocellular carcinoma. Eur J Cancer. 2011;47:2568–75.
29. Minagawa M, Ikai I, Matsuyama Y, Yamaoka Y, Makuuchi M. Staging of hepatocellular carcinoma: assessment of the Japanese TNM and AJCC/UICC TNM systems in a cohort of 13,772 patients in Japan. Ann Surg. 2007;245:909–22.
30. Ha TY, Hwang S, Moon DB, Ahn CS, Kim KH, Song GW, et al. Long-term survival analysis of liver transplantation for hepatocellular carcinoma with bile duct tumor thrombus. Transplant Proc. 2014;46:774–7.
31. Lee JH, Lee JH, Lim YS, Yeon JE, Song TJ, Yu SJ, et al. Adjuvant immunotherapy with autologous cytokine-induced killer cells for hepatocellular carcinoma. Gastroenterology. 2015;148:1383–91.
32. Breitenstein S, Dimitroulis D, Petrowsky H, Puhan MA, Müllhaupt B, Clavien PA. Systematic review and meta-analysis of interferon after curative treatment of hepatocellular carcinoma in patients with viral hepatitis. Br J Surg. 2009;96:975–81.
33. Zhou Y, Zhang Z, Zhao Y, Wu L, Li B. Antiviral therapy decreases recurrence of hepatitis B virus-related hepatocellular carcinoma after curative resection: a meta-analysis. World J Surg. 2014;38:2395–402.
34. Lau WY, Lai EC, Leung TW, Yu SC. Adjuvant intra-arterial iodine-131-labeled lipiodol for resectable hepatocellular carcinoma: a prospective randomized trial-update on 5-year and 10-year survival. Ann Surg. 2008;247:43–8.
35. Wang SN, Chuang SC, Lee KT. Efficacy of sorafenib as adjuvant therapy to prevent early recurrence of hepatocellular carcinoma after curative surgery: A pilot study. Hepatol Res. 2014;44:523–31.
36. Okita K, Izumi N, Matsui O, Tanaka K, Kaneko S, Moriwaki H, et al. Peretinoin after curative therapy of hepatitis C-related hepatocellular carcinoma: a randomized double-blind placebo-controlled study. J Gastroenterol. 2015;50:191–202.

The impact of race and ethnicity on mortality and healthcare utilization in alcoholic hepatitis

Folasade P. May[1,2*], Vineet S. Rolston[3], Elliot B. Tapper[4], Ashwini Lakshmanan[5], Sammy Saab[1,6] and Vinay Sundaram[7]

Abstract

Background: Alcoholic Hepatitis (AH) is major source of alcohol-related mortality and health care expenditures in the United States. There is insufficient information regarding the role of race and ethnicity on healthcare utilization and outcomes for patients with AH. We aimed to determine whether there are racial/ethnic differences in resource utilization and inpatient mortality in patients hospitalized with AH.

Methods: We analyzed data from the Nationwide Inpatient Sample (NIS), years 2008–2011. We calculated demographic, clinical, and healthcare utilization characteristics by race. We then performed logistic regression and generalized linear modeling with gamma distribution (log link), respectively, to determine predictors of inpatient morality and total hospital costs (THC).

Results: We identified 11,304 AH patients from 2008 to 2011. Mean age was 47.0 years, and 62.1 % were male, 61.9 % were white, 9.8 % were black, and 9.7 % were Hispanic. Mean LOS was 6.3 days and significantly longer in whites (6.5 d) than both blacks (5.4 d) and Hispanics (5.9 d). In adjusted models, inpatient mortality was lower for blacks than for whites (adj. OR = 0.50; 95 % CI = 0.32–0.78). THC was significantly higher for Hispanics than whites (fold increase = 1.25; 95 % CI = 1.01–1.49).

Conclusions: We identified differences in healthcare utilization and mortality by race/ethnicity. THC was significantly higher among Hispanics than for whites and blacks. We also demonstrated lower inpatient mortality in blacks compared to whites. These variations may implicate racial and ethnic differences in access to care, quality of care, severity of AH on presentation, or other factors.

Keywords: Liver disease, Nationwide inpatient sample, Disparities, Healthcare utilization, Alcoholic hepatitis

Background

Alcoholic hepatitis (AH) is a major cause of alcohol-related morbidity and mortality in the United States (U.S.) [1, 2]. Characterized by acute liver inflammation in the setting of chronic alcohol use, AH carries a poor prognosis with a 30-day mortality as high as 30 %, depending on the severity of disease [3–5]. AH also poses significant burden on healthcare utilization and costs in the U.S. National data demonstrate that inpatient healthcare expenditures associated with AH may exceed spending for other chronic liver disease states, including hepatitis C (HCV) and hepatocellular carcinoma (HCC) [1, 6, 7]. As effective treatment is lacking for this condition, the mortality, healthcare costs, and utilization related to AH are unlikely to improve in the near future.

There is increasing emphasis on improving health equity and addressing healthcare disparities regarding race and ethnicity in the U.S. [8]. Current literature documents racial and ethnic disparities in mortality, prevalence, and healthcare utilization in several chronic liver disease states [9–13]. For example, blacks are less

---

* Correspondence: fmay@mednet.ucla.edu
[1]Division of Digestive Diseases, Department of Medicine, David Geffen School of Medicine at UCLA, 650 Charles E. Young Drive; Suite A2-125, Los Angeles, CA 90095-6900, USA
[2]Department of Health Policy and Management, UCLA Fielding School of Public Health, Los Angeles, CA, USA
Full list of author information is available at the end of the article

likely than white Americans to undergo screening for HCV and more likely than white Americans to die from HCV-related complications [11]. Studies have similarly demonstrated Hispanic Americans to have a greater prevalence of non-alcoholic fatty liver disease and an increased risk of developing HCC when compared to caucasians and blacks [9, 10, 12, 13].

While racial/ethnic variation in healthcare outcomes and utilization has been explored in many chronic liver disease states, there is a paucity of literature regarding the impact of these factors in relation to alcoholic hepatitis [14]. In this study, we aimed to determine whether there are racial and ethnic differences in inpatient mortality and health service utilization among patients hospitalized for AH in the U.S, using a large nationwide database.

Methods

Source of data

We performed a retrospective cross-sectional study using the Nationwide Inpatient Sample (NIS), years 2008–2011 [15]. The NIS is the largest publicly available inpatient database and includes a 20 % stratified sample of all U.S. inpatient discharges occurring in a given year from approximately 1000 non-federal U.S. hospitals in 42 to 47 states, depending on the year. Each hospital included in the NIS participates in the Agency for Healthcare Research and Quality Healthcare Cost and Utilization Project. Each discharge record from the NIS contains associated patient and hospital demographic information, primary and up to 24 secondary discharge diagnoses, and up to 15 procedural codes. The study protocol was approved as exempt from review by the institutional review board of Cedars-Sinai Medical Center.

Study population

The study sample included inpatients age 18 years or older with a primary discharge diagnosis of AH. As per previously published studies utilizing administrative data to identify patients with AH, we used the International Classification of Diseases, 9th revision, Clinical Modification (ICD-9-CM) code 571.1 to identify our AH sample [2, 16].

Variables

Our main outcomes were inpatient mortality, total hospital costs (THC), length of hospital stay (LOS), and number of procedures performed (NPR). THCs were inflated to 2011 values for years 2008, 2009, and 2010 using the consumer price index (CPI) [7]. We also accounted for inpatient procedures used in the management of AH, including nasogastric intubation (NGT), mechanical ventilation (MV), hemodialysis, esophagogastroduodenoscopy (EGD), paracentesis, liver biopsy, and liver transplantation.

Additional patient-level data included patient age, sex, race/ethnicity, socioeconomic status (SES), insurance type (Medicare, Medicaid, private, self-pay, other), comorbidity, source of admission (emergency room (ER), hospital transfer, other health-related facility, other non-health facility), and disposition at discharge (home or home with aid, other health facility, and other). For SES, we used income strata. For race, categories included white, black, Hispanic, and other (Asian, Pacific islander, Native American, or another race). Hospital characteristics in the analysis included hospital region (Northeast, South, Midwest, West), hospital type (teaching, nonteaching), and hospital setting (urban, rural).

We used the Deyo modification of the Charlson index as a proxy for patient comorbidity [17, 18]. We stratified the Charlson index into 3 groups to represent the degree of comorbidity: Mild (score = 0), moderate (score = 1–3), and severe (score > 3). In addition, we used the Baveno IV consensus criteria as a measure for severity of liver disease, where patients were categorized as stage 1 (no esophageal varices or ascites), stage 2 (esophageal varices, no ascites or bleeding), stage 3 (ascites, with or without esophageal varices), or stage 4 (history of gastrointestinal bleeding with or without ascites) [19]. Stage 1 and 2 disease represented compensated cirrhosis; stage 3 and 4 disease represented decompensated cirrhosis. As greater than 90 % of patients with biopsy-proven AH have underlying liver cirrhosis, this classification system is applicable to our study population [20].

We also accounted for known conditions that might impact AH outcomes, including ascites, HCV infection, gastrointestinal bleeding, hepatic encephalopathy, and bacterial infection (ICD-9 codes are provided in Additional file 1: Table S1) [21]. For infection, we created one variable that included all ICD-9-CM codes for bacterial infections potentially treated with antibiotics, similar to methodology used in previously published studies (ICD-9 codes are provided in Additional file 1: Table S1) [16, 22].

Statistical analyses

We described patient descriptive and clinical characteristics as means with standard deviation or medians with interquartile ranges for Gaussian and non-Gaussian distributed variables, respectively. For crude statistical comparisons, we used the chi-square test for categorical variables, student's t-test and one-way analysis of variance (ANOVA) with the Tukey-Kramer method to compare continuous variables, and the Wilcoxon-Rank sum test for non-Gaussian distributed variables, all with the Bonferroni correction for multiple comparisons. For THC, LOS and NPR, we computed regional comparisons of means by quantile regression.

Following descriptive analyses, we determined significant predictors of inpatient mortality and THC among patients admitted to U.S. hospitals with AH. We used multiple imputation for missing values for hospital admission source (19 % missing), discharge disposition (14 % missing), and race (14 % missing) using 20 imputed datasets. Other missing values were less than 5 % and were not imputed [23]. For mortality, we used logistic regression, controlling for patient demographic and clinical factors, to determine the impact of race/ethnicity on inpatient mortality among patients admitted with a primary diagnosis of AH. Second, we performed a generalized linear model (GLM) with gamma distribution and log link to examine the relationship between race/ethnicity and THC. GLM was felt appropriate in the present analysis given that THC is a heavily skewed, non-integer outcome. GLM compares the log of THC across groups while controlling for covariates in the model. Thus, the antilog of the parameters of the linear regression model can be interpreted as the fold increase in THC between groups being compared. For both regression models, covariates were selected based on significance in univariate analysis at the $p < 0.05$ level or clinical experience and consistent prior data supporting their association. We used southern region as the reference geographic region as it was the region with the lowest mean value for THC based on unadjusted analysis.

Analyses were performed with STATA 13.1 software (Stata Corp, College Station, TX) with the appropriate survey estimation commands and strata weights provided in each NIS file. To represent national population estimates, we applied survey weights to the patient-level observations in the dataset. A p-value less than 0.05 on two-tailed testing was considered significant except in cases where the Bonferroni correction was indicated.

Results
Characteristics of study population
Table 1 provides demographic and clinical characteristics of the study sample of 11,304 AH patients, stratified by geographic region. Most of the patients were white (61.9 %), followed by black (9.8 %), and Hispanic (9.7 %). Mean age at admission was slightly lower in the Hispanic population (43.7 years) than in the white group (47.5 years; $p < 0.01$) and black group (48.2 y; $p < 0.01$). The majority of patients were white and male in each region.

Notably, over 50 % of blacks with AH were in the lowest quintile of income (55.4 %). In both blacks and Hispanics, Medicaid and self-pay (no insurance) were the most common insurance/payer status. There were also significant racial/ethnic differences in clinical characteristics. Blacks with AH were more likely than whites with AH to carry a diagnosis of HCV (10.0 % v 7.9 %; $p < 0.01$). Hispanics with AH were more likely than whites with AH to have a gastrointestinal bleed during hospitalization (2.9 % v. 1.8 %; $p < 0.01$).

Decompensated cirrhosis was more common in whites with AH (16.0 %) and Hispanics with AH (15.0 %) than in blacks with AH (8.6 %).

Outcomes and resource utilization
As demonstrated in Table 2, there were differences in utilization of hospital resources by race/ethnicity. Mean THC over the course of an inpatient hospitalization was significantly higher among Hispanics ($42,387) than among blacks ($33,359; $p < 0.01$). Mean LOS was longer among whites (6.5 d) compared to blacks (5.4 d) and Hispanics (5.9 d). The mean aggregate number of inpatient procedures performed was higher among whites than blacks (1.3 v. 1.1, $p < 0.01$) but similar between whites and Hispanics (1.3 v. 1.3, $p = 0.16$). Inpatient hospital mortality was lowest for blacks (2.3 %) and significantly lower in this racial group than for whites (4.5 %) (p<0.01) and Hispanics (3.9 %) (p<0.01). Only 4 liver transplants were reported in the entire sample. Given this low number, we did not compare this outcome by race/ethnicity.

Predictors of inpatient mortality
Table 3 provides significant predictors of inpatient mortality for hospitalized patients with AH in controlled models. Blacks were significantly less likely than whites to die while hospitalized for AH (adjusted OR = 0.50; 95 % CI = 0.32–0.78). Hispanics and whites had similar inpatient mortality. Additional significant predictors of inpatient mortality included increasing age, increasing Charlson index, severe cirrhosis, and greater than zero inpatient procedures performed during the current admission (Table 3).

Predictors of total hospital costs
Table 4 provides results for the predictor model for THC. When controlling for demographic and clinical factors, Hispanic ethnicity was associated with a 1.25-fold increase in THC when compared to white race. Thus, on average, a Hispanic patient admitted with AH had a THC 125 % that of a white patient admitted for the same duration of time. Despite this difference in whites and Hispanics, the THC in blacks was comparable to the THC in whites. Age, income, payer status, Charlson index, NPR, and hospitalization in the western U.S. were also significant predictors of inpatient costs.

Discussion
The cost of care and high resource utilization associated with AH is significant as demonstrated both in our study and in previous analyses [1]. However, there is currently little knowledge about variation in healthcare utilization and outcomes by race and ethnicity in this condition. This study of a nationally representative sample of

Table 1 Demographic and clinical characteristics of patients hospitalized with alcoholic hepatitis from 2008–2011; $N = 11,304$[a,b]

Parameter	White $n = 7019$ (61.9 %)	Black $n = 1103$ (9.8 %)	Hispanic $n = 1088$ (9.7 %)	Other $n = 548$ (4.9 %)	Total[a]
Male Sex (%)	4093 (58.4)	665 (60.4)	894 (82.3)	378 (69.2)	7015 (62.1)
Mean Age, y (s.d)	47.5 (11.0)	48.2 (10.5)	43.7 (11.1)	44.8 (11.6)	47.0 (11.0)
Income (%)					
0–25 %	1428 (20.4)	607 (55.4)	366 (33.9)	177 (32.8)	3062 (27.2)
26–50 %	1845 (26.3)	223 (20.0)	248 (22.8)	102 (18.8)	2874 (25.4)
51–75 %	1837 (26.2)	147 (13.3)	250 (22.4)	110 (19.7)	2703 (23.8)
76–100 %	1707 (24.3)	78 (7.0)	157 (14.7)	117 (20.9)	2278 (20.1)
Payer (%)					
Medicare	972 (13.9)	191 (17.3)	103 (9.5)	58 (10.3)	1549 (13.7)
Medicaid	1345 (19.2)	338 (30.9)	301 (28.0)	163 (29.8)	2500 (22.2)
Private	2412 (34.4)	193 (17.3)	204 (18.6)	142 (25.9)	3441 (30.5)
Self-pay	1605 (22.7)	298 (26.9)	330 (30.4)	126 (23.1)	2703 (23.8)
Other	661 (9.3)	75 (6.9)	149 (13.4)	58 (10.9)	1063 (9.4)
Admission Source (%)					
Emergency room	1449 (20.3)	168 (15.1)	409 (37.2)	105 (18.7)	2238 (19.6)
Outside hospital	63 (0.9)	2 (0.2)	15 (1.4)	8 (1.4)	94 (0.8)
Non-health facility	16 (0.2)	2 (0.2)	0 (0.0)	2 (0.4)	21 (0.2)
Other health facility	477 (6.8)	103 (9.3)	48 (4.4)	32 (5.7)	693 (6.7)
Source unknown	5014 (71.8)	828 (75.2)	616 (57.1)	401 (73.9)	8258 (73.3)
Disposition (%)					
Home/Home with aid	4821 (68.8)	849 (77.3)	656 (60.8)	392 (71.8)	7927 (70.3)
Other inpatient facility	746 (10.7)	73 (6.7)	51 (4.7)	34 (6.3)	1115 (9.9)
Other	440 (6.3)	34 (3.1)	42 (3.9)	36 (6.7)	669 (5.9)
Unknown	1012 (14.3)	147 (12.9)	339 (30.5)	86 (15.3)	1593 (13.9)
Mean Charlson Index Score (s.d.)	1.7 (1.9)	1.4 (1.8)	1.6 (1.8)	1.6 (1.9)	1.6 (1.8)
Severity of Liver Disease (%)					
No cirrhosis	4913 (70.1)	869 (78.7)	773 (67.2)	377 (69.0)	8007 (70.9)
Compensated Cirrhosis	981 (13.9)	139 (12.7)	192 (17.8)	76 (13.8)	1608 (14.2)
Decompensated Cirrhosis	1125 (16.0)	95 (8.6)	163 (15.0)	95 (17.2)	1689 (14.9)
Known Hepatitis C (%)	556 (7.9)	121 (10.0)	87 (8.2)	35 (6.3)	921 (8.1)
Sepsis (%)	199 (2.9)	27 (2.4)	24 (2.2)	13 (2.4)	294 (2.6)
Gastrointestinal Bleed (%)	126 (1.8)	22 (2.0)	31 (2.9)	13 (2.3)	241 (2.1)
Ascites (%)	2030 (28.9)	165 (15.0)	251 (23.2)	161 (29.3)	3027 (26.7)
Hepatic Encephalopathy (%)	1066 (15.1)	90 (8.1)	126 (11.5)	65 (11.9)	1602 (14.1)
Any infection (%)	1792 (25.6)	226 (20.5)	222 (20.1)	128 (23.5)	2756 (24.3)
Hospital Type/Setting (%)					
Teaching	2947 (42.4)	646 (59.6)	597 (56.4)	289 (55.4)	5283 (47.4)
Urban	6209 (89.7)	994 (91.8)	1041 (97.0)	471 (89.8)	10014 (89.9)
U.S. Hospital Region (%)					
Northeast	1610 (23.5)	293 (27.4)	250 (23.5)	123 (22.4)	2314 (20.9)
Midwest	1118 (16.0)	180 (16.3)	76 (7.1)	82 (14.9)	2387 (21.2)
South	2614 (37.0)	527 (47.3)	313 (28.6)	146 (26.2)	3969 (34.8)
West	1677 (23.5)	103 (9.1)	449 (40.9)	197 (36.6)	2634 (23.1)

Other race refers to subjects with Asian, Pacific islander, Native American, or another race
y years
[a]Race/ethnicity was unknown for 1546 individuals not included in this table
[b]Data presented as unweighted n (weighted %) or mean (s.d.)
Weighted % in columns add to 100 %

Table 2 Healthcare utilization and mortality outcomes by race/ethnicity[a,b]

	White	Black	Hispanic	Other	Total	P value W v B	P value W v H	P value B v H
THC, $								
Mean	38,965.68	33,358.73	42,386.95	42,032.85	37,978.69	<0.01	0.09	<0.01
Median	23,399.00	20,585.54	25,530.00	24,094.00	23,020.00			
(IQR)	(41,903–13,915)	(37,782–11,944)	(43,287–15,110)	(44,952–13,444)	(40,607–13,501)			
LOS, d								
Mean	6.5	5.4	5.9	6.9	6.3	<0.01	0.01	0.04
Median	4	4	4	4	4			
(IQR)	(8–3)	(7–2)	(7–2)	(8–3)	(8–3)			
NPR								
Mean	1.3	1.1	1.3	1.5	1.3	<0.01	0.21	0.16
Median	1	0	1	1	1			
(IQR)	(2–0)	(1–0)	(2–0)	(2–0)	(2–0)			
Nasogastric tube (%)	26 (0.3)	3 (0.3)	5 (0.5)	2 (0.4)	43 (0.4)	0.67	0.60	0.48
Mechanical Ventilation (%)	241 (3.4)	34 (3.1)	34 (3.1)	24 (4.5)	385 (3.4)	0.54	0.62	0.93
Hemodialysis (%)	3 (<0.1)	0 (0)	1 (<0.1)	1 (0.2)	8 (<0.1)	–	0.53	–
Liver biopsy (%)	241 (3.4)	34 (3.2)	27 (2.5)	14 (3.1)	355 (3.2)	0.68	0.10	0.32
Paracentesis (%)	1259 (17.8)	103 (9.2)	154 (14.2)	94 (17.2)	1887 (16.6)	<0.001	<0.001	<0.001
EGD (%)	1111 (15.9)	153 (13.7)	161 (14.8)	86 (15.7)	1784 (15.8)	0.06	0.40	0.43
Deaths (%)	315 (4.5)	25 (2.3)	43 (3.9)	29 (5.3)	489 (4.3)	<0.001	0.38	0.03

Other race refers to subjects with Asian, Pacific islander, Native American, or another race

W white, B black, H hispanic, THC total hospital costs, LOS length of stay, NPR number of procedures, IQR interquartile range, EGD esophagogastroduodenoscopy

[a]Total hospital costs for 2008, 2009, and 2010 are inflated to 2011 values

[b]% values are weighted to national population estimates

– there were no black subjects with hemodialysis

hospitalized patients with AH contributes several novel findings regarding the relationships between race, outcomes and resource utilization. First, we demonstrated a higher average THC among Hispanics than whites and blacks. Secondly, we identified black race as an independent predictor for lower inpatient mortality compared to white race in patients hospitalized with AH.

Hispanic patients were shown to incur the highest charges in the nation, at 1.25 times higher than whites after adjusting for other factors including SES and payer source. These results are consistent with previous findings regarding other disease states that identified an association between Hispanic ethnicity and increased in-hospital service utilization, particularly for conditions characterized by organ failure and end-of-life [24–26]. Prior studies have further demonstrated that undocumented and uninsured Americans have poor access to timely medical care, particularly Hispanics who disproportionately live below the poverty line [27], and who may face exposure to unhealthy social and physical environments and lack of access to healthcare services [28–33]. Pervasive disparities in access to preventive services and primary care [29, 30, 32], as well as presentation with late-stage disease [34–36], likely

contribute to increased resource utilization during inpatient hospitalization among Hispanics.

Differential use of the emergency room (ER) may also partially explain our findings of higher THC in Hispanics. We found that Hispanics utilized the ER as the source of admission significantly more frequently than whites or blacks. Consistent with other studies, ER-based referrals for inpatient hospitalizations are associated with higher THC [37]. Additionally, Hispanic patients who report alcohol use utilize ER services for the care of alcohol related consequences such as AH more commonly than non-Hispanics [38–40].

The finding that black patients with AH had lower adjusted mortality compared to other racial/ethnic groups is also notable. One possible explanation for this finding is that blacks do not have as severe a presentation of AH as compared to other race/ethnic groups. Previous findings from a single-center investigation demonstrated blacks (0 %) had a significantly lower proportion of patients presenting with severe AH, defined as discriminant function > 32, when compared to whites (39 %) and Hispanics (57 %) [14]. Although this previous study did not examine inpatient mortality, it can be inferred

Table 3 Predictors of inpatient mortality in patients with AH

Predictor	Died % (n = 489)	Odds Ratio (95 % CI)
Age	–	1.02 (1.01–1.03)***
Sex		
Male	322 (4.6)	Reference
Female	167 (3.9)	0.83 (0.67–1.01)
Race/Ethnicity		
White	315 (4.5)	Reference
Black	25 (2.3)	0.50 (0.32–0.78)**
Hispanic	43 (3.9)	0.89 (0.61–1.30)
Other	29 (5.3)	1.07 (0.70–1.66)
Income		
Lowest 25 %	139 (4.5)	1.21 (0.92–1.60)
25–50 %	122 (4.3)	Reference
50–75 %	117 (4.3)	1.06 (0.81–1.38)
75–100 %	97 (4.3)	0.87 (0.65–1.16)
Charlson comorbidity	–	1.41 (1.34–1.49)***
Severity of liver disease		
No cirrhosis	260 (3.3)	Reference
Stage 1–2	78 (4.9)	0.79 (0.58–1.07)
Stage 3–4	151 (9.0)	0.77 (0.59–0.99)*
Teaching Hospital		
No	234 (4.0)	0.96 (0.77–1.20)
Yes	245 (4.6)	Reference
Hospital setting		
Urban	432 (4.3)	Reference
Rural	47 (4.2)	0.89 (0.62–1.28)
Number of Procedures		
0	Reference	
1	54 (1.9)	1.53 (1.03–2.23)*
2	54 (3.8)	2.79 (1.83–4.25)***
> 2	332 (17.4)	13.3 (9.57–18.41)***

Data are presented as n (%) or odds ratios (95 % CI)
Final logistic regression model included survey weights and the following variables: sex, age, race/ethnicity, income, Charlson comorbidity score, severity of liver disease, teaching hospital status, hospital location, and number of inpatient procedures
Other race refers to subjects with Asian, Pacific islander, Native American, or another race
CI confidence interval
*P <0.05; **P <0.01; ***P <0.001

Table 4 Predictors of inpatient THC in patients with AH

Predictor	Factor (fold increase)	95 % Confidence Interval
Age	0.99	0.98–0.99*
Sex		
Male	Reference	
Female	1.03	0.94–1.15
Race/Ethnicity		
White	Reference	
Black	1.24	0.96–1.60
Hispanic	1.25	1.01–1.49*
Other	0.94	0.79–1.13
Income		
Lowest 25 %	0.93	0.76–1.13
25–50 %	Reference	
50–75 %	1.07	0.92–1.25
75–100 %	1.18	1.03–1.34*
Payer		
Medicaid	0.85	0.73–0.98*
Medicare	0.94	0.81–1.09
Private	Reference	
Self-pay	0.75	0.62–0.91**
Other	0.84	0.72–0.99*
Length of Stay	1.02	1.02–1.03***
Charlson Index	1.04	1.02–1.07***
Severity of liver disease		
No cirrhosis	Reference	
Stage 1–2	1.12	0.97–1.31
Stage 3–4	1.01	0.89–1.15
Number of Procedures		
0	Reference	
1	1.27	1.20–1.34***
2	1.74	1.53–1.99***
> 2	2.97	2.72–3.25***
Hospital Region		
Northeast	Reference	
Midwest	1.06	0.85–1.33
South	0.88	0.70–1.11
West	1.32	1.02–1.71*
Teaching Hospital		
No	Reference	
Yes	1.10	0.94–1.28
Hospital setting		
Urban	1.28	1.11–1.48***
Rural	Reference	

Parameter coefficients are presented as a fold increase with 95 % CI
Final general linear model included survey weights and the following, variables: age, sex, race/ethnicity, income, payer, length of inpatient stay, Charlson comorbidity score, severity of liver disease, hospital region, teaching hospital status, hospital location, and number of inpatient procedures
Other race refers to subjects with Asian, Pacific islander, Native American, or another race
CI confidence interval
*P <0.05; **P <0.01; ***P <0.001

that the milder disease presentation among blacks would lead to a lower rate of death during hospitalization [14]. Our study, using a nationwide database, may support this hypothesis. Another explanation for lower inpatient mortality among blacks may be related to differences in provider care patterns between blacks and non-blacks. Studies in the literature have demonstrated lower inpatient mortality in blacks compared to whites for several conditions, which may be due to variation in quality of care or disease management and, possibly, earlier discharge and/or greater out of hospital mortality among blacks [41–43]. Our data source limited our ability to investigate these hypotheses; however, future studies should explore these potential explanations.

Our data must be interpreted in the context of the study's limitations. First, NIS does not provide access to anthropometric or laboratory data. Such limitations might explain the relatively low rate of HCV seen in our AH cohort as HCVAb and HCV-RNA status may not have been known for all study subjects. It also limited us from distinguishing between non-severe AH and severe AH by calculating a discriminant function. However, we were able to account for comorbid medical conditions and severity of hepatic decompensation using the Charlson comorbidity score and Baveno IV measure. In doing so, we aimed to control for overall co-morbidity and liver disease severity, regardless of etiology. An additional limitation in our study was the inability to make conclusions about resource utilization and mortality for members of small race/ethnic groups (Asians, Pacific Islanders, Native Americans). As each of these groups was small, they were combined to create a heterogeneous 'other race' category. As a result, we were unable to analyze each of these groups separately. Lastly, as our study is a cross-sectional, observational study based on secondary data, we are unable to make conclusions about causation. These limitations are mitigated, however, by use of a large, nationally-representative database that enhances the generalizability of our results. Based on our findings, we suggest additional analyses to assess physician practice patterns in the management of AH patients, with attention to explanations for why racial and ethnic differences in mortality and resource utilization exist.

Conclusions

In conclusion, our study demonstrated significant variation in inpatient mortality and inpatient costs between whites and racial/ethnic minorities hospitalized for AH in the U.S. Hispanics admitted for AH had similar mortality to but higher associated costs than whites admitted for AH. Blacks hospitalized for AH had lower inpatient mortality but similar inpatient costs to whites hospitalized for the same condition. We suspect that the differences in morality, cost, and resource utilization observed reflect multiple factors, including differences in access to care, comorbidity, AH severity at presentation, and quality of care delivered. Further investigation is warranted regarding the specific patient-, provider-, and system-level factors driving these findings to improve clinical outcomes, improve health equity, and curtail high healthcare costs.

Abbreviations
AH: Alcoholic hepatitis; CPI: Consumer price index; EGD: Hemodialysis, esophagogastroduodenoscopy; ER: Emergency room; ICD-9 CM: International Classification of Diseases, 9th revision, Clinical Modification; IQR: Interquartile range; LOS: Length of stay; MV: Mechanical ventilation; NGT: Nasogastric intubation; NIS: Nationwide Inpatient Sample; NPR: Number of procedures; SES: Socioeconomic status; THC: Total hospital charges; US: United States

Acknowledgements
We would like to acknowledge the UCLA Institute for Digital Research and Education for their assistance with the statistical analysis included in this manuscript.

Funding
This research was supported by the NIH Training grant (T32DK07180—40) for Dr. May.

Authors' contributions
FM: study concept and design, conceptual model, analysis and interpretation of data, drafting of the manuscript, critical revision of the manuscript. ET: drafting and critical revision of the manuscript. VS: study concept and design, drafting of the manuscript, critical revision of the manuscript. AL: study concept and design, analysis and interpretation of the data, critical revision of the manuscript. SS: critical revision of the manuscript. VS: study concept and design, conceptual model, analysis and interpretation of data, drafting of the manuscript, critical revision of the manuscript, study supervision.

Competing interests
Folasade P. May, MD, PhD: None
Vineet S. Rolston, MD: None
Elliot B. Tapper, MD: None
Ashwini Lakshmanan, MD, MPH: None
Sammy Saab, MD, MPH: None
Vinay Sundaram, MD, MSC: None

Consent for publication
Not applicable.

Author details
[1]Division of Digestive Diseases, Department of Medicine, David Geffen School of Medicine at UCLA, 650 Charles E. Young Drive; Suite A2-125, Los Angeles, CA 90095-6900, USA. [2]Department of Health Policy and Management, UCLA Fielding School of Public Health, Los Angeles, CA, USA. [3]Department of Medicine, Cedars-Sinai Medical Center, Los Angeles, CA, USA. [4]Division of Gastroenterology, Beth Israel Deaconess Medical Center, Harvard Medical School, Boston, MA, USA. [5]Department of Pediatrics, Center for Fetal and Neonatal Medicine, Children's Hospital Los Angeles, Keck School of Medicine, University of Southern California, Los Angeles, CA, USA. [6]Department of Surgery, David Geffen School of Medicine at UCLA, Los Angeles, CA, USA. [7]Division of Gastroenterology and Hepatology and Comprehensive Transplant Center, Cedars-Sinai Medical Center, Los Angeles, CA, USA.

References
1. Jinjuvadia R, Liangpunsakul S, Consortium ftTRaEAHT. Trends in Alcoholic Hepatitis-related Hospitalizations, Financial Burden, and Mortality in the United States. J Clin Gastroenterol. 2015;49(6):506–11.
2. Liangpunsakul S. Clinical characteristics and mortality of hospitalized alcoholic hepatitis patients in the United States. J Clin Gastroenterol. 2011;45(8):714–9.

3. Basra S, Anand BS. Definition, epidemiology and magnitude of alcoholic hepatitis. World J Hepatol. 2011;3(5):108–13.
4. Maddrey WC, Boitnott JK, Bedine MS, Weber Jr FL, Mezey E, White Jr RI. Corticosteroid therapy of alcoholic hepatitis. Gastroenterology. 1978;75(2):193–9.
5. Thursz MR, Richardson P, Allison M, Austin A, Bowers M, Day CP, Downs N, Gleeson D, MacGilchrist A, Grant A, et al. Prednisolone or pentoxifylline for alcoholic hepatitis. N Engl J Med. 2015;372(17):1619–28.
6. Mishra A, Otgonsuren M, Venkatesan C, Afendy M, Erario M, Younossi ZM. The inpatient economic and mortality impact of hepatocellular carcinoma from 2005 to 2009: analysis of the US nationwide inpatient sample. Liver Int. 2013;33(8):1281–6.
7. Younossi ZM, Otgonsuren M, Henry L, Arsalla Z, Stepnaova M, Mishra A, Venkatesan C, Hunt S. Inpatient resource utilization, disease severity, mortality and insurance coverage for patients hospitalized for hepatitis C virus in the United States. J Viral Hepat. 2015;22(2):135–43.
8. Institute of Medicine (IOM). Crossing the Quality Chasm. Crossing the Quality Chasm: A New Health System for the 21st Century. Washington, D.C: National Academy Press; 2001.
9. Carrion AF, Ghanta R, Carrasquillo O, Martin P. Chronic liver disease in the Hispanic population of the United States. Clin Gastroenterol Hepatol. 2011;9(10):834–41. quiz e109-810.
10. El-Serag HB, Kramer J, Duan Z, Kanwal F. Racial differences in the progression to cirrhosis and hepatocellular carcinoma in HCV-infected veterans. Am J Gastroenterol. 2014;109(9):1427–35.
11. Saab S, Jackson C, Nieto J, Francois F. Hepatitis C in African Americans. Am J Gastroenterol. 2014;109(10):1576–84. quiz 1575, 1585.
12. Saab S, Manne V, Nieto J, Schwimmer JB, Chalasani NP. Nonalcoholic Fatty Liver Disease in Latinos. Clin Gastroenterol Hepatol. 2016;14(1):5–12.
13. Schneider AL, Lazo M, Selvin E, Clark JM. Racial differences in nonalcoholic fatty liver disease in the U.S. population. Obesity. 2014;22(1):292–9.
14. Levy RE, Catana AM, Durbin-Johnson B, Halsted CH, Medici V. Ethnic differences in presentation and severity of alcoholic liver disease. Alcohol Clin Exp Res. 2015;39(3):566–74.
15. Healthcare Cost and Utilization Project (HCUP). Content last reviewed September 2016. Rockville, MD: Agency for Healthcare Research and Quality. http://www.ahrq.gov/research/data/hcup/index.html.
16. Sundaram V, May FP, Manne V, Saab S. Effects of Clostridium difficile infection in patients with alcoholic hepatitis. Clin Gastroenterol Hepatol. 2014;12(10):1745–52. e1742.
17. Charlson ME, Pompei P, Ales KL, MacKenzie CR. A new method of classifying prognostic comorbidity in longitudinal studies: development and validation. J Chronic Dis. 1987;40(5):373–83.
18. Deyo RA, Cherkin DC, Ciol MA. Adapting a clinical comorbidity index for use with ICD-9-CM administrative databases. J Clin Epidemiol. 1992;45(6):613–9.
19. D'Amico G, Garcia-Tsao G, Pagliaro L. Natural history and prognostic indicators of survival in cirrhosis: a systematic review of 118 studies. J Hepatol. 2006;44(1):217–31.
20. Mathurin P, Louvet A, Duhamel A, Nahon P, Carbonell N, Boursier J, Anty R, Diaz E, Thabut D, Moirand R, et al. Prednisolone with vs without pentoxifylline and survival of patients with severe alcoholic hepatitis: a randomized clinical trial. JAMA. 2013;310(10):1033–41.
21. Louvet A, Wartel F, Castel H, Dharancy S, Hollebecque A, Canva-Delcambre V, Deltenre P, Mathurin P. Infection in patients with severe alcoholic hepatitis treated with steroids: early response to therapy is the key factor. Gastroenterology. 2009;137(2):541–8.
22. Ali M, Ananthakrishnan AN, Ahmad S, Kumar N, Kumar G, Saeian K. Clostridium difficile infection in hospitalized liver transplant patients: a nationwide analysis. Liver Transplant. 2012;18(8):972–8.
23. Little RJA, Rubin DB. Statistical analysis with missing data. 2nd ed. Hoboken: Whiley-InterScience; 2002.
24. Barnato AE, Chang C-CH, Saynina O, Garber AM. Influence of race on inpatient treatment intensity at the end of life. J Gen Intern Med. 2007;22(3):338–45.
25. Hanchate A, Kronman AC, Young-Xu Y, Ash AS, Emanuel E. Racial and ethnic differences in end-of-life costs: why do minorities cost more than whites? Arch Intern Med. 2009;169(5):493–501.
26. Propper B, Black 3rd JH, Schneider EB, Lum YW, Malas MB, Arnold MW, Abularrage CJ. Hispanic ethnicity is associated with increased costs after carotid endarterectomy and carotid stenting in the United States. J Surg Res. 2013;184(1):644–50.
27. Proctor D-WaB. Income and Poverty in the United States: 2013. In: United States Census Bureau UDoC, editor. Economics and Statistics Administration. Washington D.C: U.S. Government Printing Office; 2014. p. 60–249.
28. Rodgers JT, Purnell JQ. Healthcare navigation service in 2-1-1 San Diego: guiding individuals to the care they need. Am J Prev Med. 2012;43(6 Suppl 5):S450–6.
29. Winkleby MA, Cubbin C. Influence of individual and neighbourhood socioeconomic status on mortality among black, Mexican-American, and white women and men in the United States. J Epidemiol Community Health. 2003;57(6):444–52.
30. Adler NE, Newman K. Socioeconomic disparities in health: pathways and policies. Health Aff. 2002;21(2):60–76.
31. Hanson MD, Chen E. Socioeconomic status and health behaviors in adolescence: a review of the literature. J Behav Med. 2007;30(3):263–85.
32. Phelan JC, Link BG, Tehranifar P. Social conditions as fundamental causes of health inequalities: theory, evidence, and policy implications. J Health Soc Behav. 2010;51(Suppl):S28–40.
33. Krueger PM, Chang VW. Being poor and coping with stress: health behaviors and the risk of death. Am J Public Health. 2008;98(5):889–96.
34. Bennett CL, Ferreira MR, Davis TC, Kaplan J, Weinberger M, Kuzel T, Seday MA, Sartor O. Relation between literacy, race, and stage of presentation among low-income patients with prostate cancer. J Clin Oncol. 1998;16(9):3101–4.
35. Franks P, Fiscella K, Meldrum S. Racial disparities in the content of primary care office visits. J Gen Intern Med. 2005;20(7):599–603.
36. Lannin DR, Mathews HF, Mitchell J, Swanson MS, Swanson FH, Edwards MS. Influence of socioeconomic and cultural factors on racial differences in late-stage presentation of breast cancer. JAMA. 1998;279(22):1801–7.
37. Chandwani HS, Strassels SA, Rascati KL, Lawson KA, Wilson JP. Estimates of charges associated with emergency department and hospital inpatient care for opioid abuse-related events. J Pain Palliat Care Pharmacother. 2013;27(3):206–13.
38. Bazargan-Hejazi S, Bazargan M, Hardin E, Bing EG. Alcohol use and adherence to prescribed therapy among under-served Latino and African-American patients using emergency department services. Ethn Dis. 2005;15(2):267–75.
39. Bazargan-Hejazi S, Bing E, Bazargan M, Der-Martirosian C, Hardin E, Bernstein J, Bernstein E. Evaluation of a brief intervention in an inner-city emergency department. Ann Emerg Med. 2005;46(1):67–76.
40. Lotfipour S, Cisneros V, Anderson CL, Roumani S, Hoonpongsimanont W, Weiss J, Chakravarthy B, Dykzeul B, Vaca F. Assessment of alcohol use patterns among spanish-speaking patients. Subst Abus. 2013;34(2):155–61.
41. Andrews RM, Moy E. Racial differences in hospital mortality for medical and surgical admissions: variations by patient and hospital characteristics. Ethn Dis. 2015;25(1):90–7.
42. Onukwugha E, Mullins CD. Racial differences in hospital discharge disposition among stroke patients in Maryland. Med Decis Making. 2007;27(3):233–42.
43. Volpp KG, Stone R, Lave JR, Jha AK, Pauly M, Klusaritz H, Chen H, Cen L, Brucker N, Polsky D. Is thirty-day hospital mortality really lower for black veterans compared with white veterans? Health Serv Res. 2007;42(4):1613–31.

Usefulness of ascitic fluid lactoferrin levels in patients with liver cirrhosis

Sang Soo Lee[1,4], Hyun Ju Min[1], Ja Yun Choi[1], Hyun Chin Cho[1], Jin Joo Kim[1,4], Jae Min Lee[1,4], Hong Jun Kim[1], Chang Yoon Ha[1], Hyun Jin Kim[1,2,4], Tae Hyo Kim[1,2], Jin Hyun Kim[3] and Ok-Jae Lee[1,2]*

Abstract

Background: Although elevated levels of lactoferrin provide a biomarker for inflammatory bowel diseases and colorectal cancer, the clinical significance of these elevated levels in ascitic fluid of patients with ascites caused by liver cirrhosis is limited. The aims of our study were to investigate the usefulness of ascitic fluid lactoferrin levels for the diagnosis of spontaneous bacterial peritonitis (SBP) in patients with cirrhosis and to evaluate the association between lactoferrin levels and the development of hepatocellular carcinoma (HCC).

Methods: A total of 102 patients with ascites caused by cirrhosis were consecutively enrolled into the study, from December 2008 to December 2011. Ascitic fluid lactoferrin levels were quantified using a human lactoferrin enzyme-linked immunosorbent assay kit.

Results: The median ascitic fluid lactoferrin levels were significantly higher in patients with SBP than in those without SBP (112.7 ng/mL vs. 0.6 ng/mL; $p < 0.001$). The area under the receiver operator characteristic curve for the diagnosis of SBP was 0.898 (95 % confidence interval, 0.839–0.957, $p < 0.001$), with a sensitivity and specificity for a cut-off level of 51.4 ng/mL of 95.8 % and 74.4 %, respectively. Moreover, the incidence of HCC in the 78 patients without SBP was significantly higher in patients with high ascitic fluid lactoferrin levels (≥ 35 ng/mL) than in those with low ascitic fluid lactoferrin level (< 35 ng/mL).

Conclusions: Ascitic fluid lactoferrin level can be a useful diagnostic tool to identify SBP in patients with ascites caused by cirrhosis. Elevated ascitic fluid lactoferrin level in patients without SBP may be indicative of a developing hepatocellular carcinoma.

Keywords: Lactoferrin, Ascites, Spontaneous bacterial peritonitis, Liver cirrhosis, Hepatocellular carcinoma

Background

Lactoferrin is a 78-kDa iron-binding protein in the transferrin family [1]. Lactoferrin is found in bovine milk, as well as in human breast milk [2]. This iron-binding protein is also present in mucosal secretions, including gastrointestinal fluids, saliva, tears, semen, vaginal fluids, nasal fluid, and bronchial mucosa [3, 4]. Lactoferrin is believed to have several relevant functions, that include anticancer, antibacterial, antiviral, antifungal, antiparasitic, anti-inflammatory, anti-oxidant and immune regulatory activities [5, 6].

During an infection or inflammatory condition, lactoferrin is expressed and secreted from polymorphonuclear cells (PMNs) and lactoferrin levels are elevated in the body. Lactoferrin levels have been shown to increase in the presence of infection or inflammatory condition [7]. Therefore, an elevated lactoferrin level may provide a promising and reliable biomarker for gastrointestinal disease [8]. Lactoferrin levels are elevated not only in patients with inflammatory bowel diseases, such as ulcerative colitis and Crohn's disease, but also in patients with colorectal cancer [9–12]. Recently, several studies have provided evidence that increased systemic inflammation is associated with poor survival in various cancers [13]. In patients with hepatocellular carcinoma (HCC), these systemic inflammatory responses can be detected by routine laboratory tests, such as levels of C-reactive protein (CRP) and

* Correspondence: ojlee@gnu.ac.kr
[1]Department of Internal Medicine, Gyeongsang National University School of Medicine and Gyeongsang National University Hospital, 15, Jinju-daero 816 beon-gil, Jinju, Gyeongnam 52727, Republic of Korea
[2]Institute of Health Sciences, Gyeongsang National University, Jinju, Republic of Korea

the neutrophil-lymphocyte ratio (NLR) [14–16]. However, the association between ascitic fluid lactoferrin levels and the development of HCC in patients with ascites caused by cirrhosis has not been investigated to date.

Ascites is one of the most common complications of advanced liver disease [17]. Spontaneous bacterial peritonitis (SBP) is a clinical syndrome in which ascitic fluid becomes infected in the absence of any apparent intra-abdominal source of peritonitis [18]. The diagnosis of SBP is based on a manual count of PMN cells in ascitic fluid, with counts ≥ 250 cells/mm^3 indicative of SBP. However, this method of diagnosis is operator-dependent and, therefore, subject to human error. Moreover, lysis of the cells during transport to the laboratory can lead to false negative results.

Parsi et al. assessed the utility of ascitic fluid lactoferrin level for the diagnosis of SBP in patients with cirrhosis [19]. However, few studies have evaluated the findings of Parsi et al. to clarify the clinical usefulness of ascitic fluid lactoferrin level for the diagnosis of SBP in patients with liver cirrhosis. Therefore, the aims of our study were to investigate the usefulness of ascitic fluid lactoferrin levels for the diagnosis of SBP in patients with ascites caused by cirrhosis and to evaluate the association between lactoferrin levels and the development of HCC.

Methods
Study population
A prospective cohort study group was formed by consecutive enrollment of 182 patients with ascites caused by cirrhosis, from December 2008 to December 2011, at Gyeongsang National University Hospital in South Korea. The inclusion criteria were: (1) known diagnosis of cirrhosis, (2) age ≥ 20 years, and (3) presence of grade 2 or 3 ascites, based on the definitions of the International Ascites Club [20]. The exclusion criteria were as follows: (1) presence of HCC ($n = 75$) and (2) other causes of neutrocytic ascites, including peritoneal carcinomatosis, tuberculosis, pancreatitis, appendicitis, and hemorrhagic ascites ($n = 5$). A total of 102 patients met our inclusion and exclusion criteria and formed our study group. The Institutional Review Board of Gyeongsang National University Hospital reviewed and approved this study and all patients provided informed consent.

Definitions
Liver cirrhosis was defined by the presence of portal hypertension manifested as splenomegaly, varices, ascites, or hepatic encephalopathy, with compatible findings on diagnostic imaging, in combination with thrombocytopenia ($<100,000/\mu$l). The diagnosis of HCC was based on histology or typical radiological findings of hepatic nodules on arterial enhancement and venous wash-out, contrast-enhanced computed tomography (CT) or magnetic

resonance (MR) imaging [21]. The diagnosis of SBP was based on a PMN count ≥ 250 cells/mm^3 in ascitic fluid, with or without a positive ascitic fluid or blood culture. Ascitic fluid samples were obtained from patients with grade 2 or 3 ascites for cell count, culture and determination of lactoferrin levels.

Data collection
Clinical data including age, sex, alcohol consumption, the presence of hypertension and/or diabetes, the etiology of cirrhosis, and prior SBP history were obtained. At enrollment, laboratory tests were performed for anti-hepatitis C virus (HCV), hepatitis B virus surface antigen (HBsAg), anti-hepatitis B virus surface antibody (anti-HBs), white blood cell (WBC) count, hemoglobin level, platelet count, prothrombin time- international normalized ratio (PT-INR), total bilirubin, aspartate aminotransferase (AST), alanine aminotransferase (ALT), gamma glutamyl transpeptidase, serum albumin, creatinine, CRP, and ascitic fluid analysis, including WBC count, PMN count, and albumin levels. In addition, the Child-Pugh score was determined. The ascitic fluid samples (50 mL) were frozen at –70 °C immediately after collection until analyzed. The lactoferrin level in ascitic fluid was quantified using a human lactoferrin enzyme-linked immunosorbent assay kit according to the manufacturer's instructions (Bethyl Laboratories, Inc., Tokyo, Japan). This kit, designed as a sandwich ELISA, captures human lactoferrin present in samples by anti-lactoferrin antibody that has been pre-adsorbed on the surface of polystyrene microtiter wells. The lactoferrin levels were quantified by interpolating their absorbance (at 450 nm) from the standard curve.

Patient follow-up
All patients were closely monitored for clinical and biochemical status, with imaging examinations, by ultrasound or CT, completed every 3 to 12 months. The cumulative death rate was measured from the date of enrollment until the date of death, the last follow-up, or to the study end date of December 31, 2015. Assessment of survival included data obtained by telephone interview with patients or one of their family members. To calculate the true incidence of new HCC cases based on ascitic fluid lactoferrin levels, patients with less than 6 months of follow-up, patients diagnosed with HCC within 6 months of enrollment or patients with SBP were excluded. Based on these exclusion criteria, 24 patients removed from the calculation of the true incidence of new HCC cases due to development of SBP within 6 months of enrollment.

Statistical analysis
Data were presented as median (interquartile range) for continuous variables, and as frequency and percentage

for categorical variables. Differences between patients with and without SBP were evaluated using the chi-squared test or 2-tailed Fischer's exact test for categorical variables, and the Mann–Whitney test was used for continuous variables. Bivariate correlations were performed using Spearman's Rank Correlation to evaluate the correlation of lactoferrin levels to all other measured study variables. Receiver operator characteristic (ROC) analysis, area under the curve (AUC) and 95 % confidence interval (CI) of the AUC were used to identify the optimal cutoff value of lactoferrin level for the diagnosis of SBP. A p-value <0.05 indicated statistical significance. Statistical analyses were performed using PASW software (Version 18, SPSS Inc., Chicago, IL, USA).

Results

Patients' characteristics

Demographic and clinical characteristics of the 102 patients forming our study group are summarized in Table 1. Liver cirrhosis was caused by alcohol in 64.7 %, HBV in 17.6 %, HCV in 11.8 %, and HBV + HCV in 1.0 %, with the remaining 4.9 % of patients having a diagnosis liver of

disease from 'other' causes. SBP was diagnosed in 24 patients (22.9 %).

Median age, sex, disease etiology, Child-Pugh score, and incidence of prior SBP were comparable among patients with and without SBP. In laboratory results, median ascitic fluid lactoferrin level, ascitic WBC count, ascitic PMN count, serum WBC count, serum PMN count, and CRP level were significantly higher in patients with SBP than in those without SBP. The median ascitic fluid lactoferrin level was 0.6 in patients without SBP and 112.7 in patients with SBP (p <0.001).

Correlation of ascitic fluid lactoferrin level with laboratory parameters

The correlations between ascitic fluid lactoferrin levels with laboratory parameters are summarized in Table 2. In all patients, ascitic fluid lactoferrin levels correlated with ascitic WBC count ($r = 0.529$, p <0.001), ascitic PMN count ($r = 0.633$, $p < 0.001$), serum PMN level ($r = 0.200$, $p = 0.044$), serum platelet count ($r = -0.253$, $p = 0.018$), serum CRP level ($r = 0.355$, $p < 0.001$), serum PT-INR ($r = 0.232$, $p = 0.019$), and the Child-Pugh score ($r = 0.248$, $p = 0.012$). In

Table 1 Baseline demographic and clinical characteristics according to spontaneous bacterial peritonitis

	Total ($n = 102$)	No SBP ($n = 78$)	SBP ($n = 24$)	p-value
Age, years	54.5 (45.8–62.8)	53.0 (45.8–62.0)	55.5 (45.8–68.5)	0.376
Gender, male	73 (71.6 %)	59 (75.6 %)	14 (58.3 %)	0.123
Etiology				0.983
Alcohol	66 (64.7 %)	50 (64.1 %)	16 (66.7 %)	
HBV	18 (17.6 %)	14 (17.9 %)	4 (16.7 %)	
HCV	12 (11.8 %)	9 (11.5 %)	3 (12.5 %)	
HBV + HCV	1 (1.0 %)	1 (1.3 %)	0 (0 %)	
Others	5 (4.9 %)	4 (5.1 %)	1 (4.2 %)	
Child-Pugh score	11 (9–12)	11 (9–12)	11 (10–12)	0.089
Prior SBP	19 (18.6 %)	12 (15.4 %)	7 (29.2 %)	0.143
Ascitic fluid level				
Lactoferrin (ng/ml)	21.7 (0–100.1)	0.6 (0–54.5)	112.7 (91.5–139.8)	<0.001
WBC (cells/ml)	151 (60–416)	100.5 (48.8–181.3)	1158 (538–5651)	<0.001
PMN (cells/ml)	11.5 (4.0–98.0)	6.5 (3.0–16.3)	5695 (3660–9668)	<0.001
Serum level				
WBC (×1000/µl)	6.2 (4.7–9.8)	5.9 (5.0–8.9)	7.6 (5.5–11.8)	0.037
PMN (×1000/µl)	3.9 (2.4–6.6)	3.7 (2.3–5.6)	5.7 (3.7–9.7)	0.006
Hemoglobin (g/dL)	9.3 (8.5–10.8)	9.3 (8.4–10.7)	9.2 (8.6–10.9)	0.862
Platelet (×1000/µl)	82.0 (50.0–127.8)	90.5 (53.0–135.3)	60.0 (47.3–105.5)	0.053
Albumin (g/dL)	2.5 (2.3–2.8)	2.6 (2.3–2.8)	2.5 (2.3–2.6)	0.190
Bilirubin (g/dL)	3.8 (2.0–7.8)	3.6 (1.9–7.7)	4.4 (2.3–12.7)	0.289
PT-INR	1.61 (1.35–2.23)	1.58 (1.33–2.07)	1.97 (1.49–2.39)	0.069
CRP (mg/L)	13.9 (6.7–21.9)	11.0 (5.2–16.4)	30.7 (18.7–68.1)	<0.001

Data are presented as the median (interquartile range) for continuous data and percentages for categorical data

SBP spontaneous bacterial peritonitis, *HBV* hepatitis B virus, *HCV* hepatitis C virus, *WBC* White blood cells, *PMN* Polymorphonuclear cell, *PT-INR* prothrombin time-international normalized ratio, *CRP* C-reactive protein

Table 2 Correlation of ascitic lactoferrin level with clinical and laboratory variables in all patients (*n* = 102)

Variables	*r*	*P* value
Age (years)	0.082	0.415
WBC count in ascitic fluid (cells/mL)	0.529	<0.001
PMN count in ascitic fluid (cells/mL)	0.633	<0.001
Serum WBC count (cells/mL)	0.110	0.273
Serum PMN count (cells/mL)	0.200	0.044
Serum hemoglobin level (g/dL)	0.093	0.351
Serum platelet level (×1000/µl)	−0.253	0.018
Serum CRP	0.355	<0.001
Serum bilirubin level (g/dL)	0.132	0.187
Serum PT-INR	0.232	0.019
Serum albumin level (g/dL)	−0.023	0.820
Child-Pugh score	0.248	0.012

WBC White blood cells, *PMN* Polymorphonuclear cell, *CRP* C-reactive protein, *PT-INR* prothrombin time-international normalized ratio

ascitic fluid or blood cultures, 13 of the 24 SBP patients (54.2 %) showed positive culture results for *Escherichia coli* (5, 20.8 %), *Klebsiella pneumoniae* (4, 16.7 %), *Streptococcus species* (2, 8.3 %), *Candida albicans* (1, 4.2 %), and *Clostridium Perfringens* (1, 4.2 %). The distribution of positive findings in patients with SBP is summarized in Table 3. In the 24 patients with SBP, there was no significant difference in ascitic fluid lactoferrin level between culture positive SBP and culture negative SBP (median 126.3 ng/ml vs. 104.0 ng/ml, *p* = 0.122).

Usefulness of ascitic fluid lactoferrin levels for the diagnosis of SBP

The median ascitic fluid lactoferrin level in patients with SBP group was significantly higher than the level in patients without SBP (112.7 ng/mL vs. 0.6 ng/mL, *p* < 0.001; Fig. 1). Results of the ROC analysis are shown in Fig. 2. The area under the ROC curve for the diagnosis of SBP in the 102 patients with ascites caused by cirrhosis was 0.898 (95 % CI, 0.839–0.957, *p* < 0.001). The sensitivity and specificity for different cut-off levels of ascitic fluid lactoferrin for the diagnosis of SBP in this patient group are shown in

Table 3 Causative microorganisms of spontaneous bacterial peritonitis (*n* = 24)

Organism	Number (%)
Escherichia coli	5 (20.8 %)
Klebsiella pneumoniae	4 (16.7 %)
Streptococcus species	2 (8.3 %)
Candida albicans	1 (4.2 %)
Clostridium Perfringens	1 (4.2 %)
No growth	11 (45.8 %)

Data are presented as number (%)

Table 4. At the cut-off level of 51.4 ng/mL, the sensitivity and specificity of the test were 95.8 % and 74.4 %, respectively. At the cut-off level of 63.0 ng/mL, the sensitivity and specificity of the test were 91.7 % and 78.1 %, respectively.

Incidence of hepatocellular carcinoma

We assessed the incidence of HCC development in the patients without SBP based on ascitic fluid lactoferrin levels. Of the 78 patients without SBP, 4 patients developed HCC during the study period. The cumulative incidence of HCC at 5 years was 17.9 % and the estimated yearly incidence of HCC development was 3.6 % in the first 5 years from the time of enrollment (Fig. 3). The cumulative incidence of HCC was significantly higher in patients with ascitic fluid lactoferrin levels ≥35 ng/mL than in those with ascitic fluid lactoferrin levels <35 ng/L (log rank test, *p* < 0.001).

Discussion

Outcomes of our study provide evidence of the clinical usefulness of ascitic fluid lactoferrin levels in patients with cirrhosis to differentiate those with and without SBP. The area under the ROC for the diagnosis of SBP in the 102 patients with ascites caused by cirrhosis was 0.898 (95 % CI, 0.839–0.957, *p* < 0.001). The sensitivity and specificity of the ascitic fluid lactoferrin assay for the diagnosis of SBP in patients with ascites caused by cirrhosis were 95.8 % and 74.4 %, respectively, using a cut-off fluid level of 51.4 ng/mL. Moreover, the incidence of HCC development in patients without SBP was significantly higher for patients with high ascitic fluid lactoferrin levels, defined as a level ≥35 ng/mL.

Lactoferrin is released from PMNs during an infection or an inflammatory condition [7]. In the 102 patients with ascites caused by cirrhosis, lactoferrin levels in the ascitic fluid were significantly correlated with ascitic WBC count, ascitic PMN count, serum PMN count, serum platelet level, serum CRP, serum PT-INR, and the Child-Pugh score. Especially, high ascitic fluid lactoferrin levels were significantly correlated to inflammatory markers, including WBC, PMN, and CRP levels. It is important to note that the correlation of lactoferrin levels and inflammatory markers in blood samples and ascitic fluid could be influenced by lysis of PMN cells during transport to the laboratory, which could lead to a false negative result. Moreover, manual measurement of the ascitic fluid and PMN count is operator dependent, which makes quality control difficult. Commercially available kits for the measurement ascitic fluid lactoferrin could be used in a future development of a qualitative bedside assay. Moreover, lactoferrin is very stable and resistant to degradation at room temperature over an extended period and, therefore, a bedside assay would be feasible in making lactoferrin an important marker for SBP.

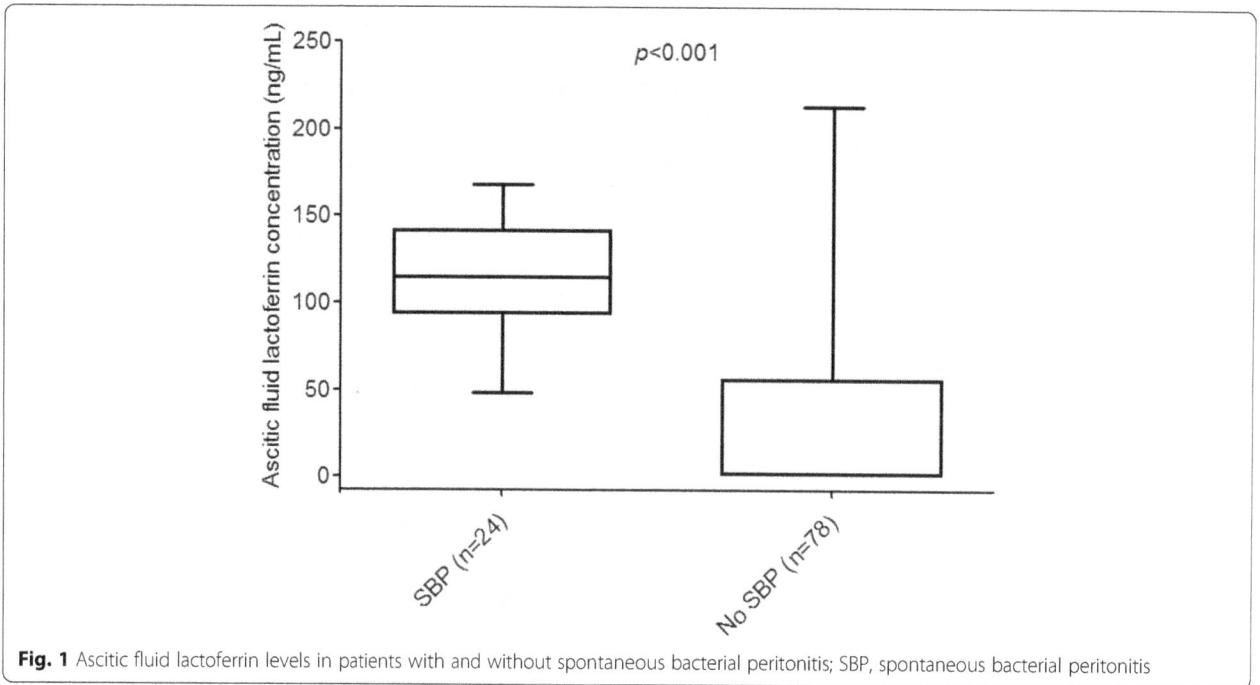

Fig. 1 Ascitic fluid lactoferrin levels in patients with and without spontaneous bacterial peritonitis; SBP, spontaneous bacterial peritonitis

Parsi et al. assessed the utility of ascitic fluid lactoferrin level for the diagnosis of SBP in patients with cirrhosis [19] as a way of eliminating the risk for false negative results and diagnostic error associated with a manual count of ascitic fluid PMN cells. We confirm Parsi et al.'s conclusion regarding the clinical usefulness of ascitic fluid lactoferrin level as a biomarker for SBP in patients with ascites. However, our cut-off ascitic fluid lactoferrin level for the diagnosis of SBP was lower than the level identified by Parsi et al. A study by Ali et al. clarified the clinical usefulness of ascitic fluid lactoferrin as a biomarker for SBP [22]. The mean ascitic fluid lactoferrin levels was significantly higher in SBP patients (180.8 ng/ml) compared with patients without SBP (42.2 ng/ml, $P = 0.001$), with an ascitic lactoferrin level of 88 ng/ml identified as a cut-off on ROC analysis to distinguish patients 'with' and 'without' SBP. This cut-off of 88 ng/ml to identify SBP was lower than the cut-off ascitic lactoferrin level identified by Parsi et al., but higher than the cut-off level in our study. This difference in the cut-off of ascitic fluid lactoferrin

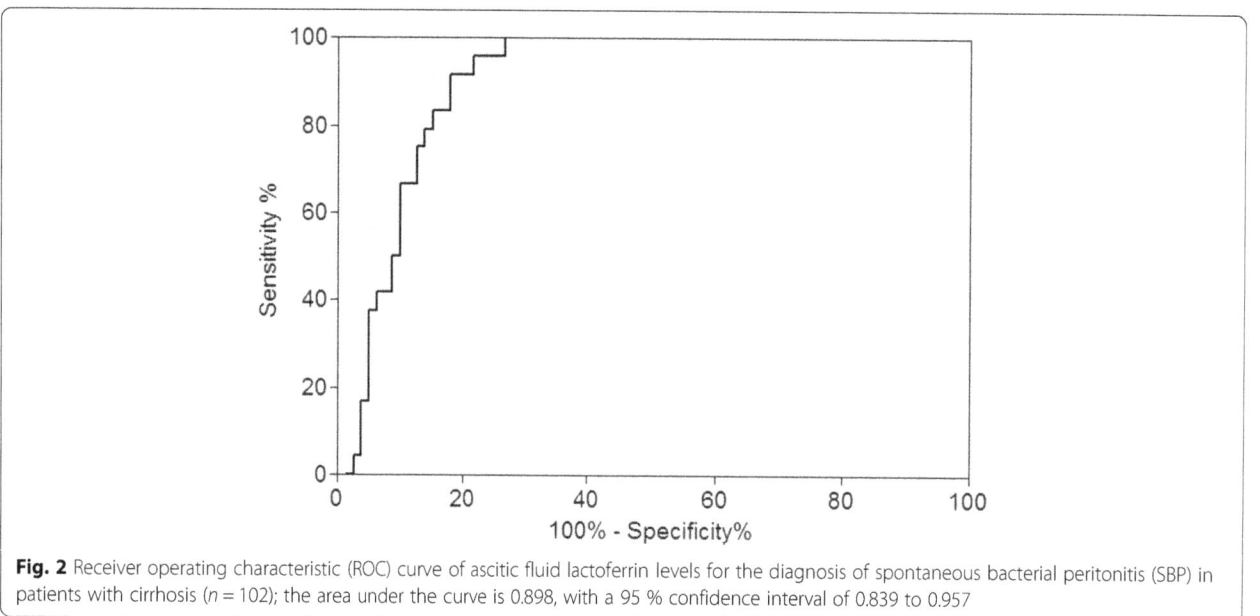

Fig. 2 Receiver operating characteristic (ROC) curve of ascitic fluid lactoferrin levels for the diagnosis of spontaneous bacterial peritonitis (SBP) in patients with cirrhosis ($n = 102$); the area under the curve is 0.898, with a 95 % confidence interval of 0.839 to 0.957

Table 4 Diagnostic accuracy of ascitic fluid lactoferrin at the different cut-off levels for detection of spontaneous bacterial peritonitis in patients with cirrhosis ($n = 102$)

Ascites lactoferrin cut-off level (ng/mL)	Sensitivity (%)	Specificity (%)
43.0	100	72.1
51.4	95.8	74.4
63.0	91.7	78.1
76.3	83.3	82.1
95.9	75.0	87.2

Data are presented as number (%)

level may be explained by the small sample sizes for SBP patients in both studies and, possibly, by differences in the etiology of cirrhosis. Thus, further multicenter studies are required to identify an optimal cut-off ascitic lactoferrin level for the diagnosis of SBP.

Recently, several studies provided evidence that increased systemic inflammation is associated with poor survival in various cancers [13]. In patients with HCC, these systemic inflammatory responses can be detected by routine laboratory tests, such as CRP level and the NLR [14–16]. In an immunohistochemistry study of liver biopsies in patients with viral and cryptogenic liver disease [23], lactoferrin was detected in 75 % of patients with chronic hepatitis. In HCV specimens, lactoferrin levels were found to increase with disease progression, suggesting that lactoferrin may play a role in modulating chronic liver inflammation [24]. However, there has been no report on the association between ascitic fluid lactoferrin levels and the development of HCC in patients with ascites caused by cirrhosis. Therefore, we hypothesized that ascitic fluid lactoferrin levels in patients with local inflammatory ascites would be higher than those in patients without local inflammatory ascites. The presence of ascitic

fluid lactoferrin is proportional to the reflux of neutrophil, and local inflammation can provide a related marker for the development of HCC. In our study, we found that ascitic fluid lactoferrin level in patients without SBP might be related to the development of HCC. HCC free survival was 100 % and 45.2 % in patients with ascitic fluid lactoferrin levels <35 ng/L and ≥35 ng/mL, respectively. Thus, patients with ascitic fluid lactoferrin levels ≥35 ng/mL require more intensive surveillance for the early detection of HCC.

To our knowledge, this is the first prospective study to investigate the usefulness of lactoferrin levels in ascitic fluid for the diagnosis of SBP in patients with ascites due to cirrhosis in Korea. However, the limitations of our study need to be acknowledged in the interpretation and application of outcomes. Foremost, this is a single center prospective study with a relatively small study group, in which only 4 patients developed HCC during the study period. However, the ascitic fluid lactoferrin levels in these 4 patients were very high at 38.7 ng/mL, 60.5 ng/mL, 99.6 ng/mL, and 128.3 ng/mL. Therefore, further studies with larger study group that include patients with ascites caused by cirrhosis and HCC are needed. We also need to consider that the 102 patients with ascites caused by cirrhosis did not present with new onset ascites. Moreover, patients with ascites presented with different Child-Pugh scores, which could have introduced biases in our analysis of prognosis.

Conclusion

Ascitic fluid lactoferrin level can be a useful indicator of SBP in patients with cirrhosis. Elevated ascitic fluid lactoferrin level in patients without SBP appears to be a promising predictor of HCC development. Therefore, larger

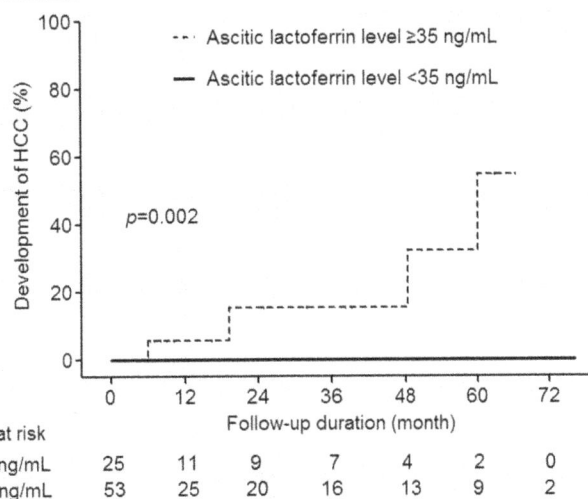

Fig. 3 Cumulative incidence of hepatocellular carcinoma in patients with ascites caused by cirrhosis based on ascitic fluid lactoferrin level

multicenter studies are required to elucidate the usefulness of lactoferrin in ascitic fluid.

Acknowledgements
We are grateful to the devoted our collaborators and research coordinators (Jeong Mi Lee, Hye Won Oh, and Ra Ri Cha

Authors' contributions
Conception and design: SSL, HJM, and OJL, Data collection: JYC, HCC, JJK, and JML, Data analysis and interpretation: SSL, HJK, HJK, CYH, THK, and JHK, Manuscript writing: SSL and JYC, Final approval of manuscript: All authors.

Competing interest
The authors declare that they have no competing interests.

Consent for publication
Not applicable.

Author details
[1]Department of Internal Medicine, Gyeongsang National University School of Medicine and Gyeongsang National University Hospital, 15, Jinju-daero 816 beon-gil, Jinju, Gyeongnam 52727, Republic of Korea. [2]Institute of Health Sciences, Gyeongsang National University, Jinju, Republic of Korea. [3]Biomedical Research Institute, Gyeongsang National University Hospital, Jinju, Republic of Korea. [4]Department of Internal Medicine, Gyeongsang National University School of Medicine and Gyeongsang National University Changwon Hospital, Jinju, Republic of Korea.

References
1. Iyer S, Lonnerdal B. Lactoferrin, lactoferrin receptors and iron metabolism. Eur J Clin Nutr. 1993;47(4):232–41.
2. Baker EN, Baker HM. Molecular structure, binding properties and dynamics of lactoferrin. Cell Mol Life Sci. 2005;62(22):2531–9.
3. Iigo M, Alexander DB, Long N, Xu J, Fukamachi K, Futakuchi M, Takase M, Tsuda H. Anticarcinogenesis pathways activated by bovine lactoferrin in the murine small intestine. Biochimie. 2009;91(1):86–101.
4. Birgens HS. Lactoferrin in plasma measured by an ELISA technique: evidence that plasma lactoferrin is an indicator of neutrophil turnover and bone marrow activity in acute leukaemia. Scand J Haematol. 1985;34(4):326–31.
5. Gibson RJ, Bowen JM. Biomarkers of regimen-related mucosal injury. Cancer Treat Rev. 2011;37(6):487–93.
6. Kanwar JR, Roy K, Patel Y, Zhou SF, Singh MR, Singh D, Nasir M, Sehgal R, Sehgal A, Singh RS, et al. Multifunctional Iron Bound Lactoferrin and Nanomedicinal Approaches to Enhance Its Bioactive Functions. Molecules. 2015;20(6):9703–31.
7. Caccavo D, Garzia P, Sebastiani GD, Ferri GM, Galluzzo S, Vadacca M, Rigon A, Afeltra A, Amoroso A. Expression of lactoferrin on neutrophil granulocytes from synovial fluid and peripheral blood of patients with rheumatoid arthritis. J Rheumatol. 2003;30(2):220–4.
8. Hayakawa T, Jin CX, Ko SB, Kitagawa M, Ishiguro H. Lactoferrin in gastrointestinal disease. Intern Med. 2009;48(15):1251–4.
9. Uchida K, Matsuse R, Tomita S, Sugi K, Saitoh O, Ohshiba S. Immunochemical detection of human lactoferrin in feces as a new marker for inflammatory gastrointestinal disorders and colon cancer. Clin Biochem. 1994;27(4):259–64.
10. Sugi K, Saitoh O, Hirata I, Katsu K. Fecal lactoferrin as a marker for disease activity in inflammatory bowel disease: comparison with other neutrophil-derived proteins. Am J Gastroenterol. 1996;91(5):927–34.
11. Hirata I, Hoshimoto M, Saito O, Kayazawa M, Nishikawa T, Murano M, Toshina K, Wang FY, Matsuse R. Usefulness of fecal lactoferrin and hemoglobin in diagnosis of colorectal diseases. World j gastroenterology. 2007;13(10):1569–74.
12. Parsi MA, Shen B, Achkar JP, Remzi FF, Goldblum JR, Boone J, Lin D, Connor JT, Fazio VW, Lashner BA. Fecal lactoferrin for diagnosis of symptomatic patients with ileal pouch-anal anastomosis. Gastroenterology. 2004;126(5):1280–6.
13. Proctor MJ, Talwar D, Balmar SM, O'Reilly DS, Foulis AK, Horgan PG, Morrison DS, McMillan DC. The relationship between the presence and site of cancer, an inflammation-based prognostic score and biochemical parameters. Initial results of the Glasgow Inflammation Outcome Study. Br J Cancer. 2010; 103(6):870–6.
14. Nagaoka S, Yoshida T, Akiyoshi J, Akiba J, Torimura T, Adachi H, Kurogi J, Tajiri N, Inoue K, Niizeki T, et al. Serum C-reactive protein levels predict survival in hepatocellular carcinoma. Liver int. 2007;27(8):1091–7.
15. Hashimoto K, Ikeda Y, Korenaga D, Tanoue K, Hamatake M, Kawasaki K, Yamaoka T, Iwatani Y, Akazawa K, Takenaka K. The impact of preoperative serum C-reactive protein on the prognosis of patients with hepatocellular carcinoma. Cancer. 2005;103(9):1856–64.
16. Xiao WK, Chen D, Li SQ, Fu SJ, Peng BG, Liang LJ. Prognostic significance of neutrophil-lymphocyte ratio in hepatocellular carcinoma: a meta-analysis. BMC Cancer. 2014;14:117.
17. Gines P, Quintero E, Arroyo V, Teres J, Bruguera M, Rimola A, Caballeria J, Rodes J, Rozman C. Compensated cirrhosis: natural history and prognostic factors. Hepatology. 1987;7(1):122–8.
18. Fernandez J, Bauer TM, Navasa M, Rodes J. Diagnosis, treatment and prevention of spontaneous bacterial peritonitis. Baillieres Best Pract Res Clin Gastroenterol. 2000;14(6):975–90.
19. Parsi MA, Saadeh SN, Zein NN, Davis GL, Lopez R, Boone J, Lepe MR, Guo L, Ashfaq M, Klintmalm G, et al. Ascitic fluid lactoferrin for diagnosis of spontaneous bacterial peritonitis. Gastroenterology. 2008;135(3):803–7.
20. Moore KP, Wong F, Gines P, Bernardi M, Ochs A, Salerno F, Angeli P, Porayko M, Moreau R, Garcia-Tsao G, et al. The management of ascites in cirrhosis: report on the consensus conference of the International Ascites Club. Hepatology. 2003;38(1):258–66.
21. Korean Liver Cancer Study Group and National Cancer Center, Korea. Practice guidelines for management of hepatocellular carcinoma 2009. Korean J Hepatol. 2009;15(3):391–423. Korean.
22. FM A, Shehata IH, Elsalam AEA ME-A. Diagnostic value of lactoferrin ascitic fluid levels in spontaneous bacterial peritonitis. Egyptian Liver Jl. 2013;3:54–61.
23. Tuccari G, Villari D, Giuffre G, Simone A, Squadrito G, Raimondo G, Barresi G. Immunohistochemical evidence of lactoferrin in hepatic biopsies of patients with viral or cryptogenetic chronic liver disease. Histol Histopathol. 2002; 17(4):1077–83.
24. Azzam HS, Goertz C, Fritts M, Jonas WB. Natural products and chronic hepatitis C virus. Liver Int. 2007;27(1):17–25.

4

Analysis of association between circulating miR-122 and histopathological features of nonalcoholic fatty liver disease in patients free of hepatocellular carcinoma

Norio Akuta[1]*, Yusuke Kawamura[1], Fumitaka Suzuki[1], Satoshi Saitoh[1], Yasuji Arase[1], Shunichiro Fujiyama[1], Hitomi Sezaki[1], Tetsuya Hosaka[1], Masahiro Kobayashi[1], Yoshiyuki Suzuki[1], Mariko Kobayashi[2], Kenji Ikeda[1] and Hiromitsu Kumada[1]

Abstract

Background: The association between circulating microRNA-122 (miR-122) and histopathological features of nonalcoholic fatty liver disease (NAFLD) remains unclear.

Methods: The association of serum miR-122 levels with histopathological features of NAFLD (steatosis, ballooning, lobular inflammation, and stage, as histological components of nonalcoholic steatohepatitis) was examined in serial liver biopsies from 36 hepatocellular carcinoma (HCC)-free Japanese patients with histopathologically-proven NAFLD. The median interval between first and second liver biopsies was 4.6 years.

Results: In patients who showed improvement of histopathological scores (steatosis, ballooning, and stage), serum miR-122 levels were significantly lower at second biopsy than first biopsy. In patients who showed no improvement, the changes at second biopsy were not different from those at first biopsy. There were significant and strong associations between serum miR-122 ratio (ratio of level at second biopsy to that at first biopsy) and changes in histopathological scores (of steatosis, lobular inflammation, and stage). There were also significant and strong associations between serum miR-122 ratio and changes in other clinical parameters, including aspartate aminotransferase and alanine aminotransferase.

Conclusions: Longitudinal examination of serial liver biopsies showed the association of serum miR-122 with histopathological features of HCC-free NAFLD patients.

Keywords: Nonalcoholic fatty liver disease, Nonalcoholic steatohepatitis, Serial liver biopsy, Longitudinal observation, microRNA-122, Circulating

Background

Non-alcoholic fatty liver disease (NAFLD) is currently the most common liver disease worldwide across different ethnicities [1–7], and associated with serious healthcare issues. NAFLD includes a wide spectrum of liver pathologies ranging from non-alcoholic fatty liver, which is usually benign, to non-alcoholic steatohepatitis (NASH), which may lead to liver cirrhosis, hepatocellular carcinoma (HCC), and liver failure without excessive alcohol intake [8]. Treatment with vitamin E and Farnesoid X nuclear receptor ligand obeticholic acid is reported to improve the histological features of NAFLD [9, 10].

NASH can only be diagnosed by the presence of histopathological components, such as steatosis, lobular inflammation, ballooning, and fibrosis. Hence, there is a need for non-invasive surrogate markers of histopathological features. The severity and progression of NAFLD is influenced by various factors, including environmental factors, and genetic and epigenetic variations [11–14].

* Correspondence: akuta-gi@umin.ac.jp
[1]Department of Hepatology, Toranomon Hospital and Okinaka Memorial Institute for Medical Research, 2-2-2 Toranomon, Minato-ku, Tokyo 105-0001, Japan
Full list of author information is available at the end of the article

Recent studies have explored the utility of circulating microRNA for assessment of NAFLD. Several reports indicated that serum levels of several microRNAs were increased in patients with NAFLD, and that serum microRNA-122 (miR-122) levels correlated with histopathological disease severity [15–18]. Based on serial follow-up of rats with experimentally-induced NAFLD, Yamada et al. [19] concluded that serum miR-122 level was indeed useful for the assessment of early NAFLD and could be superior to traditional clinical markers that are often used to monitor liver diseases. Takaki et al. [20] examined HCC tissues of mice with experimentally-induced NASH and concluded that silencing of miR-122 is an early event during hepatocarcinogenesis from NASH, and that miR-122 is potentially suitable for evaluation of the risk of HCC in patients with NASH. In a cross-sectional study based on large number of patients with histopathologically-confirmed NAFLD, we recently identified the absence of HCC and/or histopathological severity of NASH as independent predictors of high serum levels of miR-122. In another study, we followed three HCC patients with histopathologically-confirmed NAFLD and showed a decline in serum miR-122 levels before the progression of fibrosis stage [21]. However, there is no information at present on the longitudinal effect of serum miR-122 on histopathological features of NAFLD.

The aim of this single-center retrospective cohort study was to determine the long-term effects of serum miR-122 on histopathological features of NAFLD in patients free of HCC.

Methods

Patients

A total of 321 Japanese patients were diagnosed with NAFLD based on histopathological examination of liver biopsies between 1980 and 2016 at Toranomon Hospital. Of these, 39 patients underwent at least two liver biopsies and were evaluated in detail clinically over time. The need for repeated liver biopsies was determined by the attending physician. Of the 39 patients, 36 did not develop HCC during the period from the first to the second biopsy (median: 4.6 years, range: 0.5-19.0 years). The association between serum miR-122 and histopathological features of NAFLD in these 36 patients free of HCC was evaluated longitudinally.

NAFLD was diagnosed based on liver histopathological findings of steatosis in ≥5% of hepatocytes and the exclusion of other liver diseases (such as primary biliary cirrhosis, autoimmune hepatitis, drug induced liver disease, viral hepatitis, hemochromatosis, biliary obstruction, α-1-antitrypsin deficiency-associated liver disease, and Wilson disease). None of the 36 patients consumed more than 20 g/day alcohol.

The study protocol was in compliance with the Good Clinical Practice Guidelines and the 1975 Declaration of Helsinki, and was approved by the institutional review board of Toranomon Hospital. All patients provided written informed consent at the time of liver histopathological diagnosis.

Liver histopathology

Liver specimens were obtained using a 14-gauge modified Vim Silverman needle (Tohoku University style, Kakinuma Factory, Tokyo, Japan), a 16-gauge core tissue biopsy needle (Bard Peripheral Vascular Inc., Tempe, AZ) or surgical resection. The biopsy tissue sample was fixed in 10% formalin, and sections were stained with hematoxylin-eosin, Masson trichrome, silver impregnation, and periodic acid-Schiff after diastase digestion. The specimens were evaluated by four pathologists (K.K., F.K., T.F., and T.F.) who were blinded to the clinical findings. An adequate liver biopsy sample was defined as a specimen more than 1.5 cm long tissue strip and/or containing more than 11 portal tracts. Specimens with steatosis of <5%, 5–33%, 34–66%, and >66% were scored as steatosis grade 0, 1, 2, and 3, respectively. Lobular inflammation of no foci, <2 foci, 2-4 foci, and >4 foci per 200× field was scored as 0, 1, 2, and 3, respectively. Hepatocyte ballooning of none, few cells, and many cells was scored as 0, 1, and 2, respectively. NAFLD activity score represented the sum of steatosis, lobular inflammation, and hepatocyte ballooning scores (range, 0–8 points; 5–8 points as definition of NASH). Fibrosis stage of none, zone 3 perisinusoidal fibrosis (stage 1), zone 3 perisinusoidal fibrosis with portal fibrosis (stage 2), zone 3 perisinusoidal fibrosis and portal fibrosis with bridging fibrosis (stage 3), and cirrhosis (stage 4) was scored as 0, 1, 2, 3, and 4, respectively [22, 23]. Patients were also classified into four categories by histopathology according to the classification of Matteoni et al. [24] as follows; type 1: fatty liver alone, type 2: fat accumulation and lobular inflammation, type 3: fat accumulation and ballooning degeneration, type 4: fat accumulation, ballooning degeneration, and either Mallory-Denk body or fibrosis (type 3 or 4 as definition of NASH).

A decrease of one point or more in the histopathological score at the time of second biopsy (relative to the first biopsy) was classified as "improvement", no change as "no change", while an increase of one point or more was termed "progression". Changes in histopathological score (Δchange) represented the score at the second biopsy minus that at the first biopsy.

Clinical parameters

Table 1 summarizes the clinical features of 36 patients of NAFLD free of HCC recorded at the time of first and second biopsies. The normal ranges of aspartate aminotransferase (AST) and alanine aminotransferase (ALT) at our

Table 1 Clinical characteristics at the time of the first and second liver biopsies, of 36 patients with NAFLD free of hepatocellular carcinoma

	First biopsy	Second biopsy
Demographic data		
Number of patients	36	36
Gender (Male/Female)	20/16	20/16
Histological findings		
Steatosis (0/1/2/3)	0/8/20/8	1/15/15/5
Lobular inflammation (0/1/2/3)	4/14/13/5	2/20/14/0
Ballooning (0/1/2)	2/21/13	4/23/9
Stage (0/1/2/3/4)	5/13/6/11/1	2/16/5/12/1
Matteoni classification (type 1/2/3/4)	1/1/3/31	0/1/1/33
NAFLD activity score ($\leq$2/3, 4/$\geq$5)	2/12/22	4/16/16
Clinical parameters		
Age (years)	49 (24-69)	59 (26-70)
Body mass index (kg/m^2)	25.6 (20.5-36.5)	25.5 (19.1-33.6)
Serum aspartate aminotransferase (IU/l)	61 (19-152)	37 (14-132)
Serum alanine aminotransferase (IU/l)	104 (28-303)	49 (8-304)
Gamma-glutamyl transpeptidase (IU/l)	65 (17-505)	43 (9-359)
Serum albumin (g/dl)	4.1 (3.4-4.9)	4.0 (2.8-4.5)
Platelet count ($\times$10^3/mm^3)	210 (117-389)	207 (111-296)
Fasting plasma glucose (mg/dl)	94 (65-142)	106 (73-278)
Uric acid (mg/dl)	6.0 (1.8-9.5)	5.9 (1.5-9.2)
Total cholesterol (mg/dl)	209 (130-290)	202 (131-270)
Triglycerides (mg/dl)	137 (62-254)	131 (54-295)
High-density lipoprotein cholesterol (mg/dl)	44 (29-85)	45 (27-73)
Low-density lipoprotein cholesterol (mg/dl)	129 (66-205)	123 (64-175)
Non high-density lipoprotein cholesterol (mg/dl)	162 (95-228)	150 (95-219)
Serum ferritin (µg/l)	265 (<10-1,472)	202 (13-1,018)
Hyaluronic acid (µg/l)	34 (8-561)	30 (0-222)
Serum miR-122 (fold change)	1.03 (0.13-7.63)	0.66 (0.03-7.65)

Data are number of patients or median (range) values

hospital are 13-33 IU/l and 8-42 IU/l for males and 6-27 IU/l for females, respectively. Obesity was defined as body mass index (BMI) of more than 25.0 kg/m^2. Non high-density lipoprotein cholesterol was defined as total cholesterol minus high-density lipoprotein cholesterol. Changes in clinical parameters or laboratory tests represented the value at second biopsy minus that at first biopsy.

Measurement of serum miR-122

Serum samples were obtained at least twice a year after the time of histopathological diagnosis of NAFLD. The sample was frozen at −80 °C within 4 h of collection and thawed just before analysis. Circulating microRNA was extracted from 200 µl of serum samples using the QIAGEN miRNeasy serum-plasma kit (Qiagen K.K., Tokyo) according to the instructions provided by the manufacturer. RNA was reverse transcribed using TaqMan MicroRNA Reverse Transcription kit (Life Technologies Japan, Tokyo). *Caenorhabditis elegans* miR-39 (cel-miR-39) was spiked in each sample as a control for extraction and amplification steps. Table 2 provides details of the protocol used for measurement of serum miR-122, as described previously [25]. Serum miR-122 was amplified using primers and probes provided by Applied Biosystems (Foster City, CA) by the TaqMan MicroRNA assay, according to the instructions provided by the manufacturer. The relative expression of serum miR-122 was calculated using the comparative cycle threshold (CT) method ($2^{-\Delta\Delta CT}$) [26, 27] with spiked cel-miR-39 as normalized internal control. The miRNA expression levels were expressed relative to the levels of serum miR-122 measured in 286 clinical samples [21]. Serum miR-122 ratio represented serum miR-122 level at second biopsy to that at first biopsy.

Statistical analysis

Wilcoxon test was used for comparison of paired samples. Correlation analysis was evaluated by the Spearman rank correlation test. All p values less than 0.05 by the two-tailed test were considered significant. Statistical analyses were performed using the SPSS software (SPSS Inc., Chicago, IL).

Results

Histopathological changes

Table 3 summarizes the distribution of histopathological scores at the time of first and second liver biopsies. The steatosis score indicated progression, no change, and improvement in 33.3%, 55.6%, and 11.1% of the 36 patients, respectively (Table 3), with a median change per year for the entire group of 0.000/year (range, -2.393 to 0.778/year). The ballooning score indicated progression, no change, and improvement in 13.9%, 63.9%, and 22.2% of the patients, respectively (Table 3), with a median change per year of 0.000/year (range, -2.393 to 0.178/year). Analysis of the lobular inflammation score indicated that 27.8%, 33.3%, and 38.9% of the patients showed progression, no change, and improvement, respectively (Table 3), with a median change per year of 0.000/year (range, -0.1429 to 1.164/year). The stage scores indicated progression, no change, and improvement in 27.8%, 52.8%, and 19.4% of the patients, respectively, with a median change per year of 0.000/year (range, -0.714 to 0.516/year).

Table 2 Protocol used for analysis of serum miR-122

(A) Preparation of the RT reaction master mix

Component	Master mix volume per 15-μL reaction[a]
100 mM dNTPs (with dTTP)	0.15 μL
MultiScribe™ Reverse Transcriptase, 50 U/μL	1.00 μL
10× Reverse Transcription Buffer	1.50 μL
Rnase Inhibitor, 20 U/μL	0.19 μL
Nuclease-free water	4.16 μL
Total volume	7.00 μL

(B) Performance of reverse transcription

Use the following parameter values to program the thermal cycler:

Step	Time	Temperature
Hold	30 min	16 °C
Hold	30 min	42 °C
Hold	5 min	85 °C
Hold	∞	4

(C) Preparation of the qPCR reaction mix

Pipet the following components into each tube:

Component	Single reaction
TaqMan Small RNA Assay (x20)	1.00 μL
Product from RT reaction	1.33 μL
TaqMan Universal PCR Master Mix II (x2)	10.00 μL
Nuclease-free water	7.67 μL
Total volume	20.00 μL

(D) Setting up the experiment or plate documentation and running the plate

In real-time PCR system software, create an experiment or plate document on real-time PCR system using the following parameters:

•Run Mode: Standard

•Sample Volume: 20 μL

•Thermal Cycling Conditions:

	Enzyme Activation	PCR CYCLE (40 cycles)	
Step	HOLD	Denature	Anneal/extend
Temperature	95 °C	95 °C	60 °C
Time	10 min	15 s	60 s

[a]Each 15-μL RT reaction consists of 7 μL master mix, 3 μL of 5× RT primer, and 5 μL RNA sample

Association of serum miR-122 level with histopathological features

Figure 1 shows serum miR-122 levels at the time of the first and second liver biopsies, according to histopathological features. In 12 patients who showed improvement in steatosis scores, serum miR-122 levels were significantly lower at the second biopsy compared with first biopsy ($P = 0.002$, Fig. 1a). In 5 patients who showed progression of ballooning scores, serum miR-122 levels were significantly lower at second biopsy than at first biopsy ($P = 0.043$). In 8 patients who showed improvement of ballooning scores, serum miR-122 levels were significantly lower at second biopsy than at first biopsy ($P =$ 0.012, Fig. 1b). In 7 patients who showed improvement of stage scores, serum miR-122 levels were significantly lower at second biopsy compared with at first biopsy ($P = 0.018$, Fig. 1d).

Association of changes in clinical parameters with histopathological scores

Table 4 shows the association of changes in clinical parameters with histopathological scores. There was significant and strong association ($r \geq 0.5$) between ΔSteatosis and serum miR-122 ratio ($r = 0.5$, $P = 0.001$). There were also significant and strong associations between ΔLobular inflammation and ΔBMI ($r = 0.6$, $P < 0.001$), ΔAST ($r = 0.6$,

Table 3 Distribution of histological scores at the time of the first and second liver biopsies

Steatosis scores

	Scores at second biopsy				
	0	1	2	3	Total
Scores at first biopsy					
1	0	5	3	0	8
2	1	7	11	1	20
3	0	3	1	4	8
Total	1	15	15	5	36

Ballooning scores

	Scores at second biopsy			
	0	1	2	Total
Scores at first biopsy				
0	0	2	0	2
1	1	17	3	21
2	3	4	6	13
Total	4	23	9	36

Lobular inflammation scores

	Scores at second biopsy				
	0	1	2	3	Total
Scores at first biopsy					
0	0	2	2	0	4
1	0	8	6	0	14
2	2	7	4	0	13
3	0	3	2	0	5
Total	2	20	14	0	36

Stage scores

	Scores at second biopsy					
	0	1	2	3	4	Total
Scores at first biopsy						
0	1	4	0	0	0	5
1	1	8	2	2	0	13
2	0	3	2	1	0	6
3	0	1	1	8	1	11
4	0	0	0	1	0	1
Total	2	16	5	12	1	36

$P < 0.001$), ΔALT ($r = 0.5$, $P = 0.001$), ΔFerritin ($r = 0.6$, $P < 0.001$), and serum miR-122 ratios ($r = 0.6$, $P < 0.001$), respectively. There were also significant and strong associations between ΔStage and ΔBMI ($r = 0.5$, $P = 0.004$), ΔAST ($r = 0.6$, $P < 0.001$), ΔHyaluronic acid ($r = 0.5$, $P = 0.002$), and serum miR-122 ratios ($r = 0.5$, $P = 0.002$). The above results pointed to a strong association between serum miR-122 ratio and changes in histopathological scores (Fig. 2).

Association of serum miR-122 ratio with changes in other clinical parameters

We also analyzed the relationship between serum miR-122 ratios and changes in other clinical parameters. There were significant and strong associations between serum miR-122 ratio and ΔAST ($r = 0.7$, $P < 0.001$), ΔALT ($r = 0.6$, $P < 0.001$), ΔGGT ($r = 0.5$, $P = 0.003$), and ΔFerritin ($r = 0.5$, $P = 0.001$).

Discussion

There is ample evidence to suggest that many epigenetic mechanisms that are based on histone modifications, DNA methylation, microRNAs (or miRs), and ubiquitination, play a pathogenetic role in NAFLD. The miR-122 is significantly downregulated in NAFLD patients. Furthermore, inhibition of miR-122 results in downregulation of mRNA expression levels of various lipogenic genes and improvement in liver steatosis [15]. Recent studies that investigated the utility of circulating microRNA in the assessment of NAFLD found high serum levels of various microRNAs in patients with NAFLD, and reported strong association of serum miR-122 levels with histopathological disease severity [15–18]. Studies by our group also identified the lack of HCC and/or histopathological severity of NASH as independent predictors of high levels of serum miR-122 [21]. However, serum miR-122 levels tended to be low in fibrosis stage 4, and demonstrated a biphasic change with progression of fibrosis stage. Furthermore, long-term follow-up studies of HCC patients showed that serum miR-122 levels tended to decrease before the progression of fibrosis stage 4 [21]. Considered together, the above results suggest that high serum miR-122 levels could reflect potential future development of HCC, but not at present, and that low serum miR-122 levels before progression of fibrosis stage could reflect increased risk of hepatocarcinogenesis [21]. To minimize the effect of HCC on serum miR-122 levels, we excluded all patients with HCC in the present study. Using this approach, we analyzed the relation between trends in miR-122 and progression/improvement in NAFLD scores in HCC-free patients with histopathologically-confirmed NAFLD.

To our knowledge, the present observational study is the first to demonstrate the association of serum miR-122 with histological features of NAFLD. Serum miR-122 levels at the second biopsy were significantly lower than those at first biopsy in patients with improvement of histopathological scores. Furthermore, there were significantly strong associations between serum miR-122 ratio and changes in histopathological scores.

The present study has certain limitations. Our results showed that patients with improvement and progression of ballooning scores had significantly low serum miR-122 levels at second biopsy, and that serum miR-122 levels correlated with improvement in steatosis and fibrosis

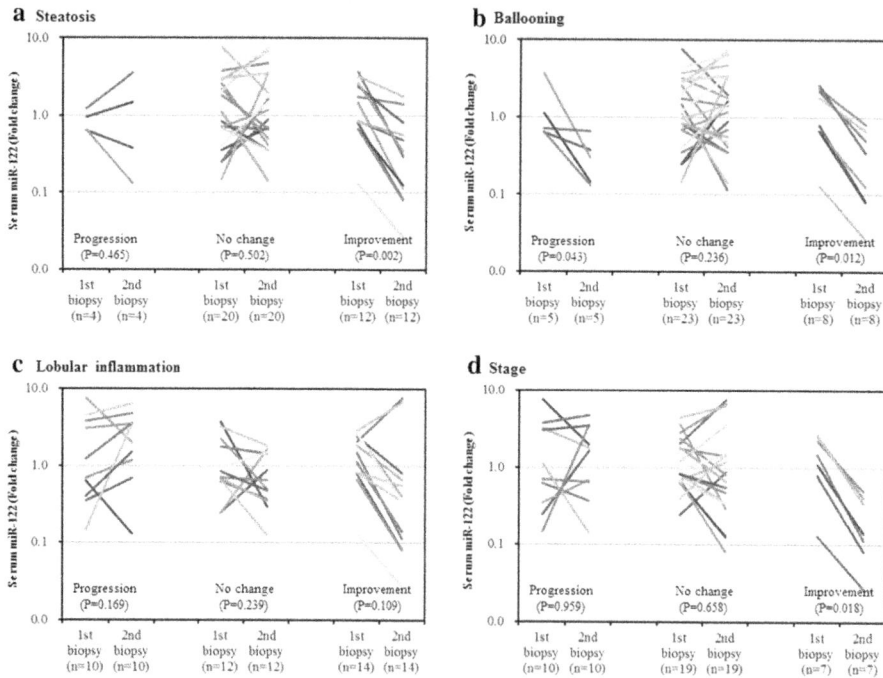

Fig. 1 Logarithmically transformed levels of serum miR-122 at the time of first and second liver biopsies, according to histopathological features [**a** Steatosis, **b** Ballooning, **c** Lobular inflammation, and **d** Stage]. In patients with improvement of steatosis, ballooning, and stage scores, serum miR-122 levels at second biopsy were significantly lower than those at first biopsy

Table 4 Correlation between changes in levels of clinical parameters and histological scores

	ΔSteatosis		ΔBallooning		ΔLobular inflammation		ΔStage	
	r	P	r	P	r	P	r	P
ΔAge	0.4	0.011	0.3	0.049	0.3	0.055	0.4	0.026
ΔBody mass index	0.3	0.045	0.3	0.045	0.6	<0.001	0.5	0.004
ΔSerum aspartate aminotransferase	0.4	0.018	0.3	0.126	0.6	<0.001	0.6	<0.001
ΔSerum alanine aminotransferase	0.4	0.018	0.3	0.108	0.5	0.001	0.3	0.054
ΔGamma-glutamyl transpeptidase	0.1	0.555	0.3	0.099	0.3	0.043	0.3	0.044
ΔSerum albumin	-0.1	0.748	-0.1	0.393	-0.3	0.110	-0.2	0.165
ΔPlatelet count	0.1	0.740	0.0	0.918	-0.2	0.145	-0.1	0.416
ΔFasting plasma glucose	0.0	0.913	0.2	0.390	0.3	0.102	0.3	0.100
ΔUric acid	-0.1	0.671	0.1	0.539	0.2	0.374	0.3	0.089
ΔTotal cholesterol	0.1	0.636	0.3	0.096	0.0	0.992	0.1	0.546
ΔTriglycerides	0.2	0.213	0.1	0.530	0.2	0.195	0.4	0.031
ΔHigh-density lipoprotein cholesterol	0.1	0.738	0.1	0.670	-0.3	0.056	-0.2	0.218
ΔLow-density lipoprotein cholesterol	0.0	0.942	0.2	0.248	0.0	0.855	0.0	0.849
ΔNon high-density lipoprotein cholesterol	0.1	0.675	0.3	0.109	0.1	0.597	0.1	0.385
ΔFerritin	0.3	0.048	0.3	0.063	0.6	<0.001	0.4	0.007
ΔHyaluronic acid	0.2	0.366	0.4	0.036	0.3	0.075	0.5	0.002
Serum miR-122 ratio[a]	0.5	0.001	0.2	0.226	0.6	<0.001	0.5	0.002

[a]Serum miR-122 ratio represented the ratio of serum miR-122 level at second biopsy to that at first biopsy

Changes (Δ) in levels of clinical parameters and histopathological scores were calculated by: value at second biopsy minus value at first biopsy

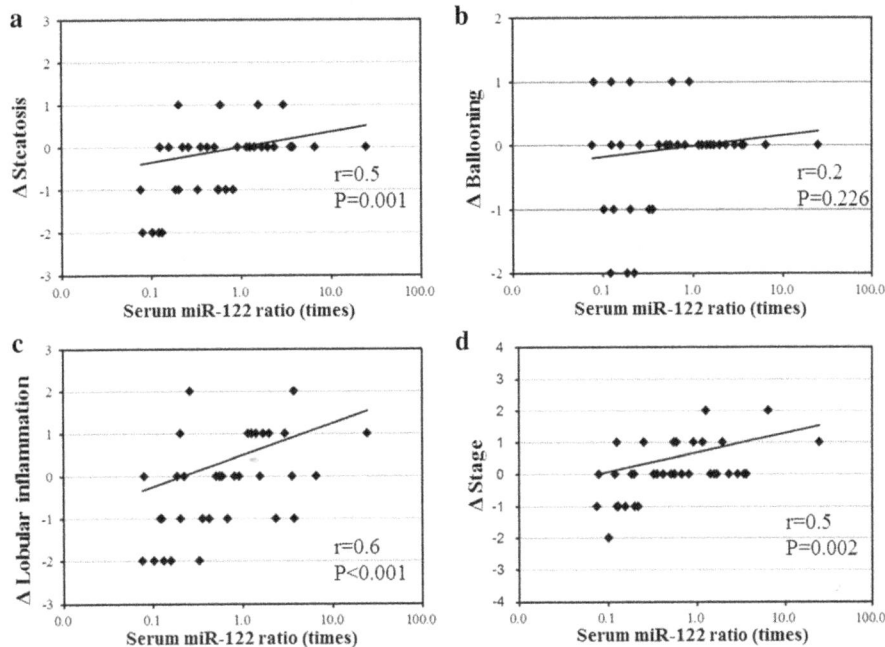

Fig. 2 Association between changes in histopathological score [**a** ΔSteatosis, **b** ΔBallooning, **c** ΔLobular inflammation, and **d** ΔStage] with logarithmically transformed serum miR-122 ratio. Changes in histopathological scores (Δ) represented the value at second liver biopsy minus value at first liver biopsy. Serum miR-122 ratio was calculated by (ratio at serum miR-122 level at second liver biopsy/ratio at serum miR-122 level at first liver biopsy). Note the strong associations (r ≥ 0.5) between serum miR-122 ratio and changes in histopathological scores [**a** ΔSteatosis, **c** ΔLobular inflammation, and **d** ΔStage]

scores but neither with progression of steatosis nor fibrosis scores. These controversial results could be statistically due to α or β error based on the small number of patients who showed progression of steatosis. Furthermore, we recently reported that steatosis with grade of fibrosis stage 4 was significantly milder than that of fibrosis stage 0-3 (such as burned-out NASH patients with progression of fatty changes and inflammatory cell infiltration resolving in fibrosis [6]). We also showed a tendency for lower miR-122 serum levels in patients with severe fibrosis stage, especially fibrosis stage 4 [21]. In the present study, only one patient showed increase in stage scores from fibrosis stage 3 at first biopsy to stage 4 at second biopsy, and the level of serum miRNA-122 decreased from 0.71 fold change at first biopsy to 0.65 fold change at second biopsy. Further large-scale longitudinal studies using serial liver biopsies are needed to determine the complex relationship between serum miR-122 and histopathological features, including burned-out NASH.

To our knowledge, there are no studies that used serial liver biopsies to investigate changes in various clinical parameters, including serum miR-122, according to the individual components of NASH (e.g., steatosis, lobular inflammation, ballooning, and fibrosis stage). Several serial-biopsy studies have investigated the histopathological changes and predictive factors of disease progression in

patients with NAFLD [28–32]. Consistent with the recently reported data [33], the present study showed significant association between changes in histopathological features and changes in levels of serum transaminase (ΔAST and ΔALT). Furthermore, there were significantly strong associations between serum miR-122 ratio and changes in other clinical parameters, including serum transaminases. One limitation of the present study, probably related to the small number of patients, is that the priority of these clinical parameters could not be determined. Further large-scale studies should be performed to identify useful surrogate markers of histopathological features.

In conclusion, longitudinal examination of serial liver biopsies showed significant association of serum miR-122 with histopathological features of NAFLD in patients free of HCC. Further studies of larger number of patients should be performed to determine the molecular mechanisms of the complex relationship between the impact of miR-122 on epigenetic risk and pathogenesis of NAFLD.

Conclusions

Longitudinal examination of serial liver biopsies showed significant association between serum miR-122 and histopathological features of NAFLD patients free of HCC.

Abbreviations
ALT: Alanine aminotransferase; AST: Aspartate aminotransferas; BMI: Body mass index; HCC: Hepatocellular carcinoma; miR-122: microRNA-122; NAFLD: Non-alcoholic fatty liver disease; NASH: Non-alcoholic steatohepatitis

Acknowledgments
The authors thank the following individuals for assistance in histopathological diagnosis: Keiichi Kinowaki, M.D., Department of Pathology, Toranomon Hospital; Fukuo Kondo, M.D., Department of Pathology, Teikyo University School of Medicine; Toshio Fukusato, M.D., Department of Pathology, Teikyo University School of Medicine; and Takeshi Fujii, M.D., Department of Pathology, Toranomon Hospital.

Funding
The authors did not receive grant support for this study.

Disclaimers
This paper has not been published or presented elsewhere in part or in entirety, and is not under consideration by another journal.

Authors' contributions
NA, YK, FS, SS, YA, SF, HS, TH, MK, YS, MK, KI, HK contributed to this work. NA, YK, YA analyzed the data. NA wrote the manuscript. NA, YK, FS, SS, YA, SF, HS, TH, MK, YS, MK, KI, HK provided the biopsy samples.

Competing interests
(1) Hiromitsu Kumada has received honorarium from MSD K.K., Bristol-Myers Squibb, Gilead Sciences., AbbVie Inc., GlaxoSmithKline K.K., and Dainippon Sumitomo Pharma. (2) Fumitaka Suzuki has received honorarium from Bristol-Myers Squibb. (3) Yoshiyuki Suzuki has received honorarium from Bristol-Myers Squibb. (4) Yasuji Arase has received honorarium from MSD K.K. (5) Kenji Ikeda has received honorarium from Dainippon Sumitomo Pharma, Eisai Co., Ltd. (6) All other authors declare no conflict of interest.

Consent for publication
Not Applicable.

Author details
[1]Department of Hepatology, Toranomon Hospital and Okinaka Memorial Institute for Medical Research, 2-2-2 Toranomon, Minato-ku, Tokyo 105-0001, Japan. [2]Liver Research Laboratory, Toranomon Hospital, Tokyo, Japan.

References
1. Angulo P. Nonalcoholic fatty liver disease. N Engl J Med. 2002;346:1221–31.
2. Williams R. Global changes in liver disease. Hepatology. 2006;44:521–6.
3. Torres DM, Harrison SA. Diagnosis and therapy of nonalcoholic steatohepatitis. Gastroenterology. 2008;134:1682–98.
4. Vuppalanchi R, Chalasani N. Nonalcoholic fatty liver disease and nonalcoholic steatohepatitis: selected practical issues in their evaluation and management. Hepatology. 2009;49:306–17.
5. Kawamura Y, Arase Y, Ikeda K, Seko Y, Imai N, Hosaka T, Kobayashi M, Saitoh S, Sezaki H, Akuta N, Suzuki F, Suzuki Y, Ohmoto Y, Amakawa K, Tsuji H, Kumada H. Large-scale long-term follow-up study of Japanese patients with non-alcoholic Fatty liver disease for the onset of hepatocellular carcinoma. Am J Gastroenterol. 2012;107:253–61.
6. Sumida Y, Nakajima A, Itoh Y. Limitations of liver biopsy and non-invasive diagnostic tests for the diagnosis of nonalcoholic fatty liver disease/nonalcoholic steatohepatitis. World J Gastroenterol. 2014;20:475–85.
7. Akuta N, Kawamura Y, Suzuki F, Saitoh S, Arase Y, Kunimoto H, Sorin Y, Fujiyama S, Sezaki H, Hosaka T, Kobayashi M, Suzuki Y, Kobayashi M, Ikeda K, Kumada H. Correlation of histopathological features and genetic variations with prognosis of Japanese patients with nonalcoholic fatty liver disease. J Hep. 2016;2:10.
8. Kleiner DE, Brunt EM. Nonalcoholic fatty liver disease: pathologic patterns and biopsy evaluation in clinical research. Semin Liver Dis. 2012;32:3–13.
9. Sanyal AJ, Chalasani N, Kowdley KV, McCullough A, Diehl AM, Bass NM, Neuschwander-Tetri BA, Lavine JE, Tonascia J, Unalp A, Van Natta M, Clark J, Brunt EM, Kleiner DE, Hoofnagle JH, Robuck PR, NASH CRN. Pioglitazone, vitamin E, or placebo for nonalcoholic steatohepatitis. N Engl J Med. 2010;362:1675–85.
10. Neuschwander-Tetri BA, Loomba R, Sanyal AJ, Lavine JE, Van Natta ML, Abdelmalek MF, Chalasani N, Dasarathy S, Diehl AM, Hameed B, Kowdley KV, McCullough A, Terrault N, Clark JM, Tonascia J, Brunt EM, Kleiner DE, Doo E, Clinical Research Network NASH. Farnesoid X nuclear receptor ligand obeticholic acid for non-cirrhotic, non-alcoholic steatohepatitis (FLINT): a multicentre, randomised, placebo-controlled trial. Lancet. 2015;385:956–65.
11. Sookoian S, Pirola CJ. The genetic epidemiology of nonalcoholic fatty liver disease: toward a personalized medicine. Clin Liver Dis. 2012;16:467–85.
12. Romeo S, Kozlitina J, Xing C, Pertsemlidis A, Cox D, Pennacchio LA, Boerwinkle E, Cohen JC, Hobbs HH. Genetic variation in *PNPLA3* confers susceptibility to nonalcoholic fatty liver disease. Nat Genet. 2008;40:1461–5.
13. Kozlitina J, Smagris E, Stender S, Nordestgaard BG, Zhou HH, Tybjærg-Hansen A, Vogt TF, Hobbs HH, Cohen JC. Exome-wide association study identifies a *TM6SF2* variant that confers susceptibility to nonalcoholic fatty liver disease. Nat Genet. 2014;46:352–6.
14. Akuta N, Kawamura Y, Arase Y, Suzuki F, Sezaki H, Hosaka T, Kobayashi M, Kobayashi M, Saitoh S, Suzuki Y, Ikeda K, Kumada H. Relationships between genetic variations of *PNPLA3*, *TM6SF2* and histological features of nonalcoholic fatty liver disease in Japan. Gut Liver. 2016;10:437–45.
15. Li YY. Genetic and epigenetic variants influencing the development of nonalcoholic fatty liver disease. World J Gastroenterol. 2012;18:6546–51.
16. Cermelli S, Ruggieri A, Marrero JA, Ioannou GN, Beretta L. Circulating microRNAs in patients with chronic hepatitis C and non-alcoholic fatty liver disease. PLoS One. 2011;6:e23937.
17. Yamada H, Suzuki K, Ichino N, Ando Y, Sawada A, Osakabe K, Sugimoto K, Ohashi K, Teradaira R, Inoue T, Hamajima N, Hashimoto S. Associations between circulating microRNAs (miR-21, miR-34a, miR-122 and miR-451) and non-alcoholic fatty liver. Clin Chim Acta. 2013;424:99–103.
18. Pirola CJ, Fernández Gianotti T, Castaño GO, Mallardi P, San Martino J, Mora Gonzalez Lopez Ledesma M, Flichman D, Mirshahi F, Sanyal AJ, Sookoian S. Circulating microRNA signature in non-alcoholic fatty liver disease: from serum non-coding RNAs to liver histology and disease pathogenesis. Gut. 2015;64:800–12.
19. Yamada H, Ohashi K, Suzuki K, Munetsuna E, Ando Y, Yamazaki M, Ishikawa H, Ichino N, Teradaira R, Hashimoto S. Longitudinal study of circulating miR-122 in a rat model of non-alcoholic fatty liver disease. Clin Chim Acta. 2015;446:267–71.
20. Takaki Y, Saito Y, Takasugi A, Toshimitsu K, Yamada S, Muramatsu T, Kimura M, Sugiyama K, Suzuki H, Arai E, Ojima H, Kanai Y, Saito H. Silencing of microRNA-122 is an early event during hepatocarcinogenesis from non-alcoholic steatohepatitis. Cancer Sci. 2014;105:1254–60.
21. Akuta N, Kawamura Y, Suzuki F, Saitoh S, Arase Y, Kunimoto H, Sorin Y, Fujiyama S, Sezaki H, Hosaka T, Kobayashi M, Suzuki Y, Kobayashi M, Ikeda K, Kumada H. Impact of circulating miR-122 for histological features and hepatocellular carcinoma of nonalcoholic fatty liver disease in Japan. Hepatol Int. 2016;10:647–56.
22. Kleiner DE, Brunt EM, Van Natta M, Behling C, Contos MJ, Cummings OW, Ferrell LD, Liu YC, Torbenson MS, Unalp-Arida A, Yeh M, McCullough AJ, Sanyal AJ, Network NSCR. Design and validation of a histological scoring system for nonalcoholic fatty liver disease. Hepatology. 2005;41:1313–21.
23. Brunt EM, Janney CG, Di Bisceglie AM, Neuschwander-Tetri BA, Bacon BR. Nonalcoholic steatohepatitis: a proposal for grading and staging the histological lesions. Am J Gastroenterol. 1999;94:2467–74.
24. Matteoni CA, Younossi ZM, Gramlich T, Boparai N, Liu YC, McCullough AJ. Nonalcoholic fatty liver disease: a spectrum of clinical and pathological severity. Gastroenterology. 1999;116:1413–9.
25. TaqMan Small RNA Assays Protocol. Applied Biosystems.
26. Kroh EM, Parkin RK, Mitchell PS, Tewari M. Analysis of circulating microRNA biomarkers in plasma and serum using quantitative reverse transcription-PCR (qRT-PCR). Methods. 2010;50:298–301.

27. Yu S, Liu Y, Wang J, Guo Z, Zhang Q, Yu F, Zhang Y, Huang K, Li Y, Song E, Zheng XL, Xiao H. Circulating microRNA profiles as potential biomarkers for diagnosis of papillary thyroid carcinoma. J Clin Endocrinol Metab. 2012;97:2084–92.
28. Adams LA, Sanderson S, Lindor KD, Angulo P. The histological course of nonalcoholic fatty liver disease: a longitudinal study of 103 patients with sequential liver biopsies. J Hepatol. 2005;42:132–8.
29. Wong VW, Wong GL, Choi PC, Chan AW, Li MK, Chan HY, Chim AM, Yu J, Sung JJ, Chan HL. Disease progression of non-alcoholic fatty liver disease: a prospective study with paired liver biopsies at 3 years. Gut. 2010;59:969–74.
30. Pais R, Charlotte F, Fedchuk L, Bedossa P, Lebray P, Poynard T, Ratziu V, LIDO Study Group. A systematic review of follow-up biopsies reveals disease progression in patients with non-alcoholic fatty liver. J Hepatol. 2013;59:550–6.
31. Ekstedt M, Franzén LE, Mathiesen UL, Thorelius L, Holmqvist M, Bodemar G, Kechagias S. Long-term follow-up of patients with NAFLD and elevated liver enzymes. Hepatology. 2006;44:865–73.
32. Fassio E, Alvarez E, Domínguez N, Landeira G, Longo C. Natural history of nonalcoholic steatohepatitis: a longitudinal study of repeat liver biopsies. Hepatology. 2004;40:820–6.
33. Seko Y, Sumida Y, Tanaka S, Mori K, Taketani H, Ishiba H, Hara T, Okajima A, Yamaguchi K, Moriguchi M, Mitsuyoshi H, Kanemasa K, Yasui K, Minami M, Imai S, Itoh Y. Serum alanine aminotransferase predicts the histological course of non-alcoholic steatohepatitis in Japanese patients. Hepatol Res. 2015;45:E53–61.

5

High serum resistin associates with intrahepatic inflammation and necrosis: an index of disease severity for patients with chronic HBV infection

Zhongji Meng[1,2†], Yonghong Zhang[3†], Zhiqiang Wei[2†], Ping Liu[1,5], Jian Kang[1], Yinhua Zhang[1], Deqiang Ma[1], Changzheng Ke[1], Yue Chen[1], Jie Luo[4*] and Zuojiong Gong[5*]

Abstract

Background: Studies have revealed that resistin plays a role as an intrahepatic cytokine with proinflammatory activities. This study investigated the association between serum resistin and fibrosis severity and the possible marker role of resistin in the inflammatory process of chronic hepatitis B.

Methods: In this study, 234 subjects with HBV infection were retrospectively selected, including 85 patients with chronic hepatitis B (CHB), 70 patients with HBV-related liver cirrhosis (LC-B), and 79 patients with HBV-related liver failure (LF-B). Serum levels of resistin, IL-1, IL-6, IL-17, IL-23, TNF-α, and TGF-β1 were assayed by ELISA. Demographic and clinical characteristics of patients were extracted from clinical databases of Taihe Hospital, Hubei University of Medicine, including serum levels of alanine aminotransferase (ALT), aspartate aminotransferase (AST), total bilirubin (TBil), and liver stiffness (LS).

Results: All the selected patients with HBV infection showed significantly increased levels of serum resistin, which was rarely detectable in the healthy controls. Serum resistin levels in patients with CHB, LC-B, and LF-B were 4.119 ± 5.848 ng/mL, 6.370 ± 6.834 ng/mL, and 6.512 ± 6.076 ng/mL, respectively. Compared with the CHB group, patients with LC-B or LF-B presented with significantly higher serum levels of resistin ($p < 0.01$). On the other hand, all of the enrolled patients had high serum levels of IL-1, IL-6, IL-17, TNF-α, and TGF-β1, but not IL-23. Interestingly, serum levels of resistin was significantly positively correlated with serum levels of TGF-β1 in LC-B patients ($R = 0.3090$, $p = 0.0290$), with IL-17 in LC-B ($R = 0.4022$, $p = 0.0038$) and LF-B patients ($R = 0.5466$, $p < 0.0001$), and with AST ($R = 0.4501$, $p = 0.0036$) and LS ($R = 0.3415$, $p = 0.0310$) in CHB patients.

Conclusions: High serum resistin associates with intrahepatic inflammation and necrosis and may be used as an index of disease severity for patients with chronic HBV infection.

Keywords: Resistin, Proinflammatory cytokines, Hepatitis B, Liver cirrhosis, Liver failure

* Correspondence: luojie_001@126.com; zjgong@163.com
†Equal contributors
[4]Department of Neurology, Taihe Hospital, Hubei University of Medicine, South Renmin Road. 32, 442000 Shiyan, Hubei, China
[5]Department of Infectious Diseases, Renmin Hospital of Wuhan University, Zhangzhidong Road. 99, 430060 Wuhan, China
Full list of author information is available at the end of the article

Background

HBV infection is the most common cause of chronic liver injury and a major cause of liver cirrhosis, hepatocellular carcinoma, and liver failure [1]. Liver failure is a severe clinical syndrome characterized by jaundice, ascites, hepatic encephalopathy, and a bleeding tendency due to impairment of liver function, leading to poor prognosis [2]. According to World Health Organization estimates, approximately 240 million people around the world suffer from chronic HBV infection (http://www.who.int/hiv/pub/hepatitis/hepatitis-b-guidelines/en/).

The outcomes of HBV infection depend on both viral and host factors, including genetic factors that determine a host's immune mechanisms [3]. It is generally accepted that HBV is not directly cytopathic; thus, HBV-related hepatocellular injuries are the results of the complex interplay among HBVs, hepatocytes, and host immune cells [3, 4]. It has been widely recognized that host immunity contributes to the pathogenesis of liver injuries and even liver failure. The immune clearance of HBV can trigger extensive liver damage that results in fibrosis and cirrhosis. Cytotoxic T-lymphocytes (CTLs), the core of cellular immunity, play a key role in the clearance of intracellular viruses, which are the major cause of cell apoptosis or necrosis [5]. Several studies have characterized intrahepatic CD4$^+$ and CD8$^+$ T lymphocytes in chronic hepatitis B (CHB) (as reviewed by Shimizu) [6]. It is generally accepted that HBV-specific CD8$^+$ T cells have important functions in controlling HBV replication in the liver without causing hepatic necroinflammation, whereas non-specific CTLs may contribute to HBV-related intrahepatic inflammation [7].

Macrophages Cells play a key role in the homeostasis of the liver, which undergo polarized activation to M1 or M2 or M2-like activation states in response to environmental signals. The M1 phenotype is characterized by the upregulation of proinflammatory cytokines and promotion of Th1 response, and strong microbicidal and tumoricidal activity. In contrast, M2 macrophages promote tissue remodeling and tumor progression, and have immunoregulatory functions (as reviewed by Antonio Sica, et al.) [8]. It is general accepted that HBV promotes intrahepatic resident and recruited macrophages M2 polarization, leading to impairment of host immunity and progression of tissue fibrosis/remodeling [9].

Th cells that produce IL-17 (Th17 cells) have recently been identified as the third subset of effector T cells, which produce IL-17A, IL-17 F, IL-22 and IL-21 [10]. High numbers of IL-17-producing CD4$^+$ T cells have been observed in both the liver and the blood of CHB patients; and the elevation in this cell population has been correlated with a high serum level of IL-27 [11]. An increase in circulating and intrahepatic IL-17-producing CD4$^+$ T cells is well correlated with ALT level and liver injury. CD4$^+$ T lymphocytes that produce IL-17 infiltrate into the livers of patients with CHB and increase the severity of liver damage [12].

Prior studies on HBV-related hepatitis flares have demonstrated that, high ALT levels usually accompanied by increased serum levels of IL-12 and Th1 phenotypic cytokines (IL-2 and IFN-γ) [13, 14], and the natural killer (NK)-cell mediated liver damage were found to be attributed to the increased serum IFN-a and IL-8 [15]. Therefore, hepatitis B flares are results of complex interplay of the virus and the innate and adaptive immune responses, and the more vigorous immune response against HBV, the higher the serum ALT (as reviewed by Chang and Liaw) [4].

Hepatic microcirculation disorders occur in all chronic liver diseases, which result in insufficient blood supply to hepatocytes. In addition, collateral circulation also depletes blood flow from the liver. As a result, a) nutrients absorbed from the intestines cannot nourish the liver; b) the therapeutic effects of certain drugs are decreased; and c) metabolic wastes accumulate. These events speed the progression of liver diseases.

Resistin is a 12.5-kd adipokine that belongs to a new family of small, cysteine-rich secretory proteins known as FIZZ (found in inflammatory zone) or resistin-like molecules [16]. In rodents, resistin is highly expressed in adipose tissue, and circulating levels of resistin are increased during diet-induced or genetic obesity [17]. It has been verified that resistin is expressed and upregulated under conditions of chronic injury in human liver tissue, and resistin can stimulate human hepatic stellate cells (HSCs) to secrete proinflammatory cytokines through activating the nuclear factor (NF)-κB signaling pathway [18]. In patients with chronic hepatitis C virus infection, low serum levels of resistin are associated with the presence of fibrosis and may therefore be a biochemical marker of fibrosis [19]. Moreover, Tsochatzis et al. found that in CHB and chronic hepatitis C (CHC) patients, resistin levels are independently associated with fibrosis severity [20]. Another study found that elevated levels of resistin were prominent in patients with hepatobiliary inflammation and were associated with breach of self-tolerance; thus, resistin may be an important marker of disease severity in autoantibody-mediated gastrointestinal inflammatory diseases [21]. Furthermore, increased serum resistin is known to be positively correlated with histological inflammatory score in nonalcoholic fatty liver disease (NAFLD), suggesting that increased resistin in NAFLD patients is related to the histological severity of this disease [22].

In the present study, patients with chronic HBV infection were retrospectively selected. The serum resistin levels and serum levels of the cytokines IL-1, IL-6, IL-17, IL-23, TNF-α, and TGF-β1 were assayed. The association between serum resistin levels and serum cytokine

Table 1 Clinical characteristics of the enrolled patients

Demographics	CHB (n = 85)	LC-B (n = 70)	LF-B (n = 79)
Male/female	64/21	42/28	65/14
Age (years), mean ± SD	39.800 ± 14.900	48.330 ± 11.050	46.400 ± 10.000
HBeAg positive/negative	47/38	26/44	30/49
HBV DNA (log10) IU/ml	6.70 ± 1.45	6.06 ± 1.17	6.45 ± 1.35
Antivirus treatment (Y/N)	62/23	56/14	68/11
ALT (IU/L)	178.894 ± 205.229	61.043 ± 117.280	186.861 ± 270.105
AST (IU/L)	116.865 ± 146.940	70.171 ± 114.080	172.730 ± 219.91
TBil (mmol/L)	41.843 ± 72.044	38.336 ± 43.166	238.420 ± 139.550

levels, liver biochemical indices, and fibrosis severity were analyzed. The possible role of resistin as a marker of the inflammatory process in patients with CHB was investigated in detail.

Methods
Patients
Patients with CHB were retrospectively selected from Aug. 2013 to Sept. 2014 at the Inpatient Department of Taihe Hospital, Hubei University of Medicine. CHB, HBV-related liver cirrhosis (LC-B), and HBV-related liver failure (LF-B) were diagnosed in accordance with published guidelines [23, 24]. Patients' serum samples were routinely stored and used for this retrospective study. The inclusion criteria were chronic infection with HBV, defined as detectable HBsAg and HBV-DNA for at least 6 months, and age ≥ 18 years. Patients were excluded if they were co-infected with the hepatitis A virus (HAV), hepatitis C virus (HCV), hepatitis D virus (HDV), hepatitis E virus (HEV), or human immunodeficiency virus (HIV); if they reported consuming significant quantities of alcohol (more than 30 g per week for men and 20 g per week for women); if they had received a liver allograft; or if a malignant disease, including HCC, had been diagnosed. Clinical databases were consulted to obtain patients' demographic and clinical characteristics, including age; sex; serum levels of alanine aminotransferase (ALT), aspartate aminotransferase (AST), and total bilirubin (TBil); and liver stiffness (LS). The study protocol was approved by the Ethics Committee of Taihe Hospital,Hubei

university of Medicine. Written informed consent was given by all the participants prior to their inclusion in this study. All data and samples used were collected during standard clinical care. Twenty serum samples from blood donors were used as healthy controls (HCs).

Quantification of serum levels of resistin
Serum levels of resistin were measured using ELISA kits (eBioscience, USA) according to the manufacturer's instructions (with resistin sensitivity < 3.1 pg/mL).

Quantification of serum levels of IL-1, IL-6, IL-17, IL-23, TNF-α and TGF-β1
Serum levels of IL-1, IL-6, IL-17, IL-23, TNF-α, and TGF-β1 were measured using ELISA kits (R&D Systems, USA) in accordance with the manufacturer's instructions. Standard curves were constructed using standard samples (IL-1β sensitivity < 1 pg/mL; IL-6 sensitivity < 0.7 pg/mL; IL-17 sensitivity < 15 pg/mL; IL-23 sensitivity < 16.3 pg/mL; TNF-α sensitivity < 5.5 pg/mL; and TGF-β1 sensitivity < 15.4 pg/mL).

Statistical analyses
Study data are presented as means ± SD. Variables were compared using a general linear model, Student's t-test, or the Mann–Whitney U test as needed. Statistical analysis was performed using SPSS for Windows. Simple linear correlation analyses were conducted using Pearson's method to assess the correlations between resistin and

Table 2 Serum levels of resistin and cytokines

Groups	HC	CHB	LC-B	LF-B
Resistin (ng/mL)	0.078 ± 0.270	4.119 ± 5.848	6.370 ± 6.834	6.512 ± 6.076
IL-1 (pg/mL)	0.077 ± 0.186	0.549 ± 1.341	0.932 ± 1.754	0.446 ± 1.104
IL-6 (pg/mL)	0.077 ± 0.186	8.830 ± 19.426	21.822 ± 50.372	29.792 ± 51.394
IL-17 (pg/mL)	2.923 ± 2.310	5.410 ± 5.634	5.164 ± 3.522	5.288 ± 5.860
IL-23 (pg/mL)	4.589 ± 3.823	8.149 ± 17.379	6.103 ± 12.005	5.874 ± 10.981
TNF-α (pg/mL)	2.489 ± 2.083	9.038 ± 8.108	27.961 ± 120.362	43.472 ± 145.516
TGF-β1 (pg/mL)	29.380 ± 3.339	46.205 ± 7.818	48.636 ± 11.555	55.537 ± 6.971

cytokines, AST, and TBil. The threshold used for statistical significance was $p < 0.05$. The statistical methods of this study were reviewed by Dr. Jing Wang from the Department of Epidemiology and Hygenic statistics, Hubei University of Medicine.

Results

Patient characteristics

After applying the criteria described above, 234 patients were selected for the present study: 85 patients with CHB, 70 patients with LC-B, and 79 patients with LF-B. Baseline characteristics of these patients are summarized in Table 1. The male/female ratios for CHB patients, LC-B patients, and LF-B patients were 64/21, 42/28, and 65/14, respectively. Most patients received NA-based antiviral treatment, in which entecavir is most used, except that some CHB patients received IFN-α treatment. Serum levels of ALT, AST, and TBil were 178.894 ± 205.229 IU/L, 116.865 ± 146.940 IU/L, and 41.843 ± 72.044 mmol/L, respectively, for CHB patients; 61.043 ± 117.280 IU/L, 70.171 ± 114.080 IU/L, and 38.336 ± 43.166 mmol/L, respectively, for LC-B patients; and 86.861 ± 270.105 IU/L, 172.730 ± 219.91 IU/L, and 238.420 ± 139.550 mmol/L, respectively, for LF-B patients (Table 2). The primary analyses of this study focused on serum levels of resistin, IL-1, IL-6, IL-17, IL-23, TNF-α and TGF-β1, which were generally determined using serum samples obtained upon patients' initial presentation in the Department of Infectious Diseases, Taihe Hospital, Hubei University of Medicine.

Patients with chronic HBV infection had significantly elevated serum resistin levels

Serum resistin was rarely detectable in the HC group (0.078 ± 0.270). In contrast, high serum resistin levels were detected in patients with CHB (4.119 ± 5.848), LC-B (6.370 ± 6.834), and LF-B (6.512 ± 6.076) (Table 1, Fig. 1). Compared with CHB patients, LC-B patients and LF-B patients had significantly higher serum levels of resistin ($p < 0.01$), whereas LC-B patients and LF-B patients did not significantly differ with respect to serum resistin levels ($p > 0.05$) (Fig. 1).

Patients with chronic HBV infection had significantly increased serum levels of IL-1, IL-6, IL-17, TNF-α, and TGF-β1, but not IL-23

With respect to cytokine detection, serum IL-1 and IL-6 were below the detection limit in HCs, whereas IL-17 (2.923 ± 2.310 pg/mL), IL-23 (4.589 ± 3.823 pg/mL), TNF-α (2.489 ± 2.083 pg/mL), and TGF-β1 (29.380 ± 3.339 pg/mL) were detected in these subjects. Compared with HCs, patients with CHB, LC-B, or LF-B had elevated levels of IL-1, IL-6, IL-17, TNF-α, and TGF-β1 (Table 1, Fig. 2). Serum IL-1 levels were higher in LC-B patients (0.932 ± 1.754 pg/mL) than in CHB patients

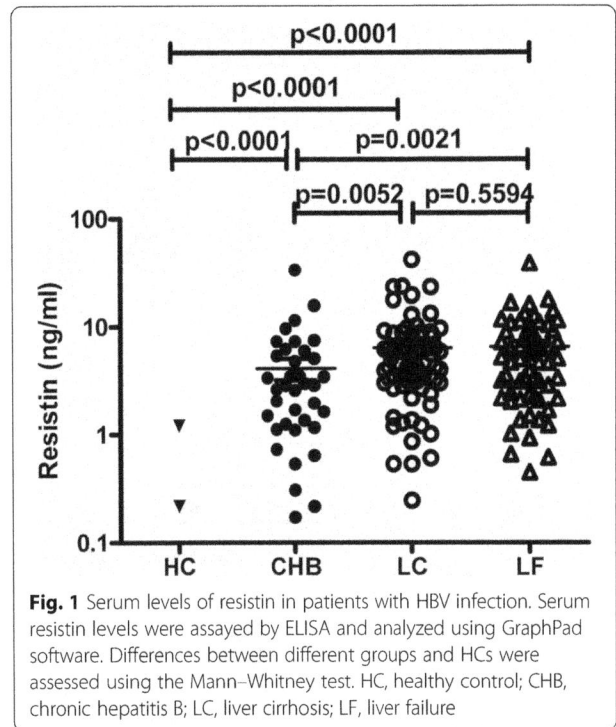

Fig. 1 Serum levels of resistin in patients with HBV infection. Serum resistin levels were assayed by ELISA and analyzed using GraphPad software. Differences between different groups and HCs were assessed using the Mann–Whitney test. HC, healthy control; CHB, chronic hepatitis B; LC, liver cirrhosis; LF, liver failure

(0.549 ± 1.341 pg/mL) and LF-B patients ($p < 0.001$) (Fig. 2a). LC-B patients (21.822 ± 50.372 pg/mL) and LF-B patients (29.792 ± 51.394 pg/mL) had markedly higher serum IL-6 levels than CHB patients ($p < 0.001$), whereas the serum IL-6 levels of LC-B patients and LF-B patients did not significantly differ ($p > 0.05$) (Fig. 2b). All patients had high serum IL-17 and TNF-α levels, with no significant differences in these cytokines among CHB patients, LC-B patients, and LF-B patients ($p > 0.05$) (Fig. 2c and e). Serum TGF-β1 levels were higher in LF-B patients (55.537 ± 6.971 pg/mL) than in CHB patients (46.205 ± 7.818 pg/mL) and LC-B patients (48.636 ± 11.555 pg/mL) ($p < 0.001$) (Fig. 2f). Average serum IL-23 levels were higher for patients than for HCs but did not significantly differ among CHB patients, LC-B patients, and LF-B patients ($p > 0.05$) (Fig. 2d).

Serum resistin was positively correlated with serum IL-17 among patients with LC-B or LF-B

Among all patients with chronic HBV infection, serum resistin was positively correlated with serum IL-17 ($R = 0.4121$, $p < 0.0001$) (Fig. 3a). Further analysis demonstrated that serum resistin was strongly positively correlated with serum IL-17 among LF-B patients ($R = 0.5466$, $p < 0.0001$) (Fig. 3d), more weakly positively correlated with serum IL-17 among LC-B patients ($R = 0.4022$, $p = 0.0038$) (Fig. 3c), and not correlated with serum IL-17 among CHB patients ($R = 0.0102$, $p = 0.9560$) (Fig. 3b).

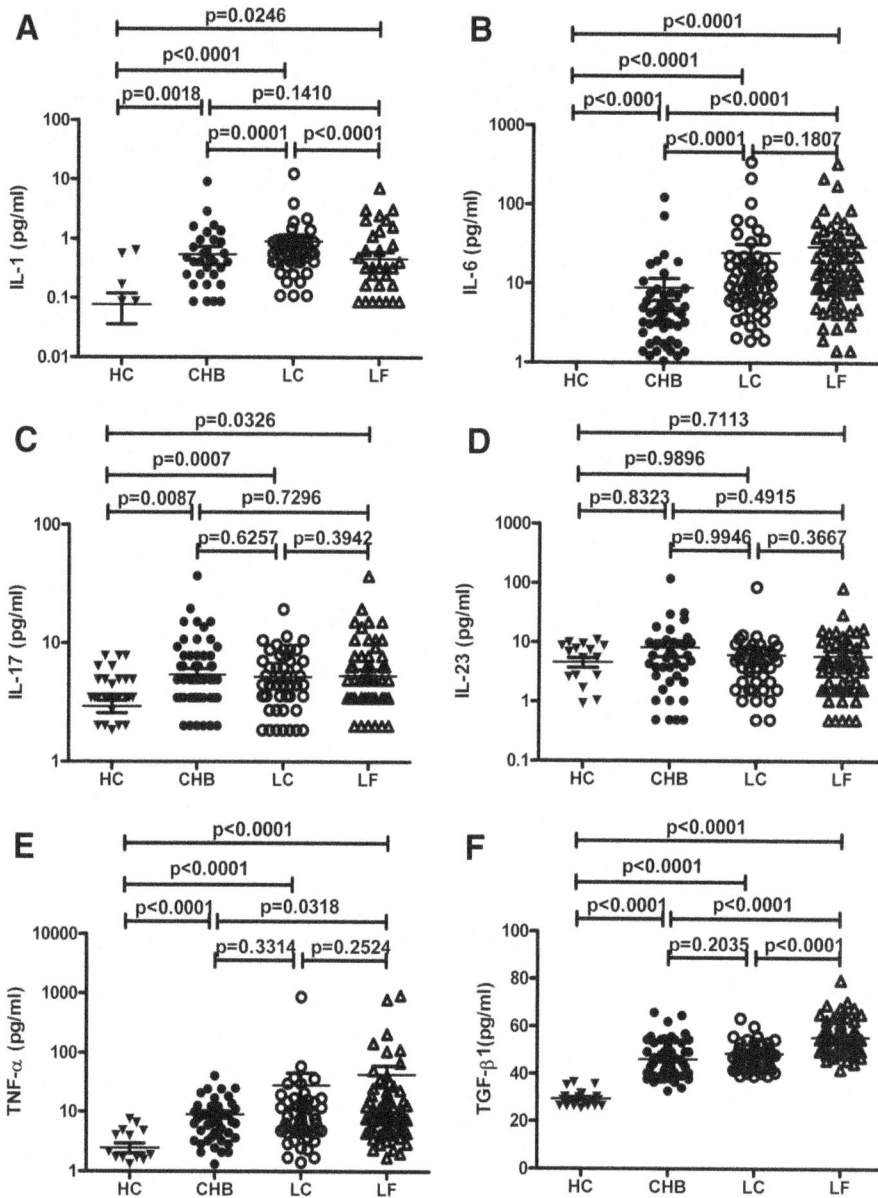

Fig. 2 Serum levels of IL-1, IL-6, IL-17, IL-23, TNF-α, and TGF-β1 in patients with HBV infection. Serum levels of IL-1 (**a**), IL-6 (**b**), IL-17 (**c**), IL-23 (**d**), TNF-α (**e**), and TGF-β1 (**f**) were assayed by ELISA and analyzed using GraphPad software. Differences between different groups and HCs were assessed using the Mann–Whitney test. HC, healthy control; CHB, chronic hepatitis B; LC, liver cirrhosis; LF, liver failure

Serum resistin was positively correlated with serum TGF-β1 in patients with LC-B

Subsequently, the relationship between serum resistin and serum TGF-β1 was analyzed. Positive correlations between serum resistin and serum TGF-β1 were observed for all patients with chronic HBV infection ($R = 0.2251$, $p = 0.0073$) (Fig. 4a). Subgroup analysis indicated that serum resistin was weakly positively correlated with serum TGF-β1 among LC-B patients ($R = 0.3090$, $p = 0.0290$) (Fig. 4b). Serum resistin was

not correlated with serum TGF-β1 among CHB patients and LF-B patients (data not shown).

Serum resistin levels were positively correlated with LS in patients with CHB

The relationship between serum resistin levels and LS was also analyzed. A weak positive correlation with LS was found among all patients with HBV infection ($R = 0.1374$, $p = 0.0445$) (Fig. 5a). In subgroup

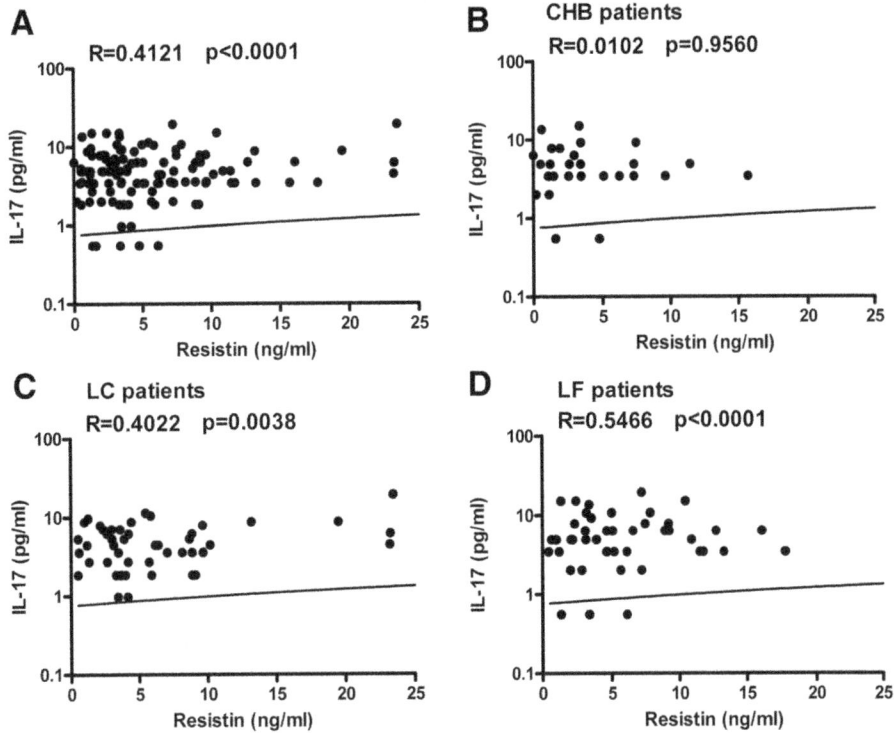

Fig. 3 The relationship between serum resistin and serum IL-17. Serum resistin levels and serum IL-17 levels were analyzed by correlation analysis using GraphPad software. The correlations between resistin levels and serum IL-17 levels among all hepatitis B patients (**a**), CHB patients (**b**), LC-B patients (**c**), and LF-B patients (**d**) are presented. CHB, chronic hepatitis B; LC, liver cirrhosis; LF, liver failure

analysis, this correlation was only found among CHB patients ($R = 0.3415$, $p = 0.0310$) (Fig. 5b). Serum resistin levels were not correlated with LS among LC-B patients or LF-B patients (data not shown).

Serum resistin was positively correlated with serum AST in patients with CHB

The relationships between serum resistin and serum ALT, AST, and TBil were also analyzed. A positive correlation between serum resistin and serum AST was observed among CHB patients ($R = 0.4501$, $p = 0.0036$)

(Fig. 6). Serum resistin was not correlated with serum AST among LC-B patients or LF-B patients; in addition, no correlations between serum resistin and serum ALT or TBil were detected either among all enrolled patients or in any examined subgroup (data not shown).

Discussion

This study revealed that patients with chronic HBV infection had significantly elevated serum resistin levels; this finding is consistent with previously reported data [20]. Patients with LC-B or LF-B had significantly higher

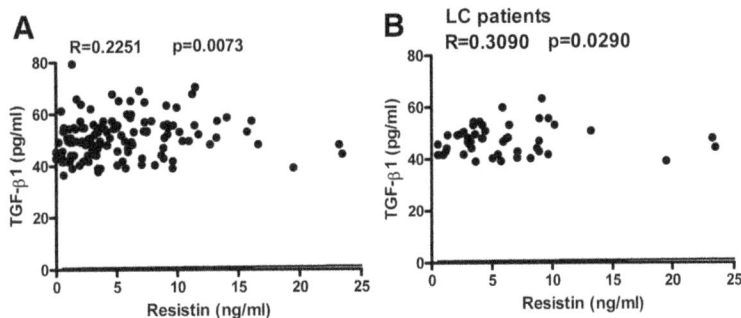

Fig. 4 The relationship between serum resistin and serum TGF-β1. Serum resistin levels and serum TGF-β1 levels were analyzed by correlation analysis using GraphPad software. The correlations between resistin levels and serum TGF-β1 levels among all hepatitis B patients (**a**) and LC-B patients (**b**) are presented. LC, liver cirrhosis

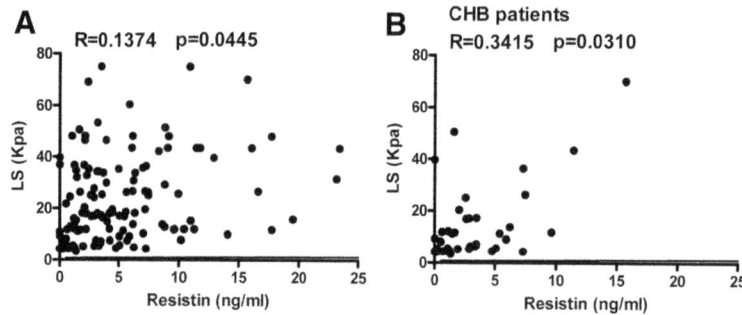

Fig. 5 The relationship between serum resistin and LS. Serum resistin levels and LS values were analyzed by correlation analysis using GraphPad software. The correlation between resistin levels and LS among all hepatitis B patients (**a**) and CHB patients (**b**) are presented. CHB, chronic hepatitis B

serum resistin levels than CHB patients ($p < 0.01$), whereas LC-B patients and LF-B patients did not significantly differ with respect to serum resistin levels ($p > 0.05$). These results suggest that serum resistin could play a role as an indicator of disease severity and/or degeneration in patients with hepatitis B. Moreover, high serum levels of IL-1, IL-6, IL-17, TNF-α, and TGF-β1 but not IL-23 were detected in CHB, LC-B, and LF-B patients. Serum IL-1 levels were higher in LC-B patients than in CHB and LF-B patients, whereas serum IL-6 and TNF-α levels were much higher for LC-B patients and LF-B patients than for CHB patients; these findings are consistent with the inflammatory roles of the proinflammatory cytokines IL-1, IL-6, and TNF-α [25].

In this study, serum resistin levels were weakly correlated with LS values determined by FibroScan among CHB patients but not among LC-B patients or LF-B patients. This result can be explained by the fact that LS

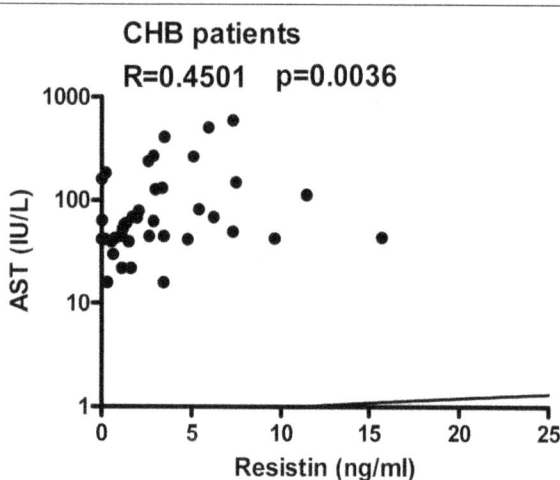

Fig. 6 The relationship between serum resistin and serum AST. Serum resistin levels and serum AST levels were analyzed by correlation analysis using GraphPad software. The correlation between resistin levels and serum AST levels among CHB patients is presented. CHB, chronic hepatitis B

depends on the extent of fibrosis due to prior intrahepatic deposits [26]. Serum markers such as procollagen peptide, matrix metalloproteinases (MMPs), tissue inhibitors of matrix metalloproteinases (TIMPs), laminins, and TGF-β1, are correlated with molecules derived directly from the ECM or produced by activated HSCs. Thus, the elevation of these serum markers suggests the activation of fibrogenesis [27, 28]. Interestingly, serum resistin levels were positively correlated with serum TGF-β1 levels, particularly among LC-B patients (Fig. 4). Furthermore, among CHB patients, serum resistin levels were positively correlated with serum AST levels (Fig. 5). These results are consistent with the general notion that resistin can act as an intrahepatic cytokine with proinflammatory activity in HSCs via a Ca^{2+}/NF-κB-dependent pathway and involvement in the pathophysiology of liver fibrosis [18].

IL-17 is a major effector cytokine secreted by Th17 cells, which play a proinflammatory role in the pathogenesis of hepatitis B and promote HBV infection-related injury [29]. In this study, all patients with CHB, LC-B, or LF-B exhibited similarly elevated serum IL-17 levels (Fig. 2c). There were no significant correlations between serum IL-17 and serum ALT, AST, or TBil (data not shown). Serum IL-17 was positively correlated with serum resistin among LC-B patients and LF-B patients but not among CHB patients (Fig. 3); these findings provide additional evidence supporting the proinflammatory role of IL-17, especially in the context of advanced liver injury.

Recently, Ming et al. found that the upregulation of the TGF-β1/IL-31 pathway is associated with disease severity in LC-B, since elevated serum TGF-β1 and IL-31 levels were positively associated with albumin, alpha-fetoprotein, creatinine, white blood cell, and platelet levels among LC-B patients [30]. Furthermore, TGF-β1/IL-31 pathway may also play an important role in the pathogenesis of liver injury during chronic HBV infection, since increased activity of the TGF-β1/IL-31 pathway has been found well correlated with the extent of liver injury, disease severity, and nonsurvival among ACLF patients, whereas reduced activity of this pathway has been detected during the recovery from liver injury in CHB cases [31]. In the current study, patients with HBV chronic infection exhibited elevated serum TGF-β1, and serum TGF-β1 levels were significantly higher in LF-B patients than in CHB patients or LC-B patients. CHB and LC-B patients did not significantly differ with respect to serum TGF-β1, although average serum TGF-β1 levels were slightly higher in LC-B patients than in CHB patients. These results provided additional data to support the potential role of TGF-β1 in the pathogenesis of liver injury in patients with chronic HBV infection, particularly patients with LF-B.

IL-23 has recently been identified as playing a critical role in a number of chronic inflammatory diseases. Xia et al. reported that both serum IL-23 level and hepatic IL-23 were positively correlated with liver injury in CHB patients [32]. In this study, average serum IL-23 levels were higher in patients than in HCs and were markedly higher in CHB patients than in HCs (8.149 vs. 4.589), with no significant differences in serum IL-23 levels among CHB patients, LC-B patients, and LF-B patients. This lack of significance may be attributable to the large deviations detected in serum IL-23 levels (which ranged from 0.49 to 118.92).

Taken together, the findings of this study demonstrated that high serum resistin was positively correlated with serum IL-17 and TGF-β1. Elevated resistin is associated with the inflammation and necrosis of liver cells and could therefore potentially be used as an index of disease severity and degeneration in patients with chronic HBV infection. However, the mechanism of resistin in the inflammatory process of chronic hepatitis B is unclear, further studies are needed to elucidate how resistin works in the progress of liver injury, and the cross-talk between resistin and IL-17 or TGF-β signaling pathways.

Conclusions

High serum resistin associates with intrahepatic inflammation and necrosis and may be used as an index of disease severity for patients with chronic HBV infection.

Abbreviations
ALT: Alanine aminotransferase; AST: Aspartate aminotransferase; CHB: Chronic hepatitis B; CTL: Cytotoxic T-lymphocyte; ELISA: Enzyme-linked immunobsorbent assay; HBV: Hepatitis B virus; HSC: Hepatic stellate cells; LC: Liver cirrhosis; LF: Liver failure; LS: Liver stiffness; NAFLD: Nonalcoholic fatty liver disease; TGF-β: Transforming growth factors beta; TNF-α: Tumor necrosis factor alpha

Acknowledgements
The authors thank Yuling He and Yingqi Huang for excellent technical assistance.

Funding
This work was partly supported by the National Key Program for Infectious Disease of China (2013ZX10002-001), the Natural Science Foundation of Hubei Province of China (2014CFB645 and 2010CDZ036), the Natural Science Foundation of Hubei Provincial Department of Education (Z20102101), and the Foundation for Innovative Research Team of Hubei University of Medicine (2014CXG05).

Authors' contributions
MZJ and ZYH1 contributed equally to this work; MZJ, ZYH, CY, LJ and GZJ participated in the design of the study and performed the statistical analysis; ZYH1, WZQ, LP, KJ, ZYH2, MDQ and KCZ carried out the ELISAs; MZ and WZQ contributed new reagents; MZ, WZQ and LP analyzed the data; MZJ, CY, LJ and GZJ conceived of the study, and participated in its design and coordination and helped to draft the manuscript. All authors read and approved the final manuscript.

Competing interests
The authors declare that they have no competing interests.

Consent for publication
Not applicable.

Author details
[1]Department of Infectious Diseases, Taihe Hospital, Hubei University of Medicine, Shiyan, China. [2]Institute of Biomedicine, Taihe Hospital, Hubei University of Medicine, Shiyan, China. [3]Institute of Wudang Chinese Medicine, Taihe Hospital, Hubei University of Medicine, Shiyan, China. [4]Department of Neurology, Taihe Hospital, Hubei University of Medicine, South Renmin Road. 32, 442000 Shiyan, Hubei, China. [5]Department of Infectious Diseases, Renmin Hospital of Wuhan University, Zhangzhidong Road. 99, 430060 Wuhan, China.

References
1. Trepo C, Chan HL, Lok A. Hepatitis B virus infection. Lancet. 2014;384(9959): 2053–63.
2. Sugawara K, Nakayama N, Mochida S. Acute liver failure in Japan: definition, classification, and prediction of the outcome. J Gastroenterol. 2012;47(8):849–61.
3. Wu JF, Chang MH. Natural history of chronic hepatitis B virus infection from infancy to adult life - the mechanism of inflammation triggering and long-term impacts. J Biomed Sci. 2015;22:92.
4. Chang ML, Liaw YF. Hepatitis B flares in chronic hepatitis B: pathogenesis, natural course, and management. J Hepatol. 2014;61(6):1407–17.
5. Balmasova IP, Yushchuk ND, Mynbaev OA, Alla NR, Malova ES, Shi Z, Gao CL. Immunopathogenesis of chronic hepatitis B. World J Gastroenterol. 2014; 20(39):14156–71.
6. Shimizu Y. T cell immunopathogenesis and immunotherapeutic strategies for chronic hepatitis B virus infection. World J Gastroenterol. 2012;18(20):2443–51.
7. Maini MK, Boni C, Lee CK, Larrubia JR, Reignat S, Ogg GS, King AS, Herberg J, Gilson R, Alisa A, et al. The role of virus-specific CD8(+) cells in liver damage and viral control during persistent hepatitis B virus infection. J Exp Med. 2000; 191(8):1269–80.
8. Sica A, Invernizzi P, Mantovani A. Macrophage plasticity and polarization in liver homeostasis and pathology. Hepatology. 2014;59(5):2034–42.
9. Bility MT, Cheng L, Zhang Z, Luan Y, Li F, Chi L, Zhang L, Tu Z, Gao Y, Fu Y, et al. Hepatitis B virus infection and immunopathogenesis in a humanized mouse model: induction of human-specific liver fibrosis and M2-like macrophages. PLoS Pathog. 2014;10(3):e1004032.
10. Zhao L, Qiu DK, Ma X. Th17 cells: the emerging reciprocal partner of regulatory T cells in the liver. J Dig Dis. 2010;11(3):126–33.
11. Zhang GL, Xie DY, Ye YN, Lin CS, Zhang XH, Zheng YB, Huang ZL, Peng L, Gao ZL. High level of IL-27 positively correlated with Th17 cells may indicate liver injury in patients infected with HBV. Liver Int. 2014;34(2):266–73.
12. Zhang JY, Zhang Z, Lin F, Zou ZS, Xu RN, Jin L, Fu JL, Shi F, Shi M, Wang HF, et al. Interleukin-17-producing CD4(+) T cells increase with severity of liver damage in patients with chronic hepatitis B. Hepatology. 2010;51(1):81–91.
13. Takehara T, Hayashi N, Katayama K, Kasahara A, Fusamoto H, Kamada T.

Hepatitis B core antigen-specific interferon gamma production of peripheral blood mononuclear cells during acute exacerbation of chronic hepatitis B. Scand J Gastroenterol. 1992;27(9):727–31.

14. Leifeld L, Cheng S, Ramakers J, Dumoulin FL, Trautwein C, Sauerbruch T, Spengler U. Imbalanced intrahepatic expression of interleukin 12, interferon gamma, and interleukin 10 in fulminant hepatitis B. Hepatology. 2002;36(4 Pt 1):1001–8.

15. Dunn C, Brunetto M, Reynolds G, Christophides T, Kennedy PT, Lampertico P, Das A, Lopes AR, Borrow P, Williams K, et al. Cytokines induced during chronic hepatitis B virus infection promote a pathway for NK cell-mediated liver damage. J Exp Med. 2007;204(3):667–80.

16. Steppan CM, Brown EJ, Wright CM, Bhat S, Banerjee RR, Dai CY, Enders GH, Silberg DG, Wen X, Wu GD, et al. A family of tissue-specific resistin-like molecules. Proc Natl Acad Sci U S A. 2001;98(2):502–6.

17. Steppan CM, Bailey ST, Bhat S, Brown EJ, Banerjee RR, Wright CM, Patel HR, Ahima RS, Lazar MA. The hormone resistin links obesity to diabetes. Nature. 2001;409(6818):307–12.

18. Bertolani C, Sancho-Bru P, Failli P, Bataller R, Aleffi S, DeFranco R, Mazzinghi B, Romagnani P, Milani S, Gines P, et al. Resistin as an intrahepatic cytokine: overexpression during chronic injury and induction of proinflammatory actions in hepatic stellate cells. Am J Pathol. 2006;169(6):2042–53.

19. Tiftikci A, Atug O, Yilmaz Y, Eren F, Ozdemir FT, Yapali S, Ozdogan O, Celikel CA, Imeryuz N, Tozun N. Serum levels of adipokines in patients with chronic HCV infection: relationship with steatosis and fibrosis. Arch Med Res. 2009; 40(4):294–8.

20. Tsochatzis E, Papatheodoridis GV, Hadziyannis E, Georgiou A, Kafiri G, Tiniakos DG, Manesis EK, Archimandritis AJ. Serum adipokine levels in chronic liver diseases: association of resistin levels with fibrosis severity. Scand J Gastroenterol. 2008;43(9):1128–36.

21. Bostrom EA, Ekstedt M, Kechagias S, Sjowall C, Bokarewa MI, Almer S. Resistin is associated with breach of tolerance and anti-nuclear antibodies in patients with hepatobiliary inflammation. Scand J Immunol. 2011;74(5):463–70.

22. Pagano C, Soardo G, Pilon C, Milocco C, Basan L, Milan G, Donnini D, Faggian D, Mussap M, Plebani M, et al. Increased serum resistin in nonalcoholic fatty liver disease is related to liver disease severity and not to insulin resistance. J Clin Endocrinol Metab. 2006;91(3):1081–6.

23. Chinese Society of Hepatology and Chinese Society of Infectious Diseases, Chinese Medical Association. The guideline of prevention and treatment for chronic hepatitis B (2010 version). Zhonghua Gan Zang Bing Za Zhi. 2011; 19(1):13–24.

24. Organization Committee of 13th Asia-Pacific Congress of Clinical Microbiology and Infection. 13th Asia-pacific congress of clinical microbiology and infection consensus guidelines for diagnosis and treatment of liver failure. Hepatobiliary Pancreat Dis Int. 2013;12(4):346–54.

25. Zhang W, Yue B, Wang GQ, Lu SL. Serum and ascites levels of macrophage migration inhibitory factor, TNF-alpha and IL-6 in patients with chronic virus hepatitis B and hepatitis cirrhosis. Hepatobiliary Pancreat Dis Int. 2002;1(4):577–80.

26. Ding D, Li H, Liu P, Chen L, Kang J, Zhang Y, Ma D, Chen Y, Luo J, Meng Z. FibroScan, aspartate aminotransferase and alanine aminotransferase ratio (AAR), aspartate aminotransferase to platelet ratio index (APRI), fibrosis index based on the 4 factor (FIB-4), and their combinations in the assessment of liver fibrosis in patients with hepatitis B. Int J Clin Exp Med. 2015;8(11):20876–82.

27. Soresi M, Giannitrapani L, Cervello M, Licata A, Montalto G. Non invasive tools for the diagnosis of liver cirrhosis. World J Gastroenterol. 2014;20(48):18131–50.

28. Liu T, Wang X, Karsdal MA, Leeming DJ, Genovese F. Molecular serum markers of liver fibrosis. Biomark Insights. 2012;7:105–17.

29. Huang Z, van Velkinburgh JC, Ni B, Wu Y. Pivotal roles of the interleukin-23/ T helper 17 cell axis in hepatitis B. Liver Int. 2012;32(6):894–901.

30. Ming D, Yu X, Guo R, Deng Y, Li J, Lin C, Su M, Lin Z, Su Z. Elevated TGF-beta1/IL-31 pathway is associated with the disease severity of hepatitis B virus-related liver cirrhosis. Viral Immunol. 2015;28(4):209–16.

31. Yu X, Guo R, Ming D, Deng Y, Su M, Lin C, Li J, Lin Z, Su Z. The transforming growth factor beta1/interleukin-31 pathway is upregulated in patients with hepatitis B virus-related acute-on-chronic liver failure and is associated with disease severity and survival. Clin Vaccine Immunol. 2015;22(5):484–92.

32. Xia L, Tian D, Huang W, Zhu H, Wang J, Zhang Y, Hu H, Nie Y, Fan D, Wu K. Upregulation of IL-23 expression in patients with chronic hepatitis B is mediated by the HBx/ERK/NF-kappaB pathway. J Immunol. 2012;188(2):753–64.

Prophylaxis of post-ERC infectious complications in patients with biliary obstruction by adding antimicrobial agents into ERC contrast media- a single center retrospective study

Hella Wobser[1]*[iD], Agnetha Gunesch[1] and Frank Klebl[1,2]

Abstract

Background: Patients with biliary obstruction are at high risk to develop septic complications after endoscopic retrograde cholangiography (ERC). We evaluated the benefits of local application of antimicrobial agents into ERC contrast media in preventing post-ERC infectious complications in a high-risk study population.

Methods: Patients undergoing ERC at our tertiary referral center were retrospectively included. Addition of vancomycin, gentamicin and fluconazol into ERC contrast media was evaluated in a case-control design. Outcomes comprised infectious complications within 3 days after ERC.

Results: In total, 84 ERC cases were analyzed. Primarily indications for ERC were sclerosing cholangitis (75%) and malignant stenosis (9.5%). Microbial testing of collected bile fluid in the treatment group was positive in 91.4%. Detected organisms were sensitive to the administered antimicrobials in 93%. The use of antimicrobials in contrast media was associated with a significant decrease in post-ERC infectious complications compared to non-use (14.3% vs. 33.3%; odds ratio [OR]: 0.33, 95% confidence interval [CI]: 0.114–0.978). After adjusting for the variables acute cholangitis prior to ERC and incomplete biliary drainage, the beneficial effect of intraductal antibiotic prophylaxis was even more evident (OR = 0.153; 95% CI: 0.039–0.598, $p = 0.007$). Patients profiting most obviously from intraductal antimicrobials were those with secondary sclerosing cholangitis.

Conclusion: Local application of a combination of antibiotic and antimycotic agents to ERC contrast media efficiently reduced post-ERC infectious events in patients with biliary obstruction. This is the first study that evaluates ERC-related infectious complications in patients with secondary sclerosing cholangitis. Our first clinical results should now be prospectively evaluated in a larger patient cohort to improve the safety of ERC, especially in patients with secondary sclerosing cholangitis.

Keywords: Endoscopic retrograde cholangiography (ERC), Intraductal antimicrobial prophylaxis, Infectious complications, Biliary obstruction, Secondary sclerosing cholangitis

* Correspondence: Hella.Wobser@ukr.de
[1]Department of Internal Medicine and Gastroenterology, University Hospital of Regensburg, Regensburg 93042, Germany
Full list of author information is available at the end of the article

Background

Infections such as cholangitis and sepsis are serious, albeit rare complications after endoscopic retrograde cholangioscopy (ERC). Post-ERC infections are reported to occur in less than 5% of all interventions [1, 2]. High hygienic standards for the intervention itself and thorough disinfection and storage of endoscope and endoscopic devices have essentially attributed to this low infectious rate [3]. Procedural improvements such as endoscopic decompression by biliary stents and immediate placement of percutaneous biliary drainage if endoscopic drainage is not possible, represent further strategies to reduce the incidence of ERC-related infectious complications [4, 5]. This is an important issue, as failure to restore an adequate drainage after injection of contrast media into obstructed bile tracts during ERC still represents the major risk factor for post-ERC infection [6, 7].

Obstruction of the bile duct system due to stones, strictures and tumors has been demonstrated to be associated with bacteriobilia [8]. Increasing intrabiliary pressure (>25 mmHg) results in biliovenous reflux and consecutively in bacteremia in case of already infected bile [9, 10]. Injection of contrast media during ERC raises the intraductal pressure, especially if a complete endoscopic drainage is not achieved thereafter. Therefore, patients with hilar tumors and sclerosing cholangitis for whom complete biliary drainage is often impossible, are at highest risk to develop post-ERC infections [11, 12].

Routine prophylactic use of systemic antibiotics was shown to reduce ERC-related bacteremia [13]. However, beneficial effects on preventing post-ERC cholangitis in unselected patients could not be demonstrated [14–16]. A recent retrospective study analyzed the benefit of systemic antibiotic prophylaxis in 11.484 patients undergoing ERC over an 11-year period [17]. At baseline all patients with biliary obstruction, immunosuppression and the need of therapeutic intervention (95% of all procedures) received routinely systemic prophylactic antibiosis. Over time, the use of prophylactic antibiotics was sequentially reduced. In the final phase, systemic antibiotic prophylaxis was restricted to patients for whom endoscopic drainage was predicted to be incomplete and to patients with immunosuppressive therapy (26% of all procedures). Despite the limited use of systemic antibiotic prophylaxis, no significant difference in infectious complications after ERC was observed. These data are in line with the current recommendations of antibiotic prophylaxis in gastrointestinal endoscopy [18, 19]. Systemic antibiotic prophylaxis should be considered before an ERC in those patients with known or suspected biliary obstruction for whom complete endoscopic drainage will presumably not be achieved. This concerns especially patients with hilar strictures and primary sclerosing cholangitis (PSC).

Of note, biliary excretion of systemically administered antibiotic agents was shown to be low in case of biliary obstruction or hepatic dysfunction [20]. Thus, antibiotic bile concentrations may be far below the minimal inhibitory concentration (MIC). Theoretically, local application of antibiotics into the ERC contrast media should result in high antibacterial concentration within the bile. Thus, this regimen is supposed to be especially effective in preventing ERC-related cholangiosepsis. Indeed, in vitro studies have demonstrated that addition of gentamicin to the ERC contrast media eliminated bacteriobilia [21]. In a high-risk study population, the combination of intravenous and intraductal antibiotic administration was shown to efficiently prevent post-ERC infectious complications [22]. Most recently, adding gentamicin to contrast media had no significant effect on the incidence of post-ERC cholangitis, however adequate drainage of biliary obstruction by stenting was obtained in all these patients [23].

Taking these rather heterogeneous and inconsistent data into account, we aimed to evaluate whether local application of antimicrobial agents into contrast media will be beneficial to reduce post-ERC infectious complications in a study population mainly predicted to incomplete endoscopic drainage.

Methods

Study population

Data acquisition

This retrospective single-center study covers an 8-year-period from January 2003 to December 2011. During this time, 1353 patients with biliary obstruction underwent ERC. Of these, 101 patients received antimicrobial agents into the ERC contrast media. 59 patients with incomplete follow up or with ERC within the preceding 70 days were excluded from this study. 13 patients underwent ERC with similar indication twice within 5 years with and without intraductal antibiotics, respectively. These were included as case- and control-ERCs into our study. 29 patients with antibiotic application into the contrast media during ERC were matched to 29 control patients without antibiotic administration in respect to indication of ERC, age and sex. In summary, our study encompasses 84 ERC cases with 42 cases receiving antibiotics into the ERC contrast media and 42 control cases without antibiotics.

Demographic data

Mean age of the predominantly male (71%) study population was 52 +/- 16.2 years. All patients presented with biliary obstruction. Malignant strictures (cholangiocellular carcinoma [n = 5], pancreatic cancer [n = 2], metastasis [n = 1]) and sclerosing cholangitis (primary sclerosing cholangitis [n = 20] and secondary sclerosing cholangitis [n = 44]) were the most prevalent causes of biliary obstruction. Other etiologies of obstructive bile tract system included choledocholithasis ($n = 4$), benign stenosis after liver transplantation ($n = 2$), acute cholangitis due to stent obstruction ($n = 3$) or benign stricture ($n = 1$) and chronic cholangitis ($n = 2$). Thus, the study population was mainly composed of high-risk patients regarding infectious post-ERC adverse events.

Definition of ERC-related infectious complications

In case of absent non-/biliary infection by the time of ERC (a) a rise in body temperature > 38 °C within 24 h after ERC (in case of body temperature < 38 °C before ERC) or (b) increase of white blood cell count and/or CRP over upper normal limits in combination with elevation of transaminases ($\Delta10$ U/l) and bilirubin ($\Delta1.5$ mg/dl) within 3 days after ERC were defined as infectious complication.

When non-/biliary infection was present by the time of ERC, (c) a rise in body temperature > 38 °C within 24 h after ERC (incase of body temperature < 38 °C before ERC) or (d) increase of white blood cell count of $\Delta2000/\mu l$ within 3 days after ERC or (e) increase of CRP $\Delta50$ mg/l within 3 days of ERC characterized infectious complication.

Definition of successful ERC

ERC was categorized as successful when (a) biliary drainage was restored and laboratory tests for alkaline phosphatase, γ-glutamyltransferase and bilirubin as well as transaminases decreased after ERC, (b) in case of sclerosing cholangitis: laboratory tests for alkaline phosphatase, γ-glutamyltransferase and bilirubin as well as transaminases decreased after ERC, even if complete biliary decompression failed, and (c) in case of stent removal/replacement: laboratory tests for alkaline phosphatase, γ-glutamyltransferase and bilirubin as well as transaminases remained at least stable.

Statistical analysis

All statistical analyses were performed with SPSS Version 22 (SPSS Inc., Chicago, IL, USA). Descriptive data of patients are presented as mean values with the interquartile range for continuous variables or percentage for categorial variables. Pearsons's chi-squared test was used to compare categorial data. Factors influencing the risk of post-ERC infectious complications were analyzed using binary logistic regression models. Due to the low patient numbers, it was predefined that only the two presumably most important risk factors for infectious complications, namely presence of acute cholangitis at ERC, and incomplete biliary drainage, would be included in the multivariate logistic regression to calculate the effect of intraductal administration of antimicrobial agents on post-ERC infectious complications. Values of $p < 0.05$ were considered to be statistically significant.

Results

Patient demographics and clinical features

Eighty-four cases of biliary obstruction undergoing ERC in our tertiary referral center were analyzed in this retrospective study to evaluate the benefit of antimicrobial agents added to the contrast media on the rate of post-ERC infectious complications. Therefore, 42 cases receiving antibiotics into ERC contrast media were matched to 42 controls without antibiotics for the parameters age, sex and etiology of biliary obstruction. Patient characteristics are shown in Table 1 for both groups.

In the treated group ($n = 42$) the following antimicrobial agents were administered to 50 ml contrast media (Optiray 300 g/ml): gentamicin 80 mg (2 ml), vancomycin 500 mg (5 ml) and fluconazole 40 mg (20 ml). Most patients in the treated group received a combination of all antimicrobial agents ($n = 29$; 69% of treated cases). Solely gentamicin was given in 7 cases (16.7%), whereas a combination of both antibiotics was administered in 6 cases (14.3%). In addition, 51.3% (43/84) of all patients received a systemic antibiotic treatment within 28 days prior to and at ERC. Of note, there was no statistical difference between the two study groups regarding frequency of systemic antibiotic treatment (24/42 patients in the treated group vs. 19/42 in the control group, $p = 0.28$). Most frequently, patients with secondary sclerosing cholangitis (SC) [29 out of 44 SC-patients, 65.9%], with primary sclerosing cholangitis (PSC) [6 out of 20 PSC-patients, 30%] and with choledocholithiasis [3 out of 4 patients, 75%] received systemic antibiotic treatment prior to and at ERC. The main indication for antibiotic treatment was acute cholangitis.

Table 1 Clinical characteristics of the study population

Patient characteristics	Intraductal antibiotic prophylaxis	No antibiotic prophylaxis	p
Mean age	51.8 ± 16.4	52.4 ± 16.2	0.26
Male (n; %)	30 (71)	30 (71)	
Etiology of biliary obstruction (n; %)			
• Sclerosing cholangitis	32 (76)	32 (76)	
• Malignant stricture	4 (10)	4 (10)	
• Choledocholithiasis	2 (5)	2 (5)	
• Benign stricture	1 (2)	1 (2)	
• Cholangitis	3 (7)	3 (7)	
Immunosuppressive medication (n; %)	11 (26)	14 (33)	0.49
Hospitalization (d)	13.9 ± 21.1	13.3 ± 16.6	0.47
Cholangitis at ERC (n; %)	27 (64)	23 (55)	0.37
Non-biliary infection (n; %)	16 (38)	13 (31)	0.49

Patients were matched in respect to age, sex and indication for ERC

Details on ERC data are shown in Table 2. There was no statistical difference between the two groups regarding the endoscopic procedures.

Microbial cultures of bile samples

Thirty-five bile samples (83.3% of the treated cases) taken from patients receiving antimicrobial agents into the contrast media were analyzed on microbial colonization (Table 3). Only three bile cultures (8.6%) were tested negative for bacterial and fungal species. The most frequently isolated bacterial organisms in the collected bile samples were *Enterococcus* spp. found in 71.4% (25/35), *E. coli* in 25.7% (9/35), *Klebsiella* spp. in 11.4% (4/35), *Pseudomonas* spp. in 11.4% (4/35) and other gram-negative bacteria in 11.4% (4/35). *Candida* spp. were isolated in 25.7% (9/35) of the bile samples. Polymicrobial infection was detected in 54% (19/35) of bile samples. The results of the antibiogram were not available for 7 bile cultures. In 3 bile samples the isolated bacteria were resistant to the administered intraductal antibiotics. All *Candida species* were sensitive to fluconazole.

Antimicrobial agents in ERC contrast media reduced ERC-related infectious complications

ERC-related infectious complications were observed in 23.8% of patients (20/84). While 33.3% (14/42) of patients not subjected to antimicrobial agents into the contrast media developed a post-ERC infectious complication, only 14.3% (6/42) patients receiving antibiotics within the ERC contrast media presented with signs and symptoms of infection (OR = 0.33, 95% CI 0.114–0.978; $p < 0.04$; Fig. 1). Hence, the risk to develop an infectious complication after ERC was 2.33-fold higher when ERC was performed without administering antimicrobial agents to the contrast media.

Among the 20 patients with post-ERC infectious complications, frequency of systemic antibiotic treatment

Table 3 Bile cultures of bile samples from patients receiving antimicrobial agents into ERC contrast media

Cultures positive for	n (%)
Enterococcus spp.	25 (71.4%)
E. coli	9 (25.7)
Klebsiella spp.	4 (11.4)
Pseudomonas spp.	4 (11.4)
Candida spp.	9 (25.7)
Other gram-negative	4 (11.4)
Polymicrobial	19 (54.0)

Note, that the sum of percentages may be greater than 100 because of polymicrobial infections

was comparable in both study groups. In the treated group, three out of the 6 patients (50%) with ERC-related infectious complications received systemic antibiotic treatment. In the control group, eight out of the 14 patients (57%) with post-ERC infections were treated with systemic antibiotics at time of ERC.

The main known factors that influence the rate of post-ERC infectious complications are acute cholangitis prior to ERC and the completeness of biliary drainage [6]. At the time of ERC, 59.5% (50/84) cases of our study population displayed acute cholangitis. Incidence of acute cholangitis was similar in both study groups ($p = 0.37$). Univariate logistic regression analysis revealed a positive correlation between acute cholangitis prior to ERC and the incidence of ERC-related infectious complications (OR = 4.214; 95% CI: 1.034–17.173; $p = 0.045$). Incomplete drainage is considered as the main reason for administering prophylactic systemic antibiotic treatment in ERC. The ERC success rate of complete drainage achieved in our study was comparatively low (41.7%). Success rate was similar in both study groups ($p = 0.07$). In contrast to previous studies, we could not detect a significant benefit of successful ERC for prevention of infectious adverse events (OR = 0.368; 95% CI: 0.101–1.337; $p = 0.13$). After adjustment for the confounders "cholangitis" and "ERC success rate", the beneficial effect of antimicrobial agents applied to contrast media for the prevention of ERC-related infectious complications was even more evident (OR = 0.153; 95% CI: 0.039–0.598; $p = 0.007$).

Secondary sclerosing cholangitis was the most eligible biliary disorder profiting from intraductal antimicrobial prophylaxis

Secondary sclerosing cholangitis (SC) was the predominant etiology of biliary obstruction in our study population (52.4% of all cases). SC represents a progressive disease characterized by fibrosis and destruction of the biliary tract system leading to biliary cirrhosis. SC in critically ill patients (SC-CIP), known to be associated

Table 2 Details of selected endoscopic procedures

Procedure	Intraductal antibiotic prophylaxis	No antibiotic prophylaxis	p
Papillotomy	16	11	0.24
Stone removal	6	3	0.29
Necrosis removal	3	1	0.3
Dilatation	12	5	0.06
Lavage	4	3	0.69
Nasobiliary drain	5	3	0.46
Stenting			0.84
• Stent insertion	4	4	
• Stent exchange	3	2	
• Stent removal	2	3	

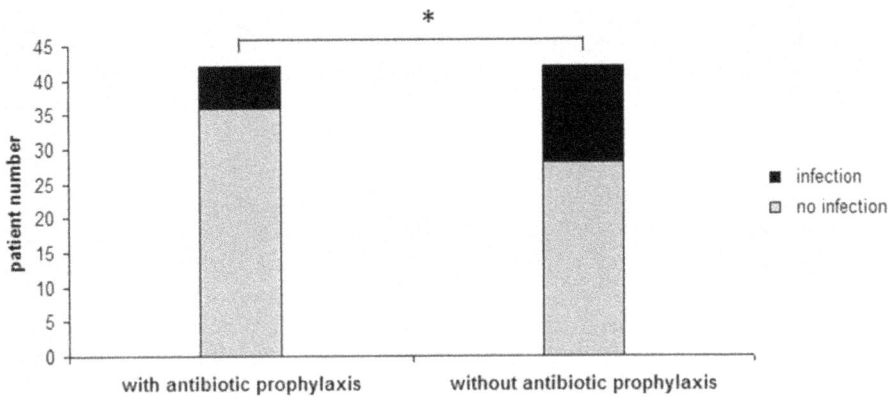

Fig. 1 ERC-related infectious complications. Patients with antibiotic prophylaxis within the contrast media developed post-ERC infectious complications significantly less frequent than patients not receiving antimicrobial agents (14.3% versus 33.3%, $p < 0.04$)

with a particularly rapid and aggressive progression to liver cirrhosis [24], was the most common cause of SC in our study population (32/44, 72.7%). Other causes of SC were ischemic cholangiopathy after liver transplantation (3/44, 6.8%), immunologic (4/44; 9.1%), toxic (2/44, 4.5%), infectious (1/44, 2.3%) and unknown (2/44, 4.5%). Subgroup analysis revealed that 65% (13/20) of the patients with post-ERC infection suffered from SC. When adding antimicrobial agents to ERC contrast media in patients with SC, we noted a significant decrease in infectious complications after ERC (2/22, 9% vs. 11/22, 50% in SC patients not given antibiotics into the contrast media; $p = 0.03$; Fig. 2). Furthermore, 77% (10/13) of the SC-patients with ERC-related infectious complications received a systemic antibiotic treatment before and at time of ERC. Moreover, 80% (8/10) of these SC-patients had no local antibiotic prophylaxis and developed post-ERC infectious complications despite a systemic antibiotic treatment.

Discussion

The presented study demonstrates several important findings that may give cause to modify the current practice of antibiotic prophylaxis to prevent ERC-related infectious complications. These include: (1) addition of antimicrobial agents into the ERC contrast media significantly reduces the incidence of post-ERC infection in patients with biliary obstruction; (2) combination of different antibiotics and antifungal regiments might be even more effective; (3) the benefit of local application of antimicrobials into obstructed bile ducts is most obvious if cholangitis is already present before ERC; (4) secondary sclerosing cholangitis represents the most eligible biliary disorder which takes particular profit from locally administered antimicrobials during ERC.

The routine administration of systemic antibiotic prophylaxis to all patients undergoing ERC has been left in favor of a selective use only in those patients with suspected or known biliary obstruction for whom complete endoscopic drainage will presumably not be achieved. This concerns

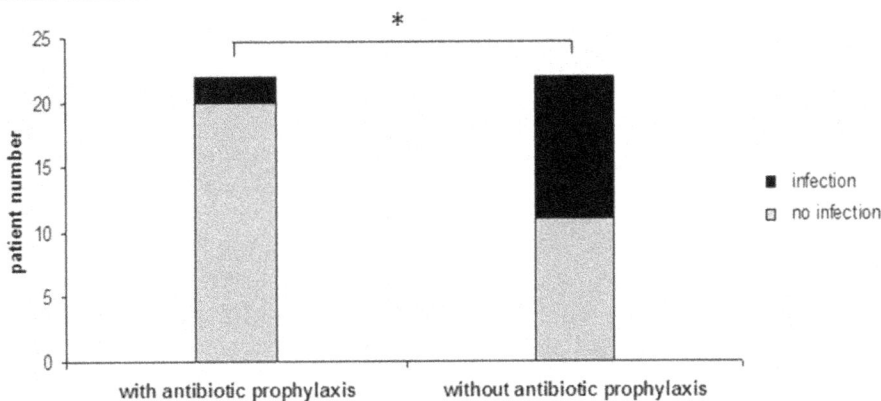

Fig. 2 Subgroup analysis of patients with sclerosing cholangitis (SC). Addition of antimicrobial agents to ERC contrast media in patients with SC resulted in a significant decrease in infectious complications after ERC (9% with antibiotics vs. 50% without antibiotics, $p = 0.03$)

particularly patients with hilar strictures and PSC [19]. Patients with post-transplant biliary strictures undergoing ERC represent other feasible candidates for systemic antibiotic prophylaxis [21]. Since systemically administered antibiotics poorly penetrate into the bile in case of biliary obstruction [20, 25, 26], a theoretical benefit of injecting antimicrobial agents directly into the bile tracts during ERC is assumable. Several studies have investigated the effect of antibiotics applied in contrast media on preventing post-ERC cholangitis with conflicting results. *In vitro* studies have proven that aminoglycosides retain their antibacterial properties when mixed to ERC contrast media. Thus, the aminoglycosides tobramycin and gentamicin efficiently eliminated common biliary bacteria such as *E. coli*, *Klebsiella pneumonia*, *Proteus vulgaris* and *Pseudomonas aeruginosa* [21, 27]. In line with these findings, we observed a significantly reduced post-ERC infection rate in patients with biliary obstruction when antimicrobial agents were added into the ERC media. Patients not receiving intraductal antibiotics into ERC contrast media exhibited a 2.33-fold increased risk to develop post-ERC cholangitis.

In contrast to our results, 3 prior prospective randomized-controlled studies could not demonstrate a beneficial effect on the rate of post-ERC infectious complications by adding antibiotics into ERC contrast media [23, 28, 29]. To explain these discrepancies, one has to take into account that only an aminoglycoside was used in the three studies, and that the analyzed study population strongly differed in matters of endoscopic procedures and subtype of biliary disorders. In the two randomized controlled studies published in 1980 and 1986 [28, 29], 51% of the study population underwent solely diagnostic ERC and did not exhibit any biliary disorder, whereas in our study all patients suffered from mainly severe obstructive biliary disease. In the most recent study [23] 114 patients with non-calculous biliary obstruction were enrolled, 57 of them receiving gentamicin 10 mg into ERC contrast media. In addition, all of them received a peri-interventional systemic antibiosis. Biliary obstruction was mainly caused by malignant strictures (79% of cases vs. 9.5% in our study), whereas in our study sclerosing cholangitis (75%) was the most prevalent cause. In contrast to our study, all patients underwent endoscopic biliary stenting (vs. 9.5% in our study). Biliary obstruction was relieved resulting in an adequate drainage in all patients, whereas in our study only in 49.3% of therapeutic ERC adequate drainage was achieved. In the mentioned study, no significant difference in the incidence of post-ERC cholangitis in each group with and without gentamicin added to contrast media (8.8% each) was detected. In contrast, in our study the incidence of post-ERC infection was significantly lower when adding antimicrobial agents into the ERC contrast media (14.3%

vs. 33% in the control group; $p = 0.045$). The absolute risk reduction was 19% when adding antimicrobial agents into the ERC contrast media. We suggest that patients with secondary sclerosing cholangitis, who presented 52.4% of our study population, are particularly prone to post-ERC infectious complications. Presumably, the ERC-related infectious risk in these patients is even more pronounced than in patients with malignant strictures. Thus, 65% (13/20) of the patients with post-ERC infection suffered from SC in our study. SC is a chronic cholestatic biliary disease characterized by PSC-like biliary lesions apparent on ERC, namely multifocal biliary strictures with interposed normal or dilated bile ducts [24]. The most frequent cause (72.7%) of SC in our study population was SC in critically ill patients (SC-CIP). SC-CIP is an emerging disease entity with unfavorable outcome, mostly observed in patients who have survived life-threatening illnesses and who received aggressive treatment on intensive-care units. The median survival of patients with SC-CIP who are not liver-transplanted was reported to be only 13 months [30]. ERC reveals severe bile-duct damage with extensive biliary casts and multiple irregular strictures. Recurrent episodes of bacterial cholangitis are typically observed in patients with SC [31, 32]. In 68.2% of our patients with SC, bile fluid was tested positive for bacteria before ERC with no statistical difference between the two study groups. However, infectious complication rate after ERC was significantly higher in patients with SC not given antibiotics into the contrast media (50% vs. 9%; $p = 0.03$). In these SC-patients, ERC-related infectious complications were observed even despite a systemic antibiotic treatment. Regarding the other subgroups of the study population, addition of antibiotics to the contrast media seemed to have no effect on the post-ERC infectious rate, although patient numbers are too small for valid statistical analysis.

Patients presenting with fever or elevated leucocytes prior to ERC were excluded from all previous studies that evaluated the benefit of intraductal antibiotics on post-ERC complications [23, 28, 29]. In contrast, 59.5% of our study population suffered already at the time of ERC from acute cholangitis (defined as bacterial colonization of the biliary system and elevated leucocytes > 12 000/µl/ CRP > 5 mg/l). Acute cholangitis at the time of ERC was present in both, the case- and control group without statistical difference. Injection of ERC contrast media into obstructed and infected bile tracts will most likely result in bacteremia [8]. This will particularly be the case when complete biliary drainage is not achieved by ERC. On the other hand, addition of antimicrobial agents to the ERC contrast media should reduce biliary bacterial growth and decrease the risk of bacteremia. Indeed, acute cholangitis, present at the time of ERC, was calculated as a risk factor for developing post-ERC infectious complications in our study. Hence, the risk of infectious complications after ERC was 2.72-fold increased when acute cholangitis was present compared to patients without cholangitis. The absolute risk reduction was 29,3% in patients with cholangitis when adding antibiotics to contrast media. In line with our data, Motte et al. identified leukocytosis and prior cholangitis as significant risk factors for septicemia following endoscopic biliary stenting of biliary obstruction [6].

Most patients in our study received a combination of antimicrobial agents into the ERC contrast media. Only 16.6% received solely gentamicin, as used in the previous studies [23, 29]. The most frequently isolated organism in bile samples taken from patients given intraductal antibiosis were gram-positive with *Enterococcus spp.* found in 71.4%. Gram-negative organisms found in the collected bile samples were *E. coli* in 25.7%, *Klebsiella spp.* in 11.4% and *Pseudomonas spp.* in 11.4%. Of note, only in 10.7% of positive bile cultures, all detected bacterial strains were sensitive to gentamicin. Combination of gentamicin with vancomycin increased the response rate to 89.3%. These data question the effectiveness of adding solely gentamicin into ERC contrast media for prevention of post-ERC infectious complications. Instead, the choice of the administered antibiotic regiments should be based on the sensitivity of the isolated bacteria and the local pattern of antibiotic resistance. Noteworthy, we found *Candida* species in 25.7% of the fungal cultures of taken bile samples. All Candida species were sensitive to fluconazole. *Candida spp.* were shown to be predominantly detected in bile fluids of patients with primary and secondary sclerosing cholangitis, immunosuppressive therapy, after placement of plastic biliary stents, and after liver transplantation [33–36]. Our data on fungal bile cultures are in line with these findings, as our study population comprises all the mentioned entities above. In conclusion, collection of bile fluid during ERC for microbiological analysis should be considered in all patients with a high risk for post-ERC infectious complications. When adding antimicrobial agents into ERC contrast media, we recommend a combination of antibiotic and antimycotic agents instead of mono-therapy suggesting a more potent effect on preventing post-ERC infectious complications.

The main limitations of our study are the retrospective study design and the rather small number of patients. Moreover, the combination of antimicrobial agents added to the contrast media was not standardized in a uniform protocol, but was recommended to the respective investigator. This explains the number of patients receiving solely gentamicin, or an antibiotic regiment without antimycotic agents. Despite these limitations, our data are of particular interest for the clinical practice of antibiotic prophylaxis in ERC. This is the first study that evaluates ERC-related infectious complications in patients with SC. Pre-procedural cholangitis and incomplete endoscopic drainage due to multifocal biliary strictures are common findings in patients with SC, defining them as a high risk-population for post-ERC infectious complications. Injection of ERC contrast media might increase the intraductal pressure and incomplete drainage of already infected bile might then facilitate bacteremia in SC. A benefit of locally applied antibiotic agents is therefore highly assumable. Our preliminary data should now be prospectively evaluated in a larger patient cohort to improve the safety of ERC, especially in patients with SC.

Conclusion
Based on our study results, we recommend the local application of antimicrobial agents into ERC contrast media especially in patients with SC in addition to the established systemic antibiotic prophylaxis.

Abbreviations
CI: Confidence interval; ERC: Endoscopic retrograde cholangiography; OR: Odds ratio; PSC: Primary sclerosing cholangitis; SC: Secondary sclerosing cholangitis; SC-CIP: Secondary sclerosing cholangitis in critically ill patients

Acknowledgements
Not applicable.

Funding
None.

Authors' contributions
HW participated in conception and design, analysis and interpretation of the data and in drafting the article. AG participated in data acquisition and data analysis and interpretation. FK conceived and supervised the study, conception and design, analysis and interpretation of the data and revised the manuscript critically. All authors read and approved the final manuscript.

Competing interests
The authors declare that they have no competing interests.

Consent for publication
Not applicable.

Author details
[1]Department of Internal Medicine and Gastroenterology, University Hospital of Regensburg, Regensburg 93042, Germany. [2]Present address: Praxiszentrum Alte Mälzerei, Regensburg, Germany.

References
1.   Andriulli A, Loperfido S, Napolitano G, Niro G, Valvano MR, Spirito F, Pilotto A, Forlano R. Incidence rates of post-ERCP complications: a systematic survey of prospective studies. Am J Gastroenterol. 2007;102:1781–8.

2. Salminen P, Laine S, Gullichsen R. Severe and fatal complications after ERCP: analysis of 2555 procedures in a single experienced center. Surg Endosc. 2008;22:1965–70.

3. Beilenhoff U, Neumann CS, Rey JF, Biering H, Blum R, Cimbro M, Kampf B, Rogers M, Schmidt V, ESGE Guidelines Committee, European Society of Gastrointestinal Endoscopy, European Society of Gastroenterology and Endoscopy Nurses and Associates. ESGE-ESGENA Guideline: cleaning and disinfection in gastrointestinal endoscopy. Endoscopy. 2008;40:939–57.

4. Dumonceau J-M, Tringali A, Blero D, Devière J, Laugiers R, Heresbach D, Costamagna G, European Society of Gastrointestinal Endoscopy. Biliary stenting: indications, choice of stents and results: European Society of Gastrointestinal Endoscopy (ESGE) clinical guideline. Endoscopy. 2012;44:277–98.

5. ASGE Standards of Practice Committee, Banerjee S, Shen B, Nelson DB, Lichtenstein DR, Baron TH, Anderson MA, Dominitz JA, Gan SI, Harrison ME, Ikenberry SO, Jagannath SB, Fanelli RD, Lee K, van Guilder T, Stewart LE. Infection control during GI endoscopy. Gastrointest Endosc. 2008;67:781–90.

6. Motte S, Deviere J, Dumonceau JM, Serruys E, Thys JP, Cremer M. Risk factors for septicemia following endoscopic biliary stenting. Gastroenterology. 1991; 101:1374–81.

7. Freeman ML. Understanding risk factors and avoiding complications with endoscopic retrograde cholangiopancreatography. Curr Gastroenterol Rep. 2003;5:145–53.

8. Subhani JM, Kibbler C, Dooley JS. Review article: antibiotic prophylaxis for endoscopic retrograde cholangiopancreatography (ERCP). Aliment Pharmacol Ther. 1999;13:103–16.

9. Yoshimoto H, Ikeda S, Tanaka M, Matsumoto S. Relationship of biliary pressure to cholangiovenous reflux during endoscopic retrograde balloon catheter cholangiography. Dig Dis Sci. 1989;34:16–20.

10. Lygidakis NJ, Brummelkamp WH. The significance of intrabiliary pressure in acute cholangitis. Surg Gynecol Obstet. 1985;161:465–9.

11. Rerknimitr R, Kladcharoen N, Mahachai V, Kullavanijaya P. Result of endoscopic biliary drainage in hilar cholangiocarcinoma. J Clin Gastroenterol. 2004;38:518–23.

12. Bangarulingam SY, Gossard AA, Petersen BT, Ott BJ, Lindor KD. Complications of endoscopic retrograde cholangiopancreatography in primary sclerosing cholangitis. Am J Gastroenterol. 2009;104:855–60.

13. Niederau C, Pohlmann U, Lübke H, Thomas L. Prophylactic antibiotic treatment in therapeutic or complicated diagnostic ERCP: results of a randomized controlled clinical study. Gastrointest Endosc. 1994;40:533–7.

14. Sauter G, Grabein B, Huber G, Mannes GA, Ruckdeschel G, Sauerbruch T. Antibiotic prophylaxis of infectious complications with endoscopic retrograde cholangiopancreatography. A randomized controlled study. Endoscopy. 1990;22:164–7.

15. Harris A, Chan AC, Torres-Viera C, Hammett R, Carr-Locke D. Meta-analysis of antibiotic prophylaxis in endoscopic retrograde cholangiopancreatography (ERCP). Endoscopy. 1999;31:718–24.

16. Bai Y, Gao F, Gao J, Zou D-W, Li Z-S. Prophylactic antibiotics cannot prevent endoscopic retrograde cholangiopancreatography-induced cholangitis: a meta-analysis. Pancreas. 2009;38:126–30.

17. Cotton PB, Connor P, Rawls E, Romagnuolo J. Infection after ERCP, and antibiotic prophylaxis: a sequential quality-improvement approach over 11 years. Gastrointest Endosc. 2008;67:471–5.

18. Allison MC, Sandoe JAT, Tighe R, Simpson IA, Hall RJ, Elliott TSJ, Endoscopy Committee of the British Society of Gastroenterology. Antibiotic prophylaxis in gastrointestinal endoscopy. Gut. 2009;58:869–80.

19. ASGE Standards of Practice Committee, Banerjee S, Shen B, Baron TH, Nelson DB, Anderson MA, Cash BD, Dominitz JA, Gan SI, Harrison ME, Ikenberry SO, Jagannath SB, Lichtenstein D, Fanelli RD, Lee K, van Guilder T, Stewart LE. Antibiotic prophylaxis for GI endoscopy. Gastrointest Endosc. 2008;67:791–8.

20. Blenkharn JI, Habib N, Mok D, John L, McPherson GA, Gibson RN, Blumgart LH, Benjamin IS. Decreased biliary excretion of piperacillin after percutaneous relief of extrahepatic obstructive jaundice. Antimicrob Agents Chemother. 1985;28:778–80.

21. Ramirez FC, Osato MS, Graham DY, Woods KL. Addition of gentamicin to endoscopic retrograde cholangiopancreatography (ERCP) contrast medium towards reducing the frequency of septic complications of ERCP. J Dig Dis. 2010;11:237–43.

22. Bernadino KP, Howell DA, Lawrence C, Ansari A, Lukens FJ, Sheth SG. Near absence of septic complications folowwing successful therapeutic ERCP justifies selective intravenous and intracontrast use of antibiotics. Gastrointest Endosc. 2005;61:AB187.

23. Norouzi A, Khatibian M, Afroogh R, Chaharmahali M, Sotoudehmanesh R. The effect of adding gentamicin to contrast media for prevention of cholangitis after biliary stenting for non-calculus biliary obstruction, a randomized controlled trial. Indian J Gastroenterol Off J Indian Soc Gastroenterol. 2013;32:18–21.

24. Ruemmele P, Hofstaedter F, Gelbmann CM. Secondary sclerosing cholangitis. Nat Rev Gastroenterol Hepatol. 2009;6:287–95.

25. Nagar H, Berger SA. The excretion of antibiotics by the biliary tract. Surg Gynecol Obstet. 1984;158:601–7.

26. Mortimer PR, Mackie DB, Haynes S. Ampicillin levels in human bile in the presence of biliary tract disease. Br Med J. 1969;3:88–9.

27. Jendrzejewski JW, McAnally T, Jones SR, Katon RM. Antibiotics and ERCP: in vitro activity of aminoglycosides when added to iodinated contrast agents. Gastroenterology. 1980;78:745–8.

28. Collen MJ, Hanan MR, Maher JA, Stubrin SE. Modification of endoscopic retrograde cholangiopancreatography (ERCP) septic complications by the addition of an antibiotic to the contrast media. Randomized controlled investigation. Am J Gastroenterol. 1980;74:493–6.

29. Pugliese V, Saccomanno S, Bonelli L, Aste H. Is it useful to add gentamycin to contrast media in endoscopic retrograde cholangiopancreatography? Prospective evaluation of 330 cases. Minerva Dietol Gastroenterol. 1986; 32:149–56.

30. Kulaksiz H, Heuberger D, Engler S, Stiehl A. Poor outcome in progressive sclerosing cholangitis after septic shock. Endoscopy. 2008;40:214–8.

31. Deltenre P, Valla D-C. Ischemic cholangiopathy. J Hepatol. 2006;44:806–17.

32. Sherlock S. Pathogenesis of sclerosing cholangitis: the role of nonimmune factors. Semin Liver Dis. 1991;11:5–10.

33. Voigtländer T, Leuchs E, Vonberg R-P, Solbach P, Manns MP, Suerbaum S, Lankisch TO. Microbiological analysis of bile and its impact in critically ill patients with secondary sclerosing cholangitis. J Infect. 2015;70:483–90.

34. Basioukas P, Vezakis A, Zarkotou O, Fragulidis G, Themeli-Digalaki K, Rizos S, Polydorou A. Isolated microorganisms in plastic biliary stents placed for benign and malignant diseases. Ann Gastroenterol Q Publ Hell Soc Gastroenterol. 2014;27:399–403.

35. Kirchner GI, Scherer MN, Obed A, Ruemmele P, Wiest R, Froh M, Loss M, Schlitt H-J, Schölmerich J, Gelbmann CM. Outcome of patients with ischemic-like cholangiopathy with secondary sclerosing cholangitis after liver transplantation. Scand J Gastroenterol. 2011;46:471–8.

36. Gotthardt DN, Weiss KH, Rupp C, Bode K, Eckerle I, Rudolph G, Bergemann J, Kloeters-Plachky P, Chahoud F, Büchler MW, Schemmer P, Stremmel W, Sauer P. Bacteriobilia and fungibilia are associated with outcome in patients with endoscopic treatment of biliary complications after liver transplantation. Endoscopy. 2013;45:890–6.

miRNA-338-3p/CDK4 signaling pathway suppressed hepatic stellate cell activation and proliferation

Bensong Duan[1†], Jiangfeng Hu[1*†], Tongyangzi Zhang[2], Xu Luo[3], Yi Zhou[3], Shun Liu[4], Liang Zhu[3], Cheng Wu[5], Wenxiang Liu[6], Chao Chen[6*] and Hengjun Gao[7,8*]

Abstract

Background: Activated hepatic stellate cell (HSC) is the main fibrogenic cell type in the injured liver. miRNA plays an important role in activation and proliferation of HSC.

Methods: Our previous study examined the expression profiles of microRNAs in quiescent and activated HSC. Real-time PCR and western blot were used to detect the expression of Collagen type I (Col 1) and Alpha-Smooth Muscle Actin (α-SMA). CCK-8 and Edu assay was used to measure the proliferation rate of HSC. Luciferase reporter gene assay was used to tested the binding between miR-338-3p and Cyclin-dependent kinase 4 (CDK4).

Results: We found overexpression of miR-338-3p could inhibit Col 1 and α-SMA, two major HSC activation markers, whereas miR-338-3p inhibitor could promote them. Besides, miR-338-3p overexpression could suppress the growth rate of HSC. Further, we found that CDK4, a pleiotropic signaling protein, was a direct target gene of miR-338-3p. Moreover, we found that overexpression of CDK4 could block the effects of miR-338-3p.

Conclusions: We found miR-338-3p is an anti-fibrotic miRNA which inhibits cell activation and proliferation. Our findings suggest that miR-338-3p/CDK4 signaling pathway participates in the regulation of HSC activation and growth and may act as a novel target for further anti-fibrotic therapy.

Keywords: Liver fibrosis, miR-338, CDK4

Background

Liver fibrosis is a common consequence of most chronic liver diseases [1]. Liver fibrosis received more attention until the hepatic stellate cell (HSC) was identified as the main ECM-producing cells in the injured liver [2]. Under the normal physiologic condition, HSCs reside in the space of disse and store a large amount of vitamin A. After suffering from liver injury, HSCs will be activated, and then proliferate, eventually transdifferentiate into myofibroblast-like cells [3].

microRNAs (miRNAs), short (~22 nt) conceding RNA molecules, can directly regulate gene expression by binding to the 3'UTR region of target mRNA to participate in lots of regulation of physiological process and diseases [4–8]. Recently, researchers focused on the role of miRNA in liver fibrosis pathophysiology to determine their regulatory effects on proliferation, differentiation of HSC [9–11]. Several abnormally expressed miRNAs were found and identified between quiescent and activated HSCs by using miRNA array or RT-PCR [12–19]. Previous studies have reported that miRNAs were critically involved in the activation of HSCs. Among them, miR-29b precursor allowed activated HSCs to switch to a more quiescent state [10]. Similarly, overexpression of miR-27a/b could lead HSCs to a quiescent phenotype [20]. microRNA-338 (miR-338), a newly identified miRNA, played a crucial role in a variety of carcinomas. Aberrant expression of miR-338 was closely related to cell proliferation, invasion, early detection and

* Correspondence: doctorhjf@foxmail.com; 15900611429@163.com; hengjun_gao@tongji.edu.cn
†Equal contributors
[1]Department of Gastroenterology, Tongji Hospital, Tongji University School of Medicine, Shanghai, China
[6]Department of Gastroenterology, First Affiliated Hospital of Chinese PLA General Hospital, Beijing, China
[7]National Engineering Center for Biochip at Shanghai, Shanghai, China
Full list of author information is available at the end of the article

clinic pathologic variables in liver cancer, colorectal cancer, gastric cancer and neuroblastoma [21–25]. In previous research, our miRNA microarray data have found altered expression of miR-338-3p during culture activation of HSC [14]. However, little is known about the role of miR-338-3p in liver fibrosis.

Cyclin-dependent kinase 4 (CDK4) is found to be involved in cell cycle regulation. Activation of cyclin D—CDK4 promotes the cell cycle progression through G1/S transition [26]. Inhibition of CDK4 shows promising efficacy on advanced breast cancer [27]. In liver tissue and hepatoma cells, CDK4/6 inhibition is a potent mediator of cytostasis [28]. However, whether the CDK4 participates in the fibrogenic process and regulates HSC activation and proliferation remains largely unknown. In this study, RT-PCR data suggested that miR-338-3p expression in fully activated HSCs were significantly decreased compared with that in quiescent HSCs. Transforming growth factor (TGF-β) is deemed to be the most potent fibrogenic cytokine. The results showed that there was a negative relationship between TGF-β and miR-338-3p. Therefore, we speculated that miR-338-3p was closely associated with HSCs function. Then, we found overexpression of miR-338-3p could suppress HSCs activation and proliferation while inhibition of miR-338-3p could promote HSCs activation and proliferation. Based on the Bioinformatics prediction, we found that CDK4 was a potential target gene of miR-338-3p. Further luciferase reporter assay and RT-PCR confirmed their complementary binding. Moreover, our results indicated that overexpression of CDK4 could partially block miR-338-3p-inhibited cell activation and proliferation.

Methods
Primary rat HSCs, cell lines and culture
The isolation method of primary rat HSCs was according to the previous literature [29]. Primary Rat HSCs, HSC-T6 and HEK293T (human embryonic kidney cell line) were kindly gifted from Dr. Gao (Tongji University, Shanghai, China). The primary cells and cell lines were cultured in DMEM (Dulbecco's modified Eagle's medium, Thermo, Waltham, MA, USA) containing 10% FBS (Fetal bovine serum, FBS, Gibco, Grand Island, NY, USA) at 37 °C in a humidified atmosphere of 5% CO_2.

Plasmid construction
Wild-type 3'UTR containing predicted miR-338-3p binding sites were amplified from HSC-T6 genomic DNA and inserted into the PGL3 luciferase reporter vector. Mutant 3'UTR was generated using the Quick Change Lighting Site-Directed Mutagenesis Kit (Agilent Technologies, Santa Clara, CA, USA). The CDK4 expression vector was obtained by cloning the CDK4-coding sequence into the pcDNA.

RT-PCR analysis
Total RNA was extracted from cultured HSCs using Trizol Reagent (Takara, Dalian, China). The primer sequences used for mRNA detection in this study were listed as follows: GAPDH (PF: CAGTGCCAGCCTCG TCTCAT, PR: AGGGGCCATCCACAGTCTTC); ColI (PF: ATCCTGCCGATGTCGCTAT, PR: CCACAAGCG TGCTGTAGGT); α-SMA (PF: CCGAGATCTCACCG ACTACC, PR: TCCAGAGCGACATAGCACAG); CDK4 (PF: GAAGAAGAAGCGGAGGAAGAGG, PR: TTAGGT TAGTGCGGGAATGAAT).

CCK-8 assay and Edu assay
Cell proliferation was performed using CCK-8 assay (Dojindo, Japan) and Edu (Ribibio, Guangzhou, China) assay. For CCK-8, HSC-T6 was transfected with the miR-338 precursor, miR-338 inhibitor (Ribibio, Guangzhou, China) or pcDNA-CDK4 in 96 well culture plates. Proliferation rates were tested at 24, 48 and 72 h after transfection. The EdU assay was conducted according to the protocol of Ribibio Edu Kit.

Luciferase assay
Luciferase assay was performed with the Dual Luciferase Reporter Assay System (Promega, Madison, WI). Transfection was carried out in 48 well plates using Fugen (Roche). There were two groups. One was co-transfected with 200 ng wild-type-CDK4-3'UTR, 20 nm miR-338 precursor, and 20 ng Renilla. Another was co-transfected with 200mutant CDK4 3'UTR without binding site of miR-338-3p, 20 nm miR-338 precursor, and 20 ng Renilla. 48 h later, Firefly and Renilla luciferase activities were tested.

Western blotting
Cells were lysed in SDS sample buffer. Antibodies against GAPDH (Biogot, 1:5000 dilution, Nanjing, China), Col1 (Abcam, 1:1500 dilution, Cambridge, MA, USA), α-sma (Sigma, 1:1000 dilution, Shanghai, China) and CDK4 (Biogot, 1:3000 dilution, Nanjing, China) were used in this study. Signals were visualized with ImageQuant LAS 4000 (GE Healthcare Life Sciences).

Statistical analysis
The statistical analysis in our study was performed by using SPSS 22.0. Data were given as mean ± SEM. Two tailed t-test was used to determine between two groups. Statistical significance level was set at $p < 0.05$.

Results
miR-338-3p was downregulated in fully activated HSCs
Based on the microarray data, multitude ectopic miR-NAs were detected in the HSCs. In our previous study, we isolated rat primary HSCs and extracted total RNA to perform miRNA microarray assay. Our attention was

focused on miR-338-3p, a new underlying member of liver fibrosis. The microarray data showed that the expression of miR-338-3p was sharply reduced by 90% at day 7 (partially activated HSCs) [14]. To validate this finding, RT-PCR was carried out to measure the endogenous miR-338-3p expression in a quiescent state and an activated state. As primary HSCs were gradually activated during culture, we assessed miR-338-3p expression at day 2, day 7 and day 14 after isolation. Our data indicated that endogenous miR-338-3p expression was obviously reduced at day 7 and day 14 (Fig. 1a). Meanwhile, collagen type I (Col1) and α-sma (α-smooth muscle actin, α-SMA), two key biomarkers of HSCs activation, was gradually increased (Fig. 1b, c). In addition, we found that treatment with transforming growth factor (TGF-β, 2 ng/ml) in quiescent HSCs (day 2), the expression of miR-338-3p was reduced rapidly (Fig. 1d). When cells were fully activated (day 14), we treated them with SB431542, a potent and specific inhibitor of TGF-β and detected the level of miR-338-3p. The results suggested that the expression of miR-338-3p was increased compared to that in control group (Fig. 1e).

Overexpression of miR-338-3p suppressed HSC activation while inhibition of it promoted HSC activation

As we discovered, miR-338-3p was significantly decreased during the process of activation, we transfected

miR-338 precursor to repair its loss at the early stage of primary HSCs. On day 7, cells transfected with miR-338 precursor showed a more original shape with less peripheral protrusions. However, the control group cells showed a more irregular shape with more peripheral protrusions (Fig. 2a). As results showed in Figs. 1b, c and 2a, it seemed that there was a negative relationship between miR-338 expression and HSCs activation. We assumed that the expression of miR-338-3p was involved in this activation process. To confirm our hypothesis, we alter the miR-338-3p expression in primary HSC by transfecting miR-338 precursor. Interestingly, the expression of Col 1 and α-sma was slightly decreased due to the upregulation of miR-338-3p (Fig. 2b). Due to the low efficiency of transfection in primary cells, HSC-T6 cell line was further used to conduct the following studies. To replicate the results, HSC-T6 cell line was transfected with miR-338 precursor or negative control. 48 h later, cells were collected and transfection efficiency was confirmed by RT-PCR (Fig. 2c). Then the expression of Col1 and α-sma in two groups was measured using RT-PCR. As expected, the data showed miR-338-3p inhibited HSCs activation. The expression of Col1 and α-sma was respectively reduced as a result of miR-338-3p overexpression (Fig. 2d, e). Furthermore, inhibition of miR-338-3p could upregulate Col1 and α-sma which

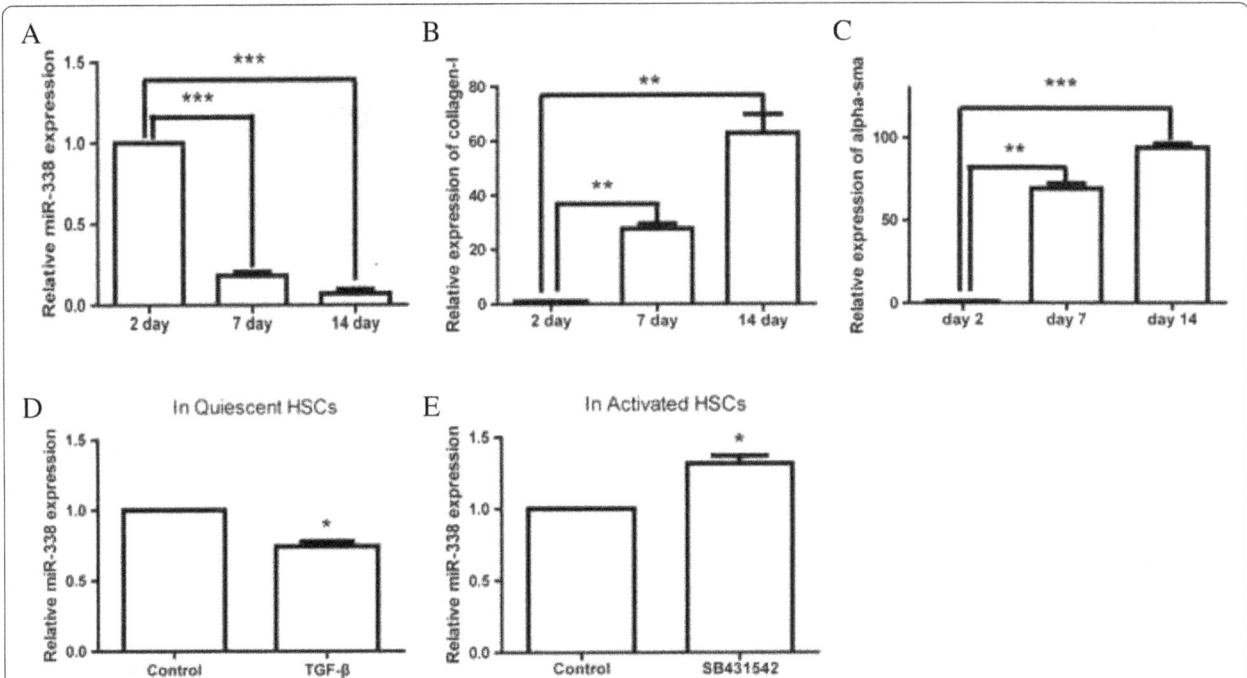

Fig. 1 Expression of miR-338-3p is reduced in HSCs during culture activation. **a** miR-338-3p expression in the HSCs during culture activation. Data shown are means ± SD ($n = 3$), ***$P < 0.001$. **b** mRNA level of Col1 in the HSCs during cell culture. Data shown are means ± SD ($n = 3$), **$P < 0.01$. **c** mRNA level of α-sma in the HSCs during cell culture. Data shown are means ± SD ($n = 3$), **$P < 0.01$, ***$P < 0.001$. **d** miR-338-3p expression of quiescent HSCs was reduced upon TGF-β treatment. Data shown are means ± SD ($n = 3$), *$P < 0.05$. **e** miR-338-3p expression of activated HSCs was increased upon SB431542 treatment. Data shown are means ± SD ($n = 3$), *$P < 0.05$

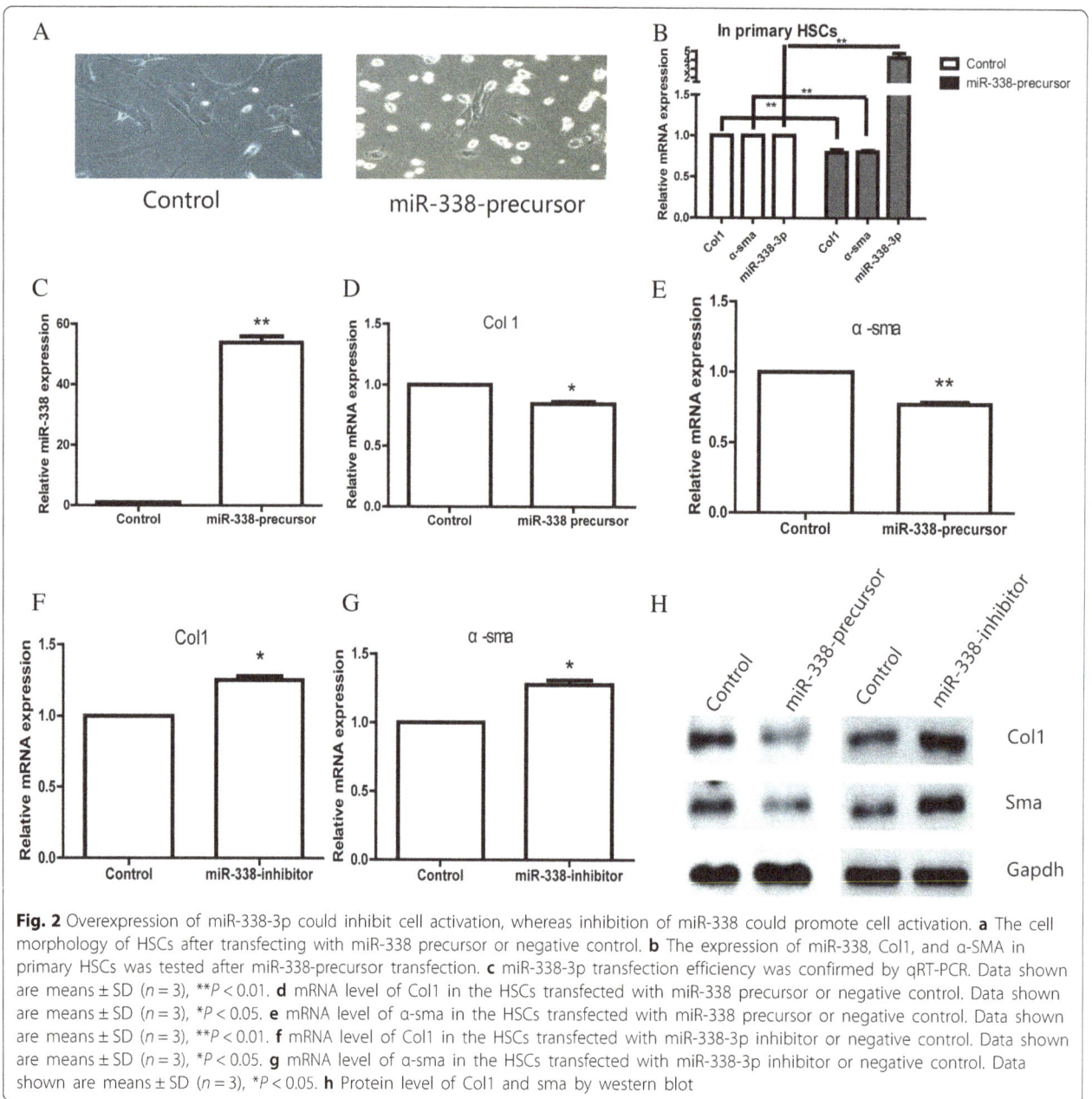

Fig. 2 Overexpression of miR-338-3p could inhibit cell activation, whereas inhibition of miR-338 could promote cell activation. **a** The cell morphology of HSCs after transfecting with miR-338 precursor or negative control. **b** The expression of miR-338, Col1, and α-SMA in primary HSCs was tested after miR-338-precursor transfection. **c** miR-338-3p transfection efficiency was confirmed by qRT-PCR. Data shown are means ± SD ($n = 3$), **$P < 0.01$. **d** mRNA level of Col1 in the HSCs transfected with miR-338 precursor or negative control. Data shown are means ± SD ($n = 3$), *$P < 0.05$. **e** mRNA level of α-sma in the HSCs transfected with miR-338 precursor or negative control. Data shown are means ± SD ($n = 3$), **$P < 0.01$. **f** mRNA level of Col1 in the HSCs transfected with miR-338-3p inhibitor or negative control. Data shown are means ± SD ($n = 3$), *$P < 0.05$. **g** mRNA level of α-sma in the HSCs transfected with miR-338-3p inhibitor or negative control. Data shown are means ± SD ($n = 3$), *$P < 0.05$. **h** Protein level of Col1 and sma by western blot

confirm their association on the other direction (Fig. 2f, g). Their expression was also confirmed at the protein level (Fig. 2h).

Overexpression of miR-338 suppressed HSC-T6 proliferation

Next, we examined the impacts of miR-338 on HSCs proliferation. HSC-T6 were transfected with miR-338 precursor, inhibitor or corresponding negative control. In the CCK-8 assay, the cell growth curves suggested that overexpression of miR-338 significantly restrained HSC-T6 proliferation in a time-dependent manner (Fig. 3a.). Moreover, cells transfected with miR-338

inhibitor showed a higher proliferative ability (Fig. 3b). Edu incorporation assay also demonstrated that miR-338 precursor reduced the proliferation of HSC-T6 (Fig. 3c-d). Besides proliferation, we also assessed the role of miR-338-3p in HSCs migration. As Fig. 3e, f showed, miR-338-3p has no effects on cell migration.

miR-338 repressed *CDK4* expression by directly binding to its 3′UTR region

Based on the prediction of Bioinformatics (TargetScan, PicTar), some genes are predicted to be the targets of miR-338-3p. Among them, we hypothesized *CDK4*, an oncogene in liver cancer, might be a putative target gene

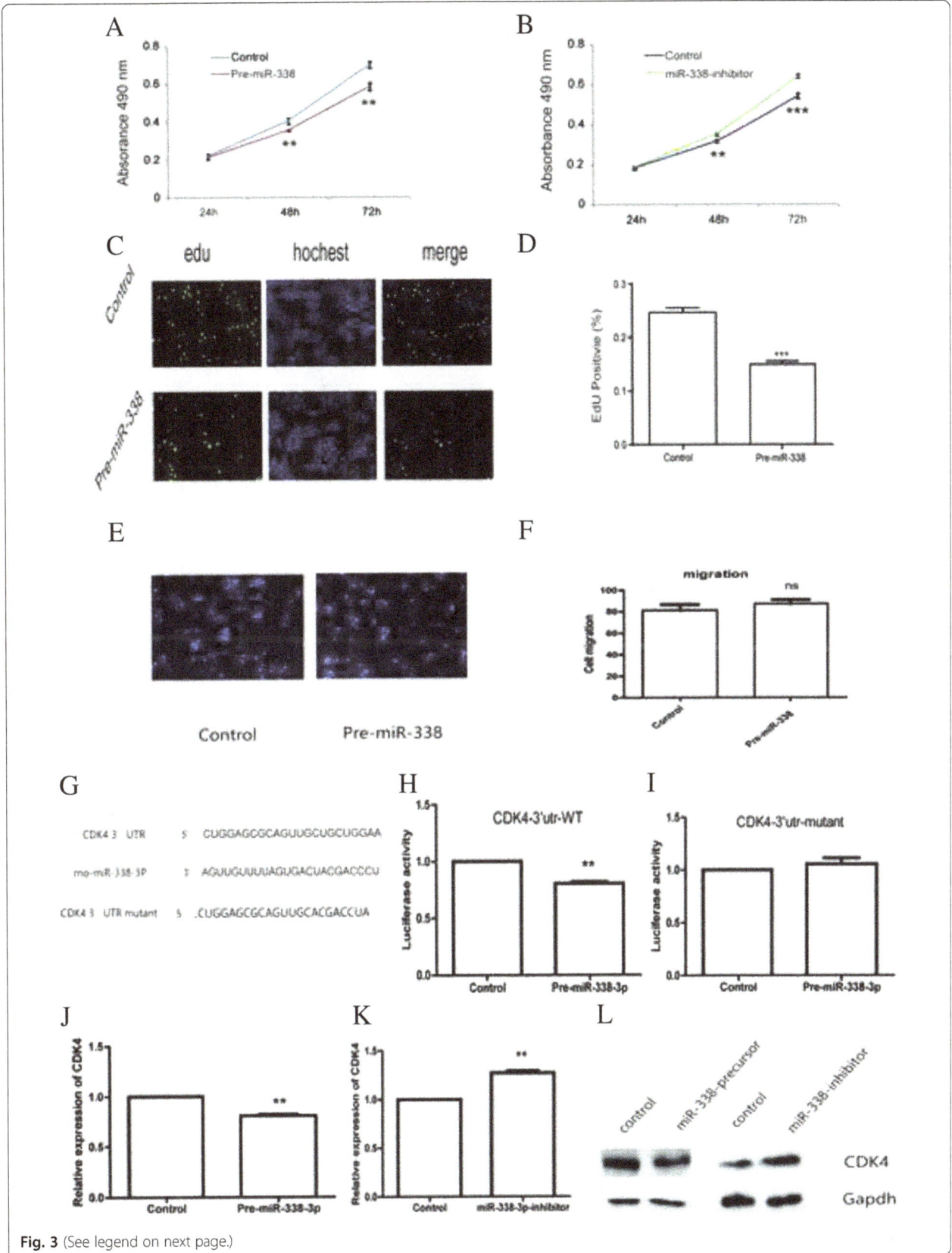

Fig. 3 (See legend on next page.)

(See figure on previous page.)

Fig. 3 miR-338-3p regulates cell proliferation and CDK4. **a** The proliferation analysis of HSC-T6 transfected with miR-338 precursor or negative control. Data shown are means ± SD ($n = 3$). **$P < 0.01$ versus the corresponding control. **b** The proliferation analysis of HSC-T6 transfected with miR-338 inhibitor or negative control. Data shown are means ± SD ($n = 3$). **$P < 0.01$ versus the corresponding control. **c** Micrograph of HSC-T6 transfected with miR-338 precursor. **d** Edu incorporation assay demonstrated that miR-338 precursor reduced the proliferation of HSC-T6. Data shown are means ± SD ($n = 3$). ***$P < 0.001$. **e**, **f** HSCs migration was measured by transwell assay. **g** The predicted sequence of binding region between miR-338-3p and *CDK4*. **h** Luciferase activity of *CDK4* 3'UTR WT reporter vector co-transfected with miR-338-3p. Data shown are means ± SD ($n = 3$). **$P < 0.01$. **i** Luciferase activity of *CDK4* 3'UTR mutant reporter vector co-transfected with miR-338-3p. Data shown are means ± SD ($n = 3$). **j** mRNA level of *CDK4* in the HSCs transfected with Pre-miR-338-3p or negative control. Data shown are means ± SD ($n = 3$). **$P < 0.01$. **k** mRNA level of *CDK4* in the HSCs transfected with miR-338-inhibitor or negative control. Data shown are means ± SD ($n = 3$). **$P < 0.01$. **l** The expression of *CDK4* was restrained by miR-338-precursor, whereas recovered by miR-338 inhibitor

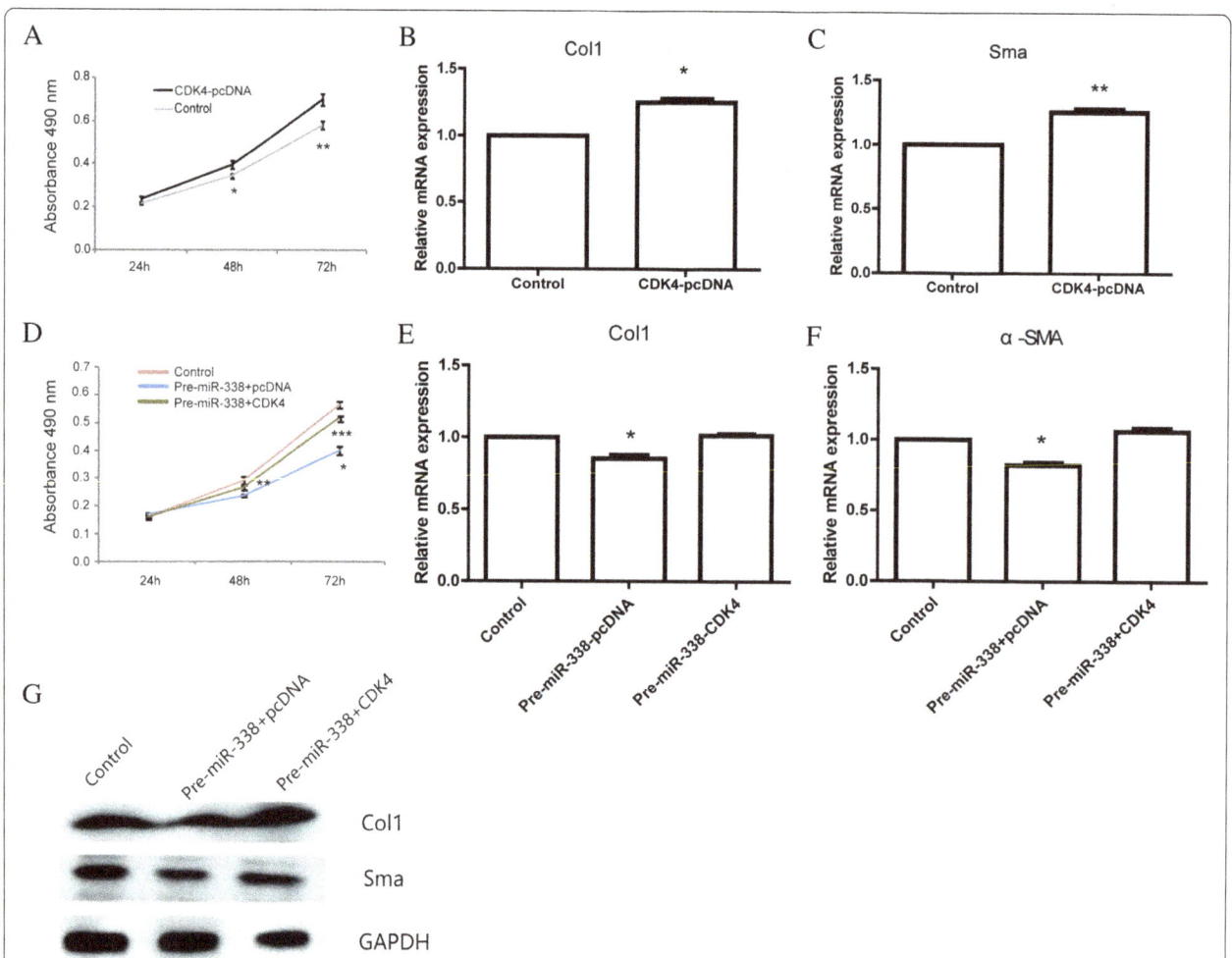

Fig. 4 Overexpression of CDK4 could partially rescue the effects of miR-338-3p upon HSCs. **a** The proliferation analysis of HSC-T6 cells transfected with *CDK4* vector or empty control. Data shown are means ± SD ($n = 3$). *$P < 0.05$, **$P < 0.01$ versus the corresponding control. **b** mRNA level of Col1 in the HSCs transfected with *CDK4* vector or empty control. Data shown are means ± SD ($n = 3$), *$P < 0.05$. **c** mRNA level of α-sma in the HSCs transfected with *CDK4* vector or empty control. Data shown are means ± SD ($n = 3$), **$P < 0.01$. **d** The proliferation analysis of HSC-T6 cells co-transfected with miR-338 precursor and *CDK4* plasmid. Data shown are means ± SD ($n = 3$). *$P < 0.05$, **$P < 0.01$, ***$P < 0.001$. **e** mRNA level of Col1 in the HSC-T6 cells co-transfected with miR-338 precursor and *CDK4* plasmid. Data shown are means ± SD ($n = 3$), *$P < 0.05$. **f** mRNA level of α-sma in the HSC-T6 cells co-transfected with miR-338 precursor and *CDK4* plasmid. Data shown are means ± SD ($n = 3$), **$P < 0.01$. **g** Protein level of Col1, α-sma in the HSC-T6 cells co-transfected with miR-338 precursor and *CDK4* plasmid

of miR-338-3p in liver fibrosis. The predicted sequence of interaction was showed in Fig. 3g. To test this prediction, 3'UTR with miR-338-3p binding sites were cloned into the PGL3 luciferase reporter vector. A mutant 3'UTR of *CDK4* with anti-sense mutation in the predicted sites was also constructed. The reporter construct was co-transfected into HEK293T with Renilla plasmid and miR-338 precursor or negative control. The wild-type *CDK4*3'UTR luciferase activity was suppressed due to miR-338-3p overexpression. By contrast, the activity of mutant-3'UTR-*CDK4* remained relatively unaffected (Fig. 3h, i). Additionally, *CDK4* expression was decreased in the miR-338 precursor group while increased in the miR-338 inhibitor group (Fig. 3j, k). miR-338-3p could also regulate *CDK4* at protein level (Fig. 4l). Taken together, these data strongly suggested that miR-338-3p repressed *CDK4* expression by directly binding to its 3'UTR region.

CDK4 rescued miR-338-inhibition of activation and proliferation of HSCs

Since miR-338 regulated cell growth, cell migration and cell invasion in liver cancer and colorectal carcinoma by targeting *CDK4* [21, 30], the role of *CDK4* in liver fibrosis remained unclear.

We conduct CCK-8 assay to determine the proliferation of HSC-T6 transfected with *CDK4* plasmid or control empty vector. The results showed that cell transfected with *CDK4* plasmid displayed a higher proliferative capacity compared with the control group (Fig. 4a). Besides, we found cells transfected with *CDK4* could promote cell activation with upregulation of Col1 and α-Sma (Fig. 4b, c). We co-transfected HSC-T6 cells with miR-338 precursor and *CDK4* plasmid to investigate whether *CDK4* would rescue the inhibition effect of miR-338 on the cell activation and proliferation or not. The results suggested that overexpression of *CDK4* partially block the repression effect of miR-338 on the activation and proliferation of HSC-T6. The growth curves of three groups (Control, Pre-miR-338/pcDNA, Pre-miR-338/CDK4) were shown in Fig. 4d. The expression of activation associated markers, Col1 andα-Sma, was showed in Fig. 4e-f.

Discussion

Liver fibrosis is a scarring response to liver damage. It's a common pathological process for most of the liver disorder. A small number of patients go on to progress cirrhosis and/or hepatocellular carcinoma. Fortunately, liver fibrosis can be reversed if the inflammation was controlled [31].

Aberrant expression of miRNAs have been involved in liver fibrosis and regarded as a potential treatment strategy. Intervening miRNAs expression could assist activated HSCs to return to a quiescent phenotype. miRNA microarray and RT-PCR was carried out to determine abnormally expressed miRNAs during HSCs activation. Our results suggested that miR-338-3p was significantly downregulated in this process. miR-338 is located on chromosome 17q25.3 with a length of 22 nt and produces two mature forms, miR-338-3p and miR-338-5p. miR-338 was first reported in neurodegeneration and gradually studied in various disease [32]. In hepatocellular carcinoma, miR-338 downregulation was associated with tumor size, TNM stage, vascular invasion and in trahepatic metastasis [21, 22]. In colorectal carcinoma, miR-338 expression was significantly increased in both blood and tissue samples. It might appear to be a potential biomarker for early detection in colorectal carcinoma [23]. In gastric carcinoma, miR-338 was epigenetically silenced and its reduction was related to pathological variables. Overexpression of miR-338 could suppress cell proliferation, migration, invasion and tumorigenicity [24]. Moreover, combined with other six miRNAs, miR-338 could be used to predict gastric cancer prognosis [33]. Despite in cancer, miR-338 was also involved in idiopathic pulmonary fibrosis [34].

This is the first study to identify the biological function of miR-338-3p in liver fibrosis. Our results demonstrated that miR-338 precursor transfection suppressed the activation and proliferation of HSC-T6, whereas inhibition of miR-338-3p promoted cell activation and proliferation.

To understand the underlying mechanism of miR-338-mediated inhibition of proliferation, we identified *CDK4*, a member of the cyclin-dependent kinase family, as a candidate target gene. *CDK4* usually work with Cyclin D to regulate the cell cycle in G1/S stage. Aberrant activation of *CDK4* was closely associated with various kinds of carcinomas. *CDK4* expression is significantly upregulated in lung cancer tissues and function as an important element for cell proliferation [35, 36]. In breast cancer, inhibition of *CDK4* can induce G1 arrest [37]. These observations suggest that inhibition of *CDK4* might be beneficial for cancer treatment. An increasing body of clinical trials targeting *CDK4* has been launched. However, the role of *CDK4* in liver fibrosis remains largely unknown. In this study, Luciferase reporter assay showed that there was a combination of miR-338 and *CDK4*. Hence, we deduced that miR-338-3p inhibited HSCs' activation and proliferation likely through silencing CDK4. Our data indicated that restoring CDK4 expression could partially rescue miR-338-inhibited cell activation and proliferation.

Conclusions

In conclusion, our study identified a new anti-fibrosis miRNA that may play an important role in the development of liver fibrosis.

Abbreviations
CDK4: Cyclin-dependent kinase 4; Col 1: Collagen type I; HSC: Hepatic stellate cell; miR-338: microRNA-338; α-SMA: Alpha-Smooth Muscle Actin

Acknowledgment
We thank Tongji University School of Medicine for technical help.

Funding
This work was supported by grants from National Natural Science Foundation of China [grants 81402756, 81101644, 11472300, 11272342]; Science and Technology Research Project from Guangxi Education Department (YB2014067). The funding body approved the study design and the methods that were used for data acquisition and analysis, but had no involvement with the interpretation of data or with the composition of the manuscript.

Authors' contributions
Conceived and designed the experiments: BD, JH, HG, CC Performed the experiments: JH, BD, TZ, XL. Analyzed the data: JH, SL, CW, YZ. Wrote the paper: JH, BD, LZ, WL. All authors read and approved the final manuscript.

Competing interests
The authors declare that they have no competing interests.

Consent for publication
Not applicable.

Author details
[1]Department of Gastroenterology, Tongji Hospital, Tongji University School of Medicine, Shanghai, China. [2]Department of Respiration, Tongji Hospital, Tongji University School of Medicine, Shanghai, China. [3]Department of Gastroenterology, Changzheng Hospital, Second Military Medical University, Shanghai, China. [4]Department of Epidemiology, School of Public Health, Guangxi Medical University, Nanning, Guangxi, China. [5]Digestive Endoscopic Center, Department of Gastroenterology, South Building General Hospital of PLA, Beijing, China. [6]Department of Gastroenterology, First Affiliated Hospital of Chinese PLA General Hospital, Beijing, China. [7]National Engineering Center for Biochip at Shanghai, Shanghai, China. [8]Department of Gastroenterology, Institute of Digestive Diseases, Tongji University School of Medicine, Shanghai, China.

References
1. Bataller R, Brenner DA. Liver fibrosis. J Clin Invest. 2005;115:209–18.
2. Gabele E, Brenner DA, Rippe RA. Liver fibrosis: signals leading to the amplification of the fibrogenic hepatic stellate cell. Front Biosci. 2003;8: d69–77.
3. Marra F. Hepatic stellate cells and the regulation of liver inflammation. J Hepatol. 1999;31:1120–30.
4. Liu Q, Wang G, Chen Y, Li G, Yang D, Kang J. A miR-590/Acvr2a/Rad51b axis regulates DNA damage repair during mESC proliferation. Stem Cell Rep. 2014;3:1103–17.
5. Yan IK, Wang X, Asmann YW, Haga H, Patel T. Circulating extracellular RNA markers of liver regeneration. PLoS One. 2016;11:e0155888.
6. Seeliger C, Balmayor ER, van Griensven M. miRNAs related to skeletal diseases. Stem Cells Dev. 2016;25(17):1261-1281.
7. Cheng CJ, Bahal R, Babar IA, Pincus Z, Barrera F, Liu C, Svoronos A, Braddock DT, Glazer PM, Engelman DM, et al. MicroRNA silencing for cancer therapy targeted to the tumour microenvironment. Nature. 2015; 518:107–10.
8. Schickel R, Boyerinas B, Park SM, Peter ME. MicroRNAs: key players in the immune system, differentiation, tumorigenesis and cell death. Oncogene. 2008;27:5959–74.
9. Yu F, Guo Y, Chen B, Dong P, Zheng J. MicroRNA-17-5p activates hepatic stellate cells through targeting of Smad7. Lab Investig. 2015;95:781–9.
10. Sekiya Y, Ogawa T, Yoshizato K, Ikeda K, Kawada N. Suppression of hepatic stellate cell activation by microRNA-29b. Biochem Biophys Res Commun. 2011;412:74–9.
11. Zhao J, Tang N, Wu K, Dai W, Ye C, Shi J, Zhang J, Ning B, Zeng X, Lin Y. MiR-21 simultaneously regulates ERK1 signaling in HSC activation and hepatocyte EMT in hepatic fibrosis. PLoS One. 2014;9:e108005.
12. Roderburg C, Urban GW, Bettermann K, Vucur M, Zimmermann H, Schmidt S, Janssen J, Koppe C, Knolle P, Castoldi M, et al. Micro-RNA profiling reveals a role for miR-29 in human and murine liver fibrosis. Hepatology. 2011;53:209–18.
13. Kitano M, Bloomston P.M. Hepatic Stellate Cells and microRNAs in Pathogenesis of Liver Fibrosis. J Clin Med. 2016;5(3):38. doi:10.3390/jcm5030038.
14. Chen C, Wu CQ, Zhang ZQ, Yao DK, Zhu L. Loss of expression of miR-335 is implicated in hepatic stellate cell migration and activation. Exp Cell Res. 2011;317:1714–25.
15. Cushing L, Kuang PP, Qian J, Shao F, Wu J, Little F, Thannickal VJ, Cardoso WV, Lu J. miR-29 is a major regulator of genes associated with pulmonary fibrosis. Am J Respir Cell Mol Biol. 2011;45:287–94.
16. Guo CJ, Pan Q, Cheng T, Jiang B, Chen GY, Li DG. Changes in microRNAs associated with hepatic stellate cell activation status identify signaling pathways. FEBS J. 2009;276:5163–76.
17. Li WQ, Chen C, Xu MD, Guo J, Li YM, Xia QM, Liu HM, He J, Yu HY, Zhu L. The rno-miR-34 family is upregulated and targets ACSL1 in dimethylnitrosamine-induced hepatic fibrosis in rats. FEBS J. 2011;278: 1522–32.
18. Hu J, Chen C, Liu Q, Liu B, Song C, Zhu S, Wu C, Liu S, Yu H, Yao D, et al. The role of the miR-31/FIH1 pathway in TGF-beta-induced liver fibrosis. Clin Sci (Lond). 2015;129:305–17.
19. Wu K, Ye C, Lin L, Chu Y, Ji M, Dai W, Zeng X, Lin Y. Inhibiting miR-21 attenuates experimental hepatic fibrosis by suppressing both ERK1 pathway in HSC and hepatocyte EMT. Clin Sci. 2016;130(16):1469-1480.
20. Ji J, Zhang J, Huang G, Qian J, Wang X, Mei S. Over-expressed microRNA-27a and 27b influence fat accumulation and cell proliferation during rat hepatic stellate cell activation. FEBS Lett. 2009;583:759–66.
21. Huang XH, Chen JS, Wang Q, Chen XL, Wen L, Chen LZ, Bi J, Zhang LJ, Su Q, Zeng WT. miR-338-3p suppresses invasion of liver cancer cell by targeting smoothened. J Pathol. 2011;225:463–72.
22. Huang XH, Wang Q, Chen JS, Fu XH, Chen XL, Chen LZ, Li W, Bi J, Zhang LJ, Fu Q, et al. Bead-based microarray analysis of microRNA expression in hepatocellular carcinoma: miR-338 is downregulated. Hepatol Res. 2009;39: 786–94.
23. Yong FL, Law CW, Wang CW. Potentiality of a triple microRNA classifier: miR-193a-3p, miR-23a and miR-338-5p for early detection of colorectal cancer. BMC Cancer. 2013;13:280.
24. Li P, Chen X, Su L, Li C, Zhi Q, Yu B, Sheng H, Wang J, Feng R, Cai Q, et al. Epigenetic silencing of miR-338-3p contributes to tumorigenicity in gastric cancer by targeting SSX2IP. PLoS One. 2013;8:e66782.
25. Chen X, Pan M, Han L, Lu H, Hao X, Dong Q. miR-338-3p suppresses neuroblastoma proliferation, invasion and migration through targeting PREX2a. FEBS Lett. 2013;587:3729–37.
26. Jia X, Liu B, Shi X, Ye M, Zhang F, Liu H. Roles of the ERK, JNK/AP-1/cyclin D1-CDK4 pathway in silica-induced cell cycle changes in human embryo lung fibroblast cells. Cell Biol Int. 2011;35:697–704.
27. O'Sullivan CC. CDK4/6 inhibitors for the treatment of advanced hormone receptor positive breast cancer and beyond: 2016 update. Expert Opin Pharmacother. 2016;17:1657-1667.
28. Rivadeneira DB, Mayhew CN, Thangavel C, Sotillo E, Reed CA, Grana X, Knudsen ES. Proliferative suppression by CDK4/6 inhibition: complex function of the retinoblastoma pathway in liver tissue and hepatoma cells. Gastroenterology. 2010;138:1920–30.
29. Riccalton-Banks L, Bhandari R, Fry J, Shakesheff KM. A simple method for the simultaneous isolation of stellate cells and hepatocytes from rat liver tissue. Mol Cell Biochem. 2003;248:97–102.
30. Sun K, Deng HJ, Lei ST, Dong JQ, Li GX. miRNA-338-3p suppresses cell growth of human colorectal carcinoma by targeting smoothened. World J Gastroenterol. 2013;19:2197–207.

31. Perez-Tamayo R. Cirrhosis of the liver: a reversible disease? Pathol Annu. 1979;14(Pt 2):183–213.

32. Saba R, Goodman CD, Huzarewich RL, Robertson C, Booth SA. A miRNA signature of prion induced neurodegeneration. PLoS One. 2008;3:e3652.

33. Li X, Zhang Y, Zhang Y, Ding J, Wu K, Fan D. Survival prediction of gastric cancer by a seven-microRNA signature. Gut. 2010;59:579–85.

34. Zhang H, Liu X, Chen S, Wu J, Ye X, Xu L, Chen H, Zhang D, Tan R, Wang Y. Tectorigenin inhibits the in vitro proliferation and enhances miR-338* expression of pulmonary fibroblasts in rats with idiopathic pulmonary fibrosis. J Ethnopharmacol. 2010;131:165–73.

35. Lingfei K, Pingzhang Y, Zhengguo L, Jianhua G, Yaowu Z. A study on p16, pRb, cdk4 and cyclinD1 expression in non-small cell lung cancers. Cancer Lett. 1998;130:93–101.

36. Wu A, Wu B, Guo J, Luo W, Wu D, Yang H, Zhen Y, Yu X, Wang H, Zhou Y, et al. Elevated expression of CDK4 in lung cancer. J Transl Med. 2011;9:38.

37. Carlson BA, Dubay MM, Sausville EA, Brizuela L, Worland PJ. Flavopiridol induces G1 arrest with inhibition of cyclin-dependent kinase (CDK) 2 and CDK4 in human breast carcinoma cells. Cancer Res. 1996;56:2973–8.

8

Exceptional serological and radiological response to sorafenib in 2 patients with advanced hepatocellular carcinoma and chronic hepatitis C viral infection

Catherine Atkin[1], Philip Earwaker[1], Arvind Pallan[2], Shishir Shetty[3], Pankaj Punia[1] and Yuk Ting Ma[1*]

Abstract

Background: In patients with advanced hepatocellular carcinoma (HCC), the multikinase inhibitor sorafenib is the only systemic treatment that has been shown to increase overall survival. However, similar to other tyrosine kinase inhibitors, most patients achieve disease stabilisation radiologically, and only 2–3% of patients achieve a partial response. Recent exploratory subgroup analyses of the large phase 3 trials have demonstrated that patients with chronic hepatitis C virus (HCV) infection associated HCC survive longer than those who are negative for HCV. The mechanism underlying this currently remains unknown. A small number of cases of complete response to sorafenib treatment have now been reported worldwide, however a prolonged response has only been reported in 2 cases, both of whom had HCV-related HCC.

Case presentation: A 55 year old gentleman was diagnosed with hepatocellular carcinoma and concomitant chronic hepatitis C viral infection. He progressed following transarterial chemoemoblisation treatment and was commenced on sorafenib treatment. His serum alphafetoprotein level normalised within 2 months of treatment and he achieved an almost complete radiological response. This response was maintained for 20 months before the patient progressed. A 75 year old lady was diagnosed with advanced hepatocellular carcinoma and concomitant chronic hepatitis C viral infection. She was commenced on sorafenib treatment but required early dose reductions due to palmar plantar erythrodysesthesia, and liver decompensation. Despite this she achieved an excellent serological and radiological response that was maintained for 24 months.

Conclusions: Our two cases show that patients with HCV-associated HCC can attain excellent responses to sorafenib treatment that is durable. Furthermore, such exceptional responses can be achieved even with dose reductions and treatment breaks.

Keywords: Sorafenib, Hepatocellular carcinoma, Hepatitis C virus infection

* Correspondence: y.t.ma@bham.ac.uk
[1]The Cancer Centre, University Hospitals Birmingham NHS Foundation Trust, Edgbaston, Birmingham B15 2TH, UK
Full list of author information is available at the end of the article

Background

Hepatocellular carcinoma (HCC) is the 5th most common cancer worldwide, and the 3rd most common cause of cancer death. It often occurs on a background of chronic liver disease, including chronic hepatitis C (HCV) or hepatitis B (HBV) viral infection, and alcoholic liver disease [1].

Sorafenib, a multikinase inhibitor, is the only systemic treatment shown to increase overall survival in those with advanced HCC [2, 3]. However only 2–3% of patients achieve a partial response to sorafenib, with most patients achieving disease stabilisation.

Here we report two cases with advanced hepatocellular carcinoma and concomitant chronic hepatitis C viral infection, who achieved almost complete radiological responses to sorafenib treatment for a prolonged period. There are only 2 other reported cases in the literature reporting prolonged responses following sorafenib treatment [4, 5].

Chronic HCV infection is one of most common causes of HCC in Western countries. Despite the recent introduction of effective antiviral HCV therapy, the incidence of HCV-associated HCC is predicted to increase over the next few years due to the epidemic of undiagnosed chronic HCV infection [1]. There is now increasing evidence to suggest that patients with HCV-related HCC may attain superior survival benefit with sorafenib compared to patients who are negative for HCV. An exploratory subgroup analysis of the SHARP trial reported that patients with HCV-related HCC treated with sorafenib had a longer median overall survival compared to those with alcohol- or HBV-related HCC (14.0 vs 10.3 vs 9.7 months, respectively) [6]. In the phase III trial comparing sunitinib and sorafenib in patients with advanced HCC, median overall survival was superior in sorafenib treated patients, particularly in those with chronic HCV infection (17.6 vs 9.2 months) [7]. Similar results were was also reported in the phase III trial comparing brivanib and sorafenib; exploratory subgroup analyses demonstrated that the HCV positive subgroup of the sorafenib arm had a longer overall survival than hepatitis C negative participants who received sorafenib (12.9 vs. 9.3 months) [8].

The precise mechanism underlying the possible higher efficacy of sorafenib in patients with chronic HCV infection currently remains unclear. In vitro, it has been shown that cellular expression of full length HCV enhances sensitivity to sorafenib. This was due to modulation of microRNA expression by the viral proteins, which in turn enhances apoptosis through downregulation of the anti-apoptotic protein Mcl-1 [9].

There is also increasing evidence outlining the mechanism by which sorafenib interacts with the hepatitis C virus. In vitro, sorafenib has been shown to inhibit HCV infection in a dose-dependent manner [10]. Multiple steps in the HCV infectious cycle appear to be affected, including inhibition of viral replication by blocking the c-Raf pathway that is normally activated by the virus, impaired secretion of HCV particles, and potent inhibition of viral entry and HCV cell-to-cell transmission [10, 11]. Further studies have researched whether sorafenib may have benefit in treating chronic HCV infection – however a small study of 33 patients being treated for HCC with sorafenib failed to show any significant change in measured viral load [12]. Similarly in our 2 cases, sorafenib treatment was not associated with any reduction in the HCV viral load.

Case presentation 1

A 55 year old gentleman was diagnosed with hepatocellular carcinoma in September 2012, following investigations for deranged liver function tests. Magnetic resonance imaging (MRI) of the abdomen demonstrated a 4.5 cm liver lesion, with arterial phase hyperenhancement and venous phase washout, with an adjacent satellite nodule and invasion into a portal vein branch. The background liver appeared cirrhotic, and the spleen was enlarged. His serum alpha fetoprotein (AFP) was 1751kU/L, and a viral hepatitis screen showed chronic hepatitis C virus (HCV) infection and evidence of previous hepatitis B viral infection. His HCV viral load at baseline was 606926 IU/mL. He had well compensated liver function (Child Pugh class A) and an Eastern Cooperative Oncology Group (ECOG) performance status of zero.

He was treated with transarterial chemoembolisation (TACE) as the invasion into his branch portal vein was non-occlusive, but his computed tomography (CT) scan 4 weeks post-TACE demonstrated disease progression, with an increase in size and enhancement of the primary liver lesion, progression of the branch portal vein invasion and multiple new abdominal, para-aortic and mediastinal lymphadenopathy (Fig. 1a).

He started treatment with sorafenib in January 2013, achieving a maintenance dose of 600 mg daily after 2 months. He achieved an excellent serological response; his serum AFP level fell from a baseline value of 348kU/L to 5kU/L within 2 months and remained suppressed thereafter. This was associated with an excellent radiological response: CT imaging after 3 months of treatment showed a significant decrease in the size of the primary liver lesion and the lymphadenopathy (Fig. 1b). Follow-up CT imaging after 6 months of treatment demonstrated disappearance of all measurable disease apart from a residual lymph node adjacent to the caudate lobe (Fig. 1c). He maintained his excellent serological and radiological response for a further 14 months, until progressive disease was seen on repeat CT imaging in

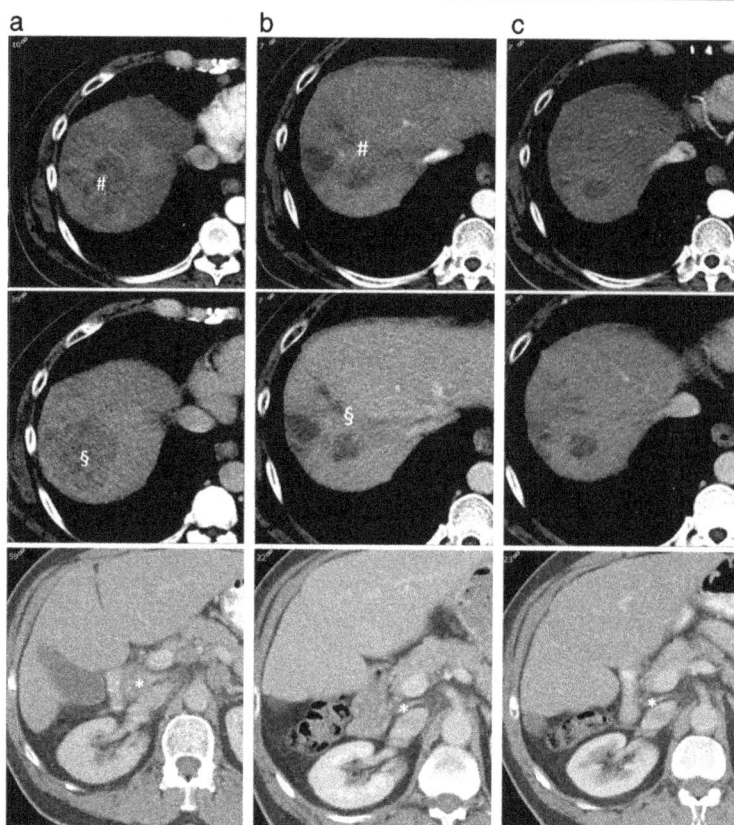

Fig. 1 Case 1 response to sorafenib. **a**. Triple phase CT of the liver 07/12/2012. Primary HCC with arterial phase enhancement (# *top panel*) and portal venous washout (§ *middle panel*) with involved lymph node between portal vein and IVC (*bottom panel* *). **b**. Triple phase CT of the liver 03/04/2013. Primary HCC with reduced arterial phase enhancement (# *top panel*) and portal venous washout (§ *middle panel*) with two cystic areas. Reduction in size of lymph node (*bottom panel* *). **c**. Triple phase CT of the liver 15/07/2013. No arterial phase enhancement (*top panel*) or portal phase washout (*middle panel*) reflecting disappearance of tumour. Residual cystic areas. Sustained reduction in size of lymph node (*bottom panel* *)

August 2014. He received a total of 20 months of treatment with sorafenib. Sorafenib had no effect on the patient's HCV viral load, which remained significantly elevated during this period. The patient entered a second line clinical trial and remained alive for a further 11 months following discontinuation of sorafenib.

Case presentation 2

A 75 year old lady was diagnosed with advanced hepatocellular carcinoma in June 2013 following investigations for low platelet count. A CT scan of the liver showed a 12 cm tumour in the left lobe with arterial phase hyperenhancement and venous phase washout, and left portal vein invasion (Fig. 2a). The background liver appeared cirrhotic. Her serum AFP level was 372 kU/L. A viral hepatitis screen confirmed chronic hepatitis C virus infection, with a low viral load (114 IU/mL). She had well compensated liver function (Child Pugh class A) and an ECOG performance status of 1.

She started sorafenib in July 2013, at a dose of 400 mg twice daily. After 7 days she developed grade 2 palmarplantar erythrodysesthesia and treatment was paused and

then restarted at reduced dose of 400 mg daily. She developed grade 2 hand-foot skin toxicity again and her sorafenib dose was thus reduced further to 200 mg daily, which was well tolerated. Repeat CT imaging after 3 months of treatment showed stable disease, however her serum AFP level had risen to 1574 kU/L. Her dose of sorafenib was cautiously increased. Over the next 2 months her serum AFP level declined rapidly to 6 kU/L.

Following this her liver synthetic function deteriorated and she decompensated with recurrent episodes of hepatic encephalopathy and ascites. Her treatment was paused for 4 months. Throughout this period her serum AFP level remained below 13kU/L. On review in March 2014 her liver synthetic function had improved (Child Pugh class B7), and she restarted low dose sorafenib. CT imaging in March showed ongoing stable disease despite the 4 month treatment break. Following resumption of sorafenib, serial CT scans showed reduction in the size of the liver lesion, with no tumour enhancement seen on her repeat imaging in December 2014 (Fig. 2b). She maintains her excellent serological and radiological response to date, 24 months after first starting sorafenib.

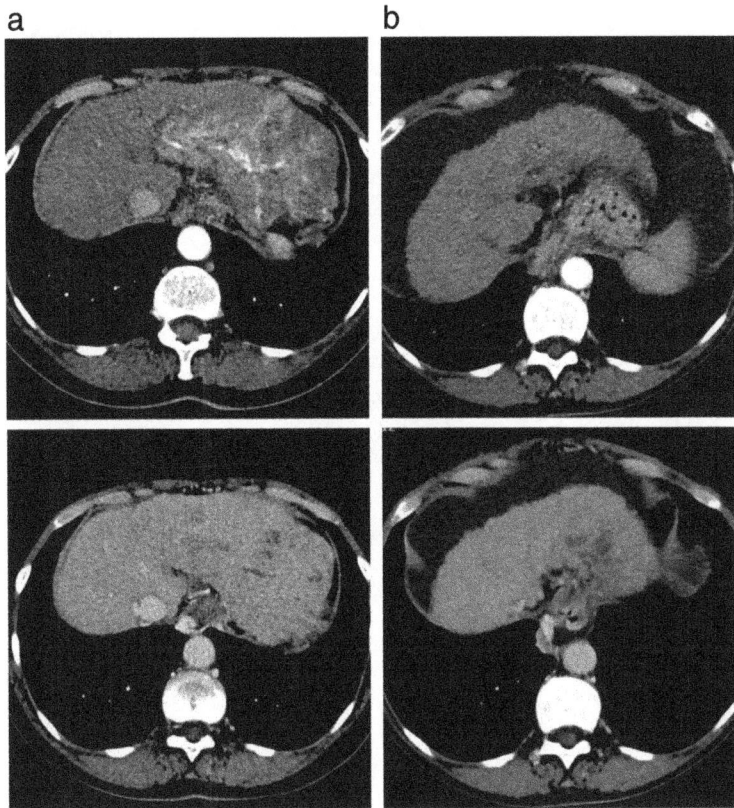

Fig. 2 Case 2 response to sorafenib. **a**. Triple phase CT of the liver 10/06/2013. Primary HCC with arterial phase enhancement (*top panel*) and portal venous washout (*bottom panel*). **b**. Triple phase CT of the liver 19/12/2014. Primary HCC with no arterial phase enhancement (*top panel*) or portal venous washout (*bottom panel*)

Her HCV viral load initially increased to 4000 IU/mL after starting sorafenib and remains elevated.

Conclusions

In patients with advanced HCC, sorafenib is the only systemic treatment that has been shown to increase overall survival [2, 3]. Sorafenib is an orally active, multikinase inhibitor that inhibits tumour angiogenesis and cell proliferation by blocking cell surface tyrosine kinases such as vascular endothelial growth factor receptor-2/3 (VEGFR-2/3) and platelet derived growth factor receptor beta, as well as downstream signalling pathways involving the serine/threonine kinases Raf-1 and B-Raf [13]. Its efficacy in treating HCC has been demonstrated in 2 randomised phase III trials [2, 3]. The SHARP trial, undertaken in patients with advanced HCC in Western countries, showed that patients with advanced hepatocellular carcinoma treated with sorafenib had a significant improvement in overall survival (10.7 months vs. 7.9 months, $p < 0.001$) and radiological time to progression (5.5 months vs. 2.8 months, $p < 0.001$) when compared to placebo [2]. The Asia-Pacific trial also showed that sorafenib significantly prolonged overall survival (6.5 months vs. 4.2 months, hazard ratio 0.68, $p = 0.014$) compared to placebo, in patients from the Asia-Pacific region [3]. In both trials a partial response was observed in only a small minority of patients (2 and 3% respectively) and no complete responses were seen.

A small number of cases of complete response to sorafenib treatment have now been reported worldwide [4, 5, 14–17], however a prolonged response (>18 months) has only been reported in 2 cases, both of whom had HCV-related HCC [4, 5]. Both of our cases also had HCV-related HCC and demonstrated prolonged responses (20 and 24 months, respectively) to sorafenib treatment. The 2 cases presented here add to the accumulating evidence that patients with HCV-related HCC may attain superior survival benefit with sorafenib compared to patients who are negative for HCV. The second case is particularly noteworthy, because the prolonged response was achieved even with dose reductions and a treatment break (due to decompensation), and highlights that even with dose reductions, significant response to sorafenib can be achieved.

Abbreviations
AFP: Alpha fetoprotein; CT: Computed tomography; ECOG: Eastern cooperative oncology group; HBV: Hepatitis B virus infection; HCC: Hepatocellular carcinoma; HCV: Hepatitis C virus infection; MRI: Magnetic resonance imaging; RNA: Ribonucleic acid; TACE: Transarterial chemoembolization; VEGFR: Vascular endothelial growth factor receptor

Acknowledgements
Not applicable.

Funding
No funding was received.

Authors' contributions
CA and PE drafted the manuscript. AP provided the radiological images for this manuscript, and was a major contributor in drafting the manuscript. SS, PP and YTM revised the manuscript critically for important intellectual content. All authors read and approved the final manuscript.

Competing interests
The authors declare that they have no competing interests.

Consent for publication
Written informed consent was obtained from both patients for publication of this case report.

Author details
[1]The Cancer Centre, University Hospitals Birmingham NHS Foundation Trust, Edgbaston, Birmingham B15 2TH, UK. [2]Department of Radiology, University Hospitals Birmingham NHS Foundation Trust, Edgbaston, Birmingham B15 2TH, UK. [3]The Liver Unit, University Hospitals Birmingham NHS Foundation Trust, Edgbaston, Birmingham B15 2TH, UK.

References
1. de Oliveria Andrade LJ, D'Oliveira A, Melo RC, De Souza EC, Costa Silva CA, Paraná R. Association between hepatitis C and hepatocellular carcinoma. J Glob Infect Dis. 2009;1:33–7.
2. Llovet JM, Ricci S, Mazzaferro V, Hilgard P, Gane E, Blanc JF, et al. Sorafenib in advanced hepatocellular carcinoma. N Engl J Med. 2008;359:378–90.
3. Cheng AL, Kang YK, Chen Z, Tsao CJ, Qin S, Kim JS, et al. Efficacy and safety of sorafenib in patients in the Asia-Pacific region with advanced hepatocellular carcinoma: a phase III randomised, double-blind, placebo-controlled trial. Lancet Oncol. 2009;10:25–34.
4. Sacco R, Bargellini I, Gianluigi G, Bertini M, Bozzi E, Altomare E, et al. Complete response for advanced liver cancer during sorafenib therapy: case report. BMC Gastroenterol. 2011;11:4.
5. Gerardi AM, Stoppino LP, Liso A, Macarini L, Landriscina M. Rapid long-lasting biochemical and radiological response to sorafenib in a case of advanced hepatocellular carcinoma. Oncol Lett. 2013;5(3):975–7.
6. Bruix J, Raoul JL, Sherman M, Mazzaferro V, Bolondi L, Craxi A, et al. Efficacy and safety of sorafenib in patients with advanced hepatocellular carcinoma: Subanalyses of a phase III trial. J Hepatol. 2012;57:821–9.
7. Cheng AL, Kang YK, Lin DY, Park JW, Kudo M, Qin S, et al. Sunitinib versus sorafenib in advanced hepatocellular cancer: results of a randomized phase III trial. J Clin Oncol. 2013;31(32):4067–75.
8. Johnson PJ, Qin S, Park JW, Poon RT, Raoul JL, Philip PA, et al. Brivanib versus sorafenib as first-line therapy in patients with unresectable, advanced hepatocellular carcinoma: results from the randomized phase III BRISK-FL study. J Clin Oncol. 2013;31(28):3517–24.
9. Braconi C, Valeri N, Gasperini P, Huang N, Taccioli C, Nuovo G, et al. Hepatitis C virus proteins modulate microRNA expression and chemosensitivity in malignant hepatocytes. Clin Cancer Res. 2010;16(3):957–66.
10. Descamps V, Helle F, Louandre C, Martin E, Brochot E, Izquierdo L, et al. The kinase-inhibitor sorafenib inhibits multiple steps of the Hepatitis C Virus infectious cycle in vitro. Antiviral Res. 2015;118:93–102.
11. Himmelsbach K, Sauter D, Baumert TF, Ludwig L, Blum HE, Hildt E. New aspects of an anti-tumour drug: sorafenib efficiently inhibits HCV replication. Gut. 2009;58:1644–53.
12. Cabrera R, Limaye AR, Horne P, Mills R, Soldevila-Pico C, Clark V, et al. The antiviral effect of sorafenib in hepatitis c-related hepatocellular carcinoma. Aliment Pharmacol Ther. 2013;37(1):91–7.
13. Wilhelm SM, Carter C, Tang L, Wilkie D, McNabola A, Rong H, et al. BAY 43–9006 exhibits broad spectrum oral antitumour activity and targets the raf/MEK/ERK pathway and receptor tyrosine kinases involved in tumor proliferation and angiogenesis. Cancer Res. 2004;64:7099–109.
14. Nakazawa T, Hidaka H, Shibuya A, Koizumi W. Rapid regression of advanced hepatocellular carcinoma associated with elevation of des-gamma-carboxy prothrombin after short-term treatment with sorafenib - a report of two cases. Case Rep Oncol. 2010;3:298–303.
15. Di Lorenzo G, Imbimbo M, Leopardo D, Marciano R, Federico P, Buonerba C, et al. A long-lasting response to sorafenib treatment in an advanced hepatocellular carcinoma patient. Int J Immunopathol Pharmacol. 2010;23(3):951–4.
16. Chelis L, Ntinos N, Souftas V, Deftereos S, Xenidis N, Chamalidou E, et al. Complete response after sorafenib therapy for hepatocellular carcinoma in an HIV-HBV co infected patient: Possible synergy with HAART ? A case report. Med Oncol. 2011;28 Suppl 1:S165–8.
17. Inuzuka T, Nishikawa H, Sekikawa A, Takeda H, Henmi S, Sakamoto A, et al. Complete response of advanced hepatocellular carcinoma with multiple lung metastases treated with sorafenib: a case report. Oncology. 2011;81 Suppl 1:152–7.

9

Novel *NBAS* mutations and fever-related recurrent acute liver failure in Chinese children

Jia-Qi Li[1], Yi-Ling Qiu[2], Jing-Yu Gong[1], Li-Min Dou[2], Yi Lu[2], A. S. Knisely[3], Mei-Hong Zhang[1], Wei-Sha Luan[1] and Jian-She Wang[2*]

Abstract

Background: Underlying causes in Chinese children with recurrent acute liver failure (RALF), including liver crises less than full acute liver failure, are incompletely understood. We sought to address this by searching for genes mutated in such children.

Methods: Five unrelated Chinese boys presenting between 2012 and 2015 with RALF of unexplained etiology were studied. Results of whole exome sequencing were screened for mutations in candidate genes. Mutations were verified in patients and their family members by Sanger sequencing. All 5 boys underwent liver biopsy.

Results: *NBAS* was the only candidate gene mutated in more than one patient (biallelic mutations, 3 of 5 patients; 5 separate mutations). All *NBAS* mutations were novel and predictedly pathogenic (frameshift insertion mutation c.6611_6612insCA, missense mutations c.2407G > A and c.3596G > A, nonsense mutation c.586C > T, and splicing-site mutation c.5389 + 1G > T). Of these mutations, 3 lay in distal (C-terminal) regions of *NBAS*, a novel distribution. Unlike the 2 patients without *NBAS* mutations, the 3 patients with confirmed *NBAS* mutations all suffered from a febrile illness before each episode of liver crisis (fever-related RALF), with markedly elevated alanine aminotransferase and aspartate aminotransferase activities 24-72 h after elevation of body temperature, succeeded by severe coagulopathy and mild to moderate jaundice.

Conclusions: As in other countries, so too in China; *NBAS* disease is a major cause of fever-related RALF in children. The mutation spectrum of *NBAS* in Chinese children seems different from that described in other populations.

Keywords: *NBAS*, Recurrent acute liver failure, Acute liver failure, Whole exome sequencing

Background

Acute liver failure (ALF) is a rare but often fatal emergency for children, especially infants. Together with non-genetic causes such as viral infections, drug or toxin exposure, and autoimmune hepatitis, identified hereditary metabolic disorders account for half the instances of ALF in children [1–5]. Although recent work in Europe has implicated several genes in recurrent ALF (RALF) in infancy [6–10], the etiology of some instances of pediatric RALF remains unexplained. Furthermore, the causes of RALF in non-European populations are largely unexplored.

Biallelic mutations in *NBAS* (NM_015909) were first identified as causing fever-related RALF (infantile liver failure syndrome 2; MIM616483) by Haack et al. [8]. *NBAS* was previously linked to SOPH (short stature, optic nerve atrophy, and Pelger–Huët anomaly of granulocytes; MIM614800) syndrome in an isolated Russian Yakut population, but without liver failure [11]. Further observations expanded the phenotype spectrum of *NBAS* disease to involve brain, connective tissues other than bone, and the immune system as well [12–15].

Using whole-exome sequencing (WES), we evaluated 5 Chinese children with RALF. Here we describe our work and its implications.

* Correspondence: jshwang@shmu.edu.cn
[2]The Center for Pediatric Liver Diseases, Children's Hospital of Fudan University, Shanghai 201102, China

Methods

Enrollment criteria

The probands were Chinese children evaluated for RALF from 2012 to 2015 by JSW, to whose clinic instances of pediatric liver disease from throughout China are referred (1096 new pediatric liver-disease patients seen during these 4y). Their parents and siblings also took part.

Participation required informed consent (for children, informed parental consent) under a protocol approved by Children's Hospital and Jinshan Hospital of Fudan University according to the ethical guidelines of the 1975 Declaration of Helsinki. RALF of indeterminate etiology was defined as present when a child had >1 episode of liver injury, including at least 1 episode of ALF (Pediatric Acute Liver Failure Study Group criteria) [3]. That is, no child had evidence of chronic liver disease; all children had biochemical evidence of acute liver injury; all children

had hepatic-based coagulopathy, with a prothrombin time (PTT) ≥15 s or an international normalized ratio (INR) >1.5 not corrected by vitamin K in the presence of hepatic encephalopathy, or a PTT ≥20s or an INR >2.0 regardless of the presence or absence of clinical hepatic encephalopathy; and all other causes possibly responsible for liver crises were excluded through comprehensive evaluation. Liver biopsy was performed when coagulopathy permitted.

Clinical features of probands

Five unrelated boys with RALF of indeterminate etiology were enrolled in this study, including 4 of Han and 1 of Miao ancestry. The major clinical features of these probands are shown in Table 1. All parents were non-consanguine, except those of patient 4. Patient 1, initially diagnosed with liver crisis aged 6mo 18d, is the product of a 4th pregnancy (ectopic pregnancy, surgically treated;

Table 1 Clinical features of patients 1–5

Clinical features	Patient				
	1	2	3	4	5
Ethnic group	Han	Han	Han	Miao	Han
Consanguineous parents	No	No	No	Yes	No
Birth weight (SDS)	−0.08	0.69	−0.85	NA	0.44
Age, initial RALF episode	6mo18d	7mo21d	6mo1d	6y10mo	2y2mo
Age at last assessment	6y11mo	4y8mo	2y4mo	12y11mo	4y8mo
Episodes of ALF	5	1	10	1	1
Episodes of liver crisis without ALF	3	2	1	1	4
Age at last ALF	6y11mo	2y2mo	2y4mo	6y10mo	2y2mo
Age at last liver crisis	3y1mo	4y1mo	1y7mo	9y1mo	3y10mo
Febrile illness before each episode of RALF	+	+	+	−	−
Hepatomegaly	+	+	+	+	+
Splenomegaly	+	+	+	+	+
Hepatomegaly between episodes/crises	−	−	+	NA	+
Splenomegaly between episodes/crises	−	−	−	NA	+
Body length (SDS)	−1.42	−1.47	0.31	−1.34	1.66
Age at LBX	5y11mo	2y3mo	6mo13d	9y1mo	3y10mo
Clinical status at LBX	During 7th crisis (DS)	After 2nd crisis	During 1st crisis (DS)	During 2nd crisis (DS)	During 5th crisis (DS)
ALT /AST (IU/L) at LBX	1091/307	27/12	200/24	43/22	84/48
Results of LBX	Steatosis	Centrilobular fibrosis	Steatosis; centrilobular fibrosis	Unremarkable	Inflammation
NBAS mutations	c.6611_6612insCA + c.3596G > A	c.3596G > A + c.586C > T	c.5389 + 1G > T + c.2407G > A	−	−

NA Not available, RALF Recurrent acute liver failure, ALF Acute liver failure, ALT Alanine transaminase (expected range 0–40 IU/L), AST Aspartate transaminase (expected range, 0–40 IU/L), LBX Liver biopsy, DS Downswing (resolution of crisis), SDS Standard deviation score. y Year, mo Month, d Day. All probands were male. All were born at term. None was dysmorphic. Patient 3 suffered from recurrent infections; immunologic evaluation identified no specific deficiency. Clinical-biochemistry evidence of hepatobiliary injury was seen in none between liver crises or bouts of ALF

2 induced abortions) complicated by intrahepatic chole-stasis manifest as pruritus that halted after delivery. The parents are otherwise well. Patient 2, initially diagnosed in liver crisis aged 7mo 21d, is the product of a 1st pregnancy. A younger brother is well. Their mother has a 3y history of hyperthyroidism. Their father is healthy. Patient 3, initially diagnosed in ALF aged 6mo 1d, is the product of a 3rd pregnancy. A sister and brother died in fever-related liver crisis aged respectively 4mo and 8mo. Material from them suitable for genetic analysis was unavailable. Patient 4, initially diagnosed in ALF aged 6y 10mo, is the product of a 5th pregnancy (2 induced abortions, 2 live births). One sister has moyamoya disease; the other is healthy. Their parents are consanguineous. Patient 5, initially diagnosed in ALF aged 2y 2mo, is the product of a first and only pregnancy. The parents are healthy. All patients were normally grown, without dysmorphism. Patients 1–3 always had febrile illnesses before liver crises or episodes of ALF. Patient 5, with one episode of liver crisis without a febrile illness, had febrile illnesses before 3 liver crises and before one episode of ALF. No febrile illness preceded liver crisis or ALF in patient 4.

Liver biopsy

All 5 patients underwent percutaneous core needle liver biopsy. In patient 1, biopsy was conducted during resolution of the 4th episode of ALF (5y 11mo). Alanine transaminase (ALT) and aspartate aminotransferase (AST) values ("transaminases") 1d before liver biopsy were abnormal (ALT/AST = 1091/307 IU/L; 0–40 expected for each). Patient 2 underwent liver biopsy 2mo after his 2nd liver crisis (2y 3mo); transaminases 2d before biopsy were normal (ALT/AST = 27/12). Patient 3 underwent liver biopsy during resolution of his 1st episode of ALF (6mo 13d). Transaminases were abnormal 4d before biopsy (ALT/AST = 200/24) and were normal 3d after biopsy (ALT/AST = 30/27). In patient 4, whose biopsy occurred during resolution of ALF (9y 1mo), ALT and AST 2d after liver biopsy were 43 and 22. Patient 5 underwent biopsy during resolution of his 5th liver crisis (3y 10mo). Transaminases 1d before liver biopsy were abnormal (ALT/AST = 84/48).

Whole Exome sequencing

Peripheral blood samples were obtained from the probands, their parents, and their siblings. Genomic DNA was extracted routinely from peripheral blood leukocytes. Sequencing was conducted at Genesky Biotechnologies, Shanghai.

Exomes (probands; sister of patient 4) were captured using an Agilent SureSelect Human All Exon v5 kit (Agilent Technologies, Wokingham, UK). Sequencing (150 bp paired-end reads) was performed using the Illumina hiseq2500 platform following the manufacturer's instructions (Illumina, CA). Read alignment was performed with Burrows-Wheeler Aligner (http://bio-bwa.sourceforge.net/) and Picard (https://broadinstitute.github.io/picard/). Varscan (http://varscan.sourceforge.net/) and GATK (https://software.broadinstitute.org/gatk/best-practices/) were used for variants calling. Total sequencing depth was 100X. Mean coverage of the exome ranged from 35X to 50X, with >92% of the exome covered at least 2X and >80% covered at >10X. Sequencing statistics are shown in Additional file 1.

Exome sequencing analysis

Detailed variant filtering strategies for each patient are outlined in Additional file 2. Variants occurring with allele frequency ≥ 1% in the Thousand Genomes Project (http://www.1000genomes.org/home) and NHLBI Exome Sequencing Project (http://evs.gs.washington.edu/EVS/) databases or ≥4.5% in the Genesky in-house database were filtered out. Potential disease-causing mutations predicted by Polyphen-2 (http://genetics.bwh.harvard.edu/pph2/), SIFT (http://sift.jcvi.org/), and MutationTaster [16] (http://www.mutationtaster.org/) then were selected as suspected pathogenic variations. Suspected pathogenic variations in genes known to be associated with ALF (Additional file 3) and present in accord with inheritance modes identified candidate genes. Suspected pathogenic variations in genes not known to be associated with ALF but present in accord with recessive inheritance also identified candidate genes.

Sanger sequencing

Polymerase chain reaction (PCR) amplification was carried out using primers specific for NBAS exons 8, 22, 31, 43, and 50 (Additional file 4). PCR conditions are available on request. The amplified products were sequenced using an ABI 3730xl DNA Analyzer (Applied Biosystems, Foster City, CA) and analyzed using CodonCode Aligner software (http://www.codoncode.com). NM_015909 was used as the NBAS reference sequence.

Results

Identification of biallelic NBAS mutations in 3 RALF patients

Five Chinese boys with RALF of undetermined etiology were identified from 2012 to 2015 among patients at our institutions. All underwent WES (patients 1–5), as did the healthy sister of patient 4. Filtering criteria yielded 9, 11, 13, 11, and 1 candidate genes in patients 1 through 5 respectively (Additional file 5). The only gene shared by 2 or more patients was NBAS. Two predictedly pathogenic variations of NBAS were detected in patient 1, patient 2, and patient 3, while no NBAS variant was detected in either patient 4 or patient 5. Sanger sequencing in parents proved compound heterozygosity in patients 1, 2, and 3 (Fig. 1).

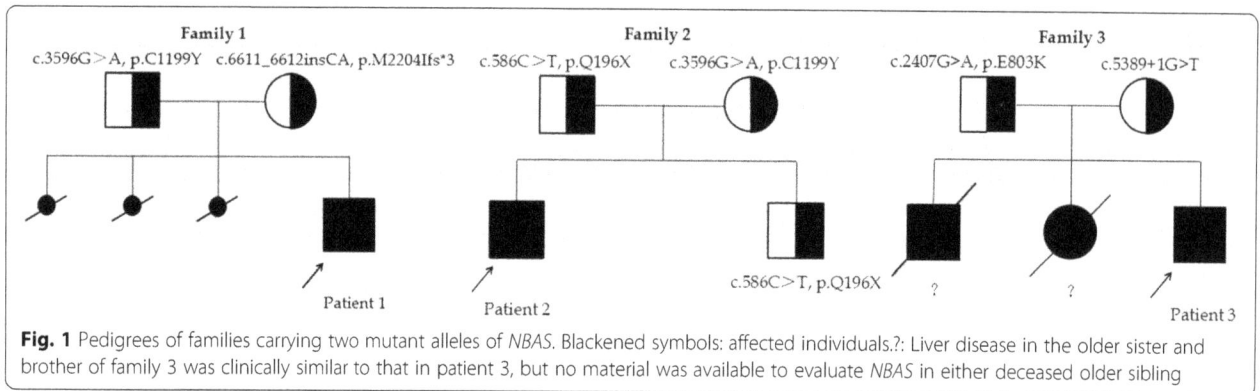

Fig. 1 Pedigrees of families carrying two mutant alleles of *NBAS*. Blackened symbols: affected individuals.?: Liver disease in the older sister and brother of family 3 was clinically similar to that in patient 3, but no material was available to evaluate *NBAS* in either deceased older sibling

Patient 1 harbored mutations c.3596G > A, p.C1199Y (missense) and c.6611_6612insCA, p.M2204Ifs*3 (frameshift); patient 2, mutations c.3596G > A, p.C1199Y (missense) and c.586C > T, p.Q196X (nonsense); and patient 3, c.2407G > A, p.E803K (missense) and c.5389 + 1G > T (splice-site). Two missense mutations (c.3596G > A, p. C1199Y [2 patients] and c.2407G > A, p. E803K), were both predicted to be pathogenic by Polyphen-2, SIFT, and MutationTaster [16] analyses. Patients 1 and 2 each harboured the c.3596G > A mutation. The missense mutation c.2407G > A is described (6 heterozygous instances, Exome Aggregation Consortium (ExAc) Server [http://exac.broadinstitute.org/]). The other 4 mutations are not recorded in public databases (Thousand Genomes Project; NHLBI Exome Sequencing Project; ExAc) or in the Genesky in-house database; we consider them novel.

Clinical manifestations in 3 *NBAS* mutant patients

Unlike the 2 patients without *NBAS* mutation, those harbouring *NBAS* mutations always had a febrile illness before a liver crisis or episode of ALF. Our 3 *NBAS*-disease patients clinically resembled one another: all suffered from a febrile illness, likely infective (viral / bacterial) before each episode of RALF (fever-related RALF), with markedly elevated ALT (77–9382 IU/L; normal 0–40) and AST (213–17,344 IU/L; normal 0–40) activities 24-72 h after elevation of body temperature, succeeded by severe coagulopathy (maximum INR = 6.89; normal 0.8–1.2) and mild to moderate jaundice that were ascribed to ALF. Hypoglycemia and hepatic encephalopathy were transiently observed in patients 1 and 3. Total bile acid concentrations in all 3 patients were increased (18.2–517.2 umol/ L; normal 0–10). Serum alkaline phosphatase and γ-glutamyltranspeptidase activities were normal or only mildly increased, as were blood ammonia values. Ages during episodes of ALF and liver crises are shown in Additional file 6. The details of episodes of RALF in patient 3 are shown in Additional file 7. Similar details for patients 1 and 2 are not available, as they received care at several hospitals other than ours. Biomarkers of hepatobiliary injury

completely recovered between liver crises. Not all episodes of fever led to hepatic crisis. All patients used antipyretics and hepatoprotectives (e.g., ademetionine 1, 4-butanedisulfonate; reduced glutathione). In patient 1, however, during his 7th episode of RALF (4th of ALF) biomarkers returned to normal without hepatoprotectives. The 3 *NBAS*-disease patients were free from facial dysmorphism and had no broken bones. No radiogrammes were exposed in patients 1 and 2; a left lower limb radiogram in patient 3 was assessed as normal. Formal cognitive evaluation and investigations for Pelger-Huët anomaly were not conducted in any patient. Motor development was normal for all 3. Lymphocyte panels and immunoglobulin values were unremarkable in patients 1 and 3; these were not evaluated in patient 2. Ophthalmoscopy found no abnormality in patient 3 and was not conducted in patients 1 and 2.

Liver biopsy in 5 RALF patients

Light microscopy was undertaken in patients 1–5, with ultrastructural study in patients 1–4. Hepatocyte cytoplasm contained small vacuoles in patients 1 and 3, confirmed as steatosis by transmission electron microscopy. Patients 2 and 3 had centrilobular fibrosis that was worse in patient 3. In patient 4, the liver was unremarkable. Inflammation and minimal portal-tract fibrosis were seen in patient 5. Ultrastructural findings were non-specific, with questionably increased glycogen stores in patients 1–4, dilated endoplasmic reticulum (ER) and abnormal mitochondria in patient 2, dense mitochondrial matrix in patient 3, and swollen mitochondria, questionably decreased in number, in patient 4.

Discussion

Mutations in *NBAS* were first identified as an important cause of infantile and later-onset recurrent liver failure in 2015 [8]. NBAS is a subunit of the syntaxin 18 complex, implicated in Golgi-to-endoplasmic reticulum (ER) retrograde transport [17]. NBAS also plays an important role in nonsense-mediated mRNA decay, which regulates gene expression in response to cellular and environmental stress [18]. *NBAS* had earlier been implicated in the developmental disorder SOPH syndrome [11], in which liver disease is not a feature. And a patient with *NBAS* disease manifest as SOPH syndrome with fever-associated liver crises that fell short of RALF is described [19]. Correlations between *NBAS* mutations and clinical manifestations are incomplete.

With this report, 23 *NBAS*-disease children with recurrent liver crises are described: 14 from European countries [12, 14, 19], 3 from the United States [12, 14], 3 from Lebanon (siblings; parental consanguinity known) [13], and our 3 Han Chinese. These patients' phenotypes range from isolated RALF to RALF in association with multisystemic disease. Our Han Chinese patients all had isolated RALF.

RALF patients usually exhibit recurrent vomiting, progressive lethargy and pyrexia 1 or 2d before medical assessment, which finds high serum transaminases; mild to moderate jaundice and severe coagulopathy then develop [8]. Our 3 *NBAS*-disease patients clinically resembled other reported children with isolated RALF [8]. All suffered from a febrile illness before each liver crisis (fever-related RALF) and at presentation had substantially elevated serum AST and ALT values, followed by mild to moderate jaundice and severe coagulopathy. However, of

interest as at slight variance from published descriptions is that in our patients the frequency and severity of ALF did not lessen with increasing age (Additional file 6), and that vomiting did not usually precede rises in transaminase values.

That in *NBAS* disease raised body temperature itself might both mark and initiate a liver crisis has been suggested [14], with the corollary and experience that early and effective control of fever might prevent or alleviate liver crisis. However, in our patients peak body temperature and length of fever were not, episode for episode of RALF, positively correlated with the severity of ensuing liver crises (Additional file 7). Expression profiling has identified ER stress in cultured fibroblasts from patients with *NBAS* disease [8]. ER stress accelerates lipogenesis in the liver [20, 21] and activates the unfolded protein response, which can trigger cellular destruction through apoptosis [22, 23]. Small-vacuole steatosis in liver, although not specific for ER stress, is consistent with that etiology. Widespread loss of hepatocytes, however, as might be expected if apoptosis is triggered, was not identified even in liver biopsied during ALF with hypertransaminasemia (patient 1). Findings on microscopy did not contribute to diagnosis.

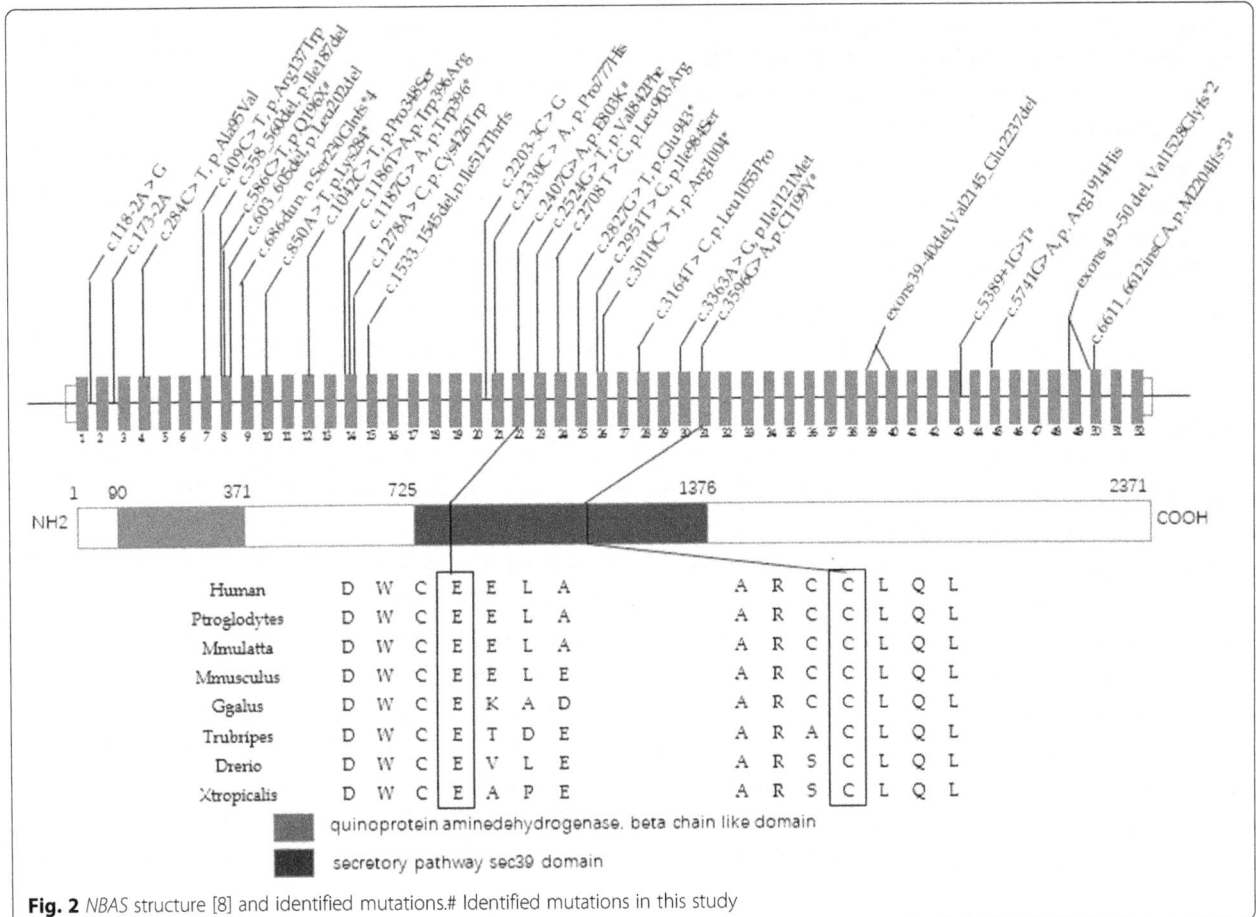

Fig. 2 *NBAS* structure [8] and identified mutations.# Identified mutations in this study

The identified *NBAS* mutations in reported patients with liver crises comprise 5 nonsense, 14 missense, and 7 deletion/insertion mutations, with 4 splice-site variants. These are clustered into 3 regions in the first half of the gene, exons 2–4, exons 7–15 and exons 21–26 (Fig. 2). However, among the mutations identified in our patients, none of which has before been associated with RALF, 3 lie in the second half of the gene (c.6611_6612insCA, p.M2204Ifs*3; c.5389 + 1G > T; c.3596G > A, p. C1199Y, exons 50, 43, and 31 respectively). That patients 1 and 2, not identifiably related, share mutation c3596G > A, p.C1199Y may be of relevance to a special *NBAS* mutation in Han Chinese.

Conclusions

In summary, we have identified *NBAS*-related RALF in 3 Han Chinese children. Their disorder clinically resembled that in western European (and North American, and Lebanese) children with *NBAS*-related RALF, although several of the mutations in our patients lay in a region of *NBAS* not previously found involved. RALF in each of these patients was fever-related, suggesting that to search for *NBAS* lesions in Han Chinese children with fever-related RALF may be worthwhile. That 2 of the 5 patients with RALF whom we studied – one of whom was born to consanguine parents – had no demonstrable mutations in *NBAS* or in other genes hitherto implicated in RALF implies that heritable causes of RALF remain to be discovered.

Additional files

Additional file 1: Sequencing statistics for patients 1–5.

Additional file 2: Variant filtering strategy for patients 1–5. A. Filtering procedure for suspected pathogenic genes for a single sample. B. Filtering procedure for candidate gene list. ALF, acute liver failure.

Additional file 3: Reported genes associated with acute liver failure.

Additional file 4: Specific primers for *NBAS* exons 8, 22, 31, 43, and 50.

Additional file 5: Candidate genes for patients 1–5.

Additional file 6: Ages during episodes of ALF and liver crises. P, patient. ALF, acute liver failure. N1, episodes of ALF. N2, episodes of acute liver crisis. The age of last following up for patients 1–3 is 6y 11 m, 4y 8 m, and 2y4m, respectively. With the increasing age, the episodes of ALF and RALF were not decreased.

Additional file 7: Details of RALF in patient 3. ALT, alanine aminotransferase; AST, aspartate aminotransferase; GGT, gamma-glutamyl transpeptidase; INR, international normalized ratio; TB, total bilirubin; TBA, total bile acids.

Abbreviations
ALF: Acute liver failure; ALT: Alanine transaminase; AST: Aspartate aminotransferase; ER: Endoplasmic reticulum; INR: International normalized ratio; PTT: Prothrombin time; RALF: Recurrent acute liver failure; SOPH: Short stature, optic nerve atrophy, and Pelger–Huët anomaly of granulocytes; WES: Whole exome sequencing

Acknowledgments
The authors are grateful for the support of the families of the RALF patients whom we have studied, and thank referring physicians, nurses, and technical staff.

Funding
This research work was supported by the National Natural Science Foundation of China, Grant 81570468.

Authors' contributions
JSW designed the research; JQL performed the experiments; JSW, JQL and YLQ drafted the manuscript; JSW, JQL, YLQ, and LMD were involved in the acquisition, anlysis and interpretation of clinical and whole exome sequencing data; JYG, YL and MHZ were involved in the acquisition, anlysis and interpretation of clinical data; ASK performed anlysis and interpretation of pathologic data; JQL and JSW edited and revised the manuscript; ASK and WSL did critical revision of manuscript. All authors read and approved the final manuscript.

Competing interests
Not applicable.

Consent for publication
Written informed consent for publication of their clinical details was obtained from the guardians of all patients.

Author details
[1]Department of Pediatrics, Jinshan Hospital of Fudan University, Shanghai 201508, China. [2]The Center for Pediatric Liver Diseases, Children's Hospital of Fudan University, Shanghai 201102, China. [3]Institut für Pathologie, Medizinische Universität Graz, Auenbruggerplatz 25, A-8036 Graz, Austria.

References
1. Shanmugam NP, Bansal S, Greenough A, Verma A, Dhawan A. Neonatal liver failure: aetiologies and management-state of the art. Eur J Pediatr. 2011;170:573–81.
2. Dhawan A. Etiology and prognosis of acute liver failure in children. Liver Transpl. 2008;14(Suppl 2):80–4.
3. Squires RJ, Shneider BL, Bucuvalas J, Alonso E, Sokol RJ, Narkewicz MR, et al. Acute liver failure in children: the first 348 patients in the pediatric acute liver failure study group. J Pediatr. 2006;148:652–8.
4. Durand P, Debray D, Mandel R, Baujard C, Branchereau S, Gauthier F, et al. Acute liver failure in infancy: a 14-year experience of a pediatric liver transplantation center. J Pediatr. 2001;139:871–6.
5. Devictor D, Desplanques L, Debray D, Ozier Y, Dubousset AM, Valayer J, et al. Emergency liver transplantation for fulminant liver failure in infants and children. Hepatology. 1992;16:1156–62.
6. Engelmann G, Meyburg J, Shahbek N, Al-Ali M, Hairetis MH, Baker AJ, et al. Recurrent acute liver failure and mitochondriopathy in a case of Wolcott-Rallison syndrome. J Inherit Metab Dis. 2008;31:540–6.
7. Casey JP, McGettigan P, Lynam-Lennon N, McDermott M, Regan R, Conroy J, et al. Identification of a mutation in *LARS* as a novel cause of infantile hepatopathy. Mol Genet Metab. 2012;106:351–8.
8. Haack TB, Staufner C, Kopke MG, Straub BK, Kolker S, Thiel C, et al. Biallelic mutations in *NBAS* cause recurrent acute liver failure with onset in infancy. Am J Hum Genet. 2015;97:163–9.
9. Brassia A, Ottolenghi C, Boutron A, Bertrand AM, Valmary-Degano S, Cervoni JP, et al. Dihydrolipoamide dehydrogenase deficiency: a still overlooked cause of recurrent acute liver failure and Reye-like syndrome. Mol Genet Metab. 2013;109:28–32.
10. Schmidt WM, Rutledge SL, Schule R, Mayerhofer B, Zuchner S, Boltshauser E, et al. Disruptive *SCYL1* mutations underlie a syndrome characterized by recurrent episodes of liver failure, peripheral neuropathy, cerebellar atrophy, and ataxia. Am J Hum Genet. 2015;97:855–61.

11. Maksimova N, Hara K, Nikolaeva I, Chun-Feng T, Usui T, Takagi M, et al. Neuroblastoma amplified sequence gene is associated with a novel short stature syndrome characterised by optic nerve atrophy and Pelger-Huet anomaly. J Med Genet. 2010;47:538–48.

12. Garcia Segarra N, Ballhausen D, Crawford H, Perreau M, Campos-Xavier B, van Spaendonck-Zwarts K, et al. *NBAS* mutations cause a multisystem disorder involving bone, connective tissue, liver, immune system, and retina. Am J Med Genet A. 2015;167A:2902–12.

13. Capo-Chichi J, Mehawej C, Delague V, Caillaud C, Khneisser I, Hamdan FF, et al. Neuroblastoma amplified sequence (*NBAS*) mutation in recurrent acute liver failure: confirmatory report in a sibship with very early onset, osteoporosis and developmental delay. Eur J Med Genet. 2015;58:637–41.

14. Staufner C, Haack TB, Kopke MG, Straub BK, Kolker S, Thiel C, et al. Recurrent acute liver failure due to *NBAS* deficiency: phenotypic spectrum, disease mechanisms, and therapeutic concepts. J Inherit Metab Dis. 2016;39:3–16.

15. Balasubramanian M, Hurst J, Brown S, Bishop NJ, Arundel P, DeVile C, et al. Compound heterozygous variants in *NBAS* as a cause of atypical osteogenesis imperfecta. Bone. 2017;94:65–74.

16. Schwarz JM, Cooper DN, Schuelke M, Seelow D. MutationTaster2: mutation prediction for the deep-sequencing age. Nat Methods. 2014;11:361–2.

17. Aoki T, Ichimura S, Itoh A, Kuramoto M, Shinkawa T, Isobe T, et al. Identification of the neuroblastoma-amplified gene product as a component of the syntaxin 18 complex implicated in Golgi-to-endoplasmic reticulum retrograde transport. Mol Biol Cell. 2009;20:2639–49.

18. Longman D, Hug N, Keith M, Anastasaki C, Patton EE, Grimes G, et al. *DHX34* and *NBAS* form part of an autoregulatory NMD circuit that regulates endogenous RNA targets in human cells, zebrafish and *Caenorhabditis elegans*. Nucleic Acids Res. 2013;41:8319–31.

19. Kortum F, Marquardt I, Alawi M, et al. Acute liver failure meets SOPH syndrome: a case report on an intermediate phenotype. Pediatrics. 2017;139:1.

20. Choi SH, Ginsberg HN. Increased very low density lipoprotein (VLDL) secretion, hepatic steatosis, and insulin resistance. Trends Endocrinol Metab. 2011;22:353–63.

21. Kammoun HL, Chabanon H, Hainault I, Luquet S, Magnan C, Koike T, et al. GRP78 expression inhibits insulin and ER stress-induced SREBP-1c activation and reduces hepatic steatosis in mice. J Clin Invest. 2009;119:1201–15.

22. Zhang X. Role of endoplasmic reticulum stress in the pathogenesis of nonalcoholic fatty liver disease. World J Gastroenterol. 2014;20:1768–76.

23. Dara L, Ji C, Kaplowitz N. The contribution of endoplasmic reticulum stress to liver diseases. Hepatology. 2011;53:1752–63.

miR-363-5p as potential prognostic marker for hepatocellular carcinoma indicated by weighted co-expression network analysis of miRNAs and mRNA

Jun Zhang[*], Jia Fan, Chongming Zhou and Yanyu Qi

Abstract

Background: This study aimed to investigate potential miRNAs and genes associated with the prognosis of hepatocellular carcinoma (HCC).

Methods: Weighted co-expression network analysis was utilized to analyze the mRNA and miRNA sequencing data of HCC from TCGA (The Cancer Genome Atlas) database. Significant network modules were identified, and then functions of genes in the gene network modules and target genes of miRNAs in the miRNA network modules were explored. Additionally, correlations between network modules and prognostic factors of HCC were analyzed.

Results: In total, 10 mRNA network modules were identified, three of which were significantly related to tumor stage, NAFLD (non-alcoholic fatty liver disease) and patient age. Four miRNA network modules were identified, of which one was associated with tumor stage. Targets of hsa-miR-363-5p were found distributed in the gene network modules, such as RGPD5, RGPD6, ZNF445 and ZNF780B. Kaplan–Meier test revealed that low expression of hsa-miR-363-5p was associated with better overall survival of HCC patients.

Conclusion: hsa-miR-363-5p may be a potential prognostic marker for HCC.

Keywords: Hepatocellular carcinoma, microRNA, Weighted co-expression network analysis, Prognosis

Background

Hepatocellular carcinoma (HCC) is the most common primary liver malignancy with increasing incidence worldwide, which is mainly associated with chronic hepatitis B virus (HBV) and/or hepatitis C virus (HCV) infections, as well as alcohol consumption [1, 2]. There are few effective treatments for advanced HCC partly because the cell- and molecular-based mechanisms that contribute to the pathogenesis of this tumor type remain unclear.

Aberrant expression of microRNA (miRNA) has been detected in a variety of human malignancies and proved to be important influencing factors in cancer-associated genomic regions. Recently, remarkable studies have revealed the vital roles of miRNA in HCC pathogenesis.

Several miRNAs are upregulated in HCC tissues compared to that in normal tissues, such as miR-21, miR-122, and miR-223 [3, 4], whereas some miRNAs were downregulated, such as miR-122a, miR-22 and miR-152 [5–7]. A series of miRNAs have been identified as tumor suppressors in HCC. For instance, the putative tumor suppressor miR-124 regulates cell aggressiveness of HCC by targeting ROCK2 and EZH2 [8]. miRNA-26a suppresses tumor growth and metastasis of HCC by modulating the interleukin-6-Stat3 pathway [9]. Overexpression of miR-101 blocks epithelial-mesenchymal transition and angiogenesis of HCC via decreasing multiple genes (e.g. COX2, EZH2 and STMN1) [10]. Furthermore, there are some studies identified the associations between several miRNAs and clinical outcomes of HCC patients. For instance, the high level of miR-425-3p is associated with time to progression and progression free survival [11]. Upregulation of miR-494 contributes to

* Correspondence: zhangzhzhzh@hotmail.com
Department of Oncology, The third people's hospital of Chengdu, Chengdu 610031, China

the lower survival rate of HCC patients [12]. However, there are still numerous of miRNAs and their targets that are associated with HCC prognosis remain to be identified.

Weighted gene co-expression network analysis (WGCNA) was used to explore the biological functions of genes based on RNA sequencing or microarray data in different samples [13]. In this study, in order to identify the potential key miRNAs and genes associated with the prognosis of HCC, weighted co-expression network analysis was performed on the mRNA and miRNA. The results may provide novel information for the study of HCC prognosis, and provide novel potential biomarkers for the clinical therapy of HCC.

Methods

Sequencing and clinical data

The clinical data of 377 patients with HCC were extracted from The Cancer Genome Atlas (TCGA, http://cancer genome.nih.gov/). Among the 377 patients, mRNA sequencing data for 371 patients and miRNA sequencing data for 372 patients of level 3 were available. Both mRNA and miRNA sequencing data were generated using the Illumina HiSeq platform..

Data preprocessing

First, mRNAs and miRNAs with verbose <3 were removed using the goodSamplesGenes function in Weighted Gene Co-expression Network Analysis (WGCNA) (Version 1.43–10) package of R (Version 3.1.0) [14]. Meanwhile, abnormally low expressed mRNAs and miRNAs with RPKM (reads per kilobase of exon per million reads mapped) < 10 or deviation of average linkage distance and the main cluster >40% were removed, via an average linkage method. Subsequently, Pearson correlation coefficient between all of genes as well as miRNAs was calculated using the multiple testing, and the false positive rate < 5% was controlled by q-value [15].

Weighted Gene co-expression network analysis (WGCNA)

Euclidean distance and Pearson's correlation matrices were used to calculate the correlation between gene pairs and miRNA pairs, and the correlation between gene i and gene j (or miRNA i and miRNA j) was defined as $s_{i,j} = |cor (\mu_i, \mu_j)|$., where μi and μj represent expression value vector of i and j, respectively, and cor represents the Pearson correlation coefficient between the two expression value vectors. The calculated Pearson's correlation matrices were transformed into matrices of connection strengths using a power function $a_{i,j} = s_{i,j}^{\beta}$. The β value is set as weighting coefficient only when the correlation coefficient between log(k) and log(p(k)) reaches 0.8, where p(k) represents the proportion of nodes with connectivity k. After the adjacency

parameter was determined, the correlation matrix was transformed into an adjacency matrix, which was subsequently transformed into a topological overlap matrix. The topological overlap matrix (TOM) [16] was computed as follow:

$$\varpi_{ij} = \frac{1_{ij} + \alpha_{ij}}{k_i, k_j + 1 - \alpha_{ij}},$$

where $1_{ij} = \Sigma_\mu \alpha_{i\mu} \alpha_{j\mu}$ indicates the product sums of the adjacency coefficients of the nodes connected to both i and j. $k_\cup = \Sigma_\mu \alpha_{\cup\mu}$ indicates the sum of the adjacency coefficients of the nodes only connected to i. Similarly, $k_j = \Sigma_\mu \alpha_{j\mu}$ indicates the sum of the adjacency coefficient of the nodes only connected to j. If two nodes are neither connected each other nor share any neighbors, $\varpi_{ij} = 0$. The formula $d_{ij}^\varpi = 1 - \varpi_{ij}$ was used to calculate the dissimilarity degree between any two nodes.

Identification of significant network modules

Genes were performed hierarchical clustering using the dissimilarity coefficient as the distance measure. Each branch corresponds to a module. Modules were identified by using a mixed dynamic TreeCut (Version 1.62) algorithm criterion [17]. The eigengenes in each module, which is stipulated as the first principal component of a given module and can be considered as a representative gene expression profile in a module, was calculated in turn when modules cannot be identified with the dynamic TreeCut algorithm criterion, then the merged close modules were clustered into new modules. The network significance approach determined the module related to prognostic factors based on module significance (MS). The MS indicated the average gene significance (GS) of all the genes in the module. Significant miRNA network modules were identified using the same methods as gene network module identification.

Analysis of correlations between network modules and prognostic factors

Correlations between mRNA/miRNA network modules and seven prognostic factors of HCC [(gender, age, tumor stage, alcohol consumption, hepatitis B virus (HBV), hepatitis C virus (HCV) and non-alcoholic fatty liver disease (NAFLD)] were analyzed by calculating the Pearson correlation coefficient [18], and $p < 0.01$ was set as the cut-off criterion.

Functional enrichment analysis of genes and miRNAs

Gene Ontology (GO) functional enrichment analysis of genes in the modules was conducted based on the Database for Annotation, Visualization and Integrated Discovery (DAVID, https://david.ncifcrf.gov/) [19, 20]. The p-value of each GO term was calculated by Fisher's

Exact Test [21], and only terms with *p*-value <0.05 were considered significant.

Furthermore, before GO enrichment analysis of miRNA targets, target genes of miRNAs in the modules were predicted based on the information in TargetScan (http://www.targetscan.org/), miRanda (http://www.microrna.org/microrna/home.do), and miRwalk (http://zmf.umm.uni-heidelberg.de/apps/zmf/mirwalk2/). Only the miRNA-gene pairs that were common in the three databases and met with false discovery rate (FDR) < 0.05 were chosen for further analysis. Afterwards, the target genes of miRNAs were underwent GO enrichment analysis, and only terms with *p*-value <0.05 were considered significant.

Results

Data preprocessing

For the mRNA sequencing data, after data preprocessing, 362 mRNAs were removed due to low expression or data missing, and a total of 20,169 mRNAs were remained for further analysis. Subsequently, hierarchically clustering of mRNA expression data for the 371 patients was carried out (Fig. 1a). Deviation between data of some patient samples and the main cluster was more than 40%, thus, 3.5E + 6 was set as the cut-off criteria. Finally, data of 22 patient samples were removed due to deviation >40% or RPKM <10, thus, mRNA data of 349 patients remained for further analysis.

For the miRNA sequencing data, 854 miRNAs remained after data preprocessing. The hierarchically clustering of miRNA expression data for the 372 patients showed that deviation between data of some patient samples and the main cluster was more than 40%, thus, 2.25E + 5 was set as the cut-off threshold (Fig. 1b). Finally, a total of 320 patient sample data remained for further analysis.

mRNA expression module analysis of WGCNA

In total, 10 mRNA network modules were identified using WGCNA. Because module identification does not make use of prior biological knowledge about the mRNA, the biological meaning of each module is initially unknown and hence the modules were assigned a

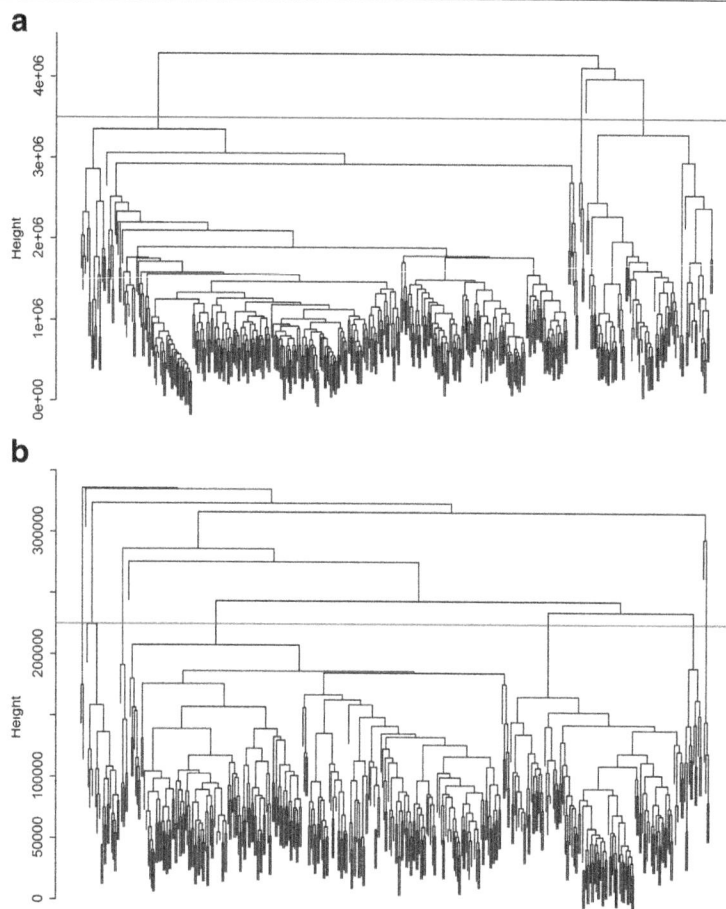

Fig. 1 The cluster dendrogram of co-expression network modules for mRNAs (**a**) and miRNAs (**b**). The *red line* represents the cut-off of data filtering in the step of data preprocessing

color label (plum, antique white, coral, ivory, light cyan, medium purple, brown, dark magenta, pale violet and dark grey). (Fig. 2a).

To reveal the functions of the mRNAs in each of the modules, GO enrichment analysis was performed. According to the results, the mRNAs in the dark magenta module ($n = 8695$) were enriched for mRNA that coded for proteins involved in alternative splicing; in the dark grey module ($n = 6199$), they were involved with sensory transduction; in the coral module ($n = 1488$), they were involved with oxidoreductase (Table 1).

Correlations between gene network modules and clinical prognostic data were analyzed. Module dark magenta was found to be significantly correlated with tumor stage of HCC ($r = 0.2$, $p = 4e-5$); module antique white was related to NAFLD ($r = 0.18$, $p = 2e-4$); and module coral was associated with age ($r = 0.13$, $p = 0.008$) (Fig. 2b).

Additionally, GO enrichment analysis of the three gene modules that correlated with prognosis of

HCC was conducted. The results showed that module dark magenta was significantly related to several functions like alternative splicing and transcription (Table 2).

Weighted Gene co-expression network analysis (WGCNA) of miRNA

According to the module analysis of miRNA co-expression networks, four miRNA network modules were identified, and assigned the color labels brown, blue, turquoise and grey. The correlation analysis of modules and clinical prognostic data revealed that module blue was markedly associated with tumor stage of HCC ($r = 0.22$, $p = 2e-5$) (Fig. 3).

As the most significant module related to tumor stage, 111 miRNAs contained in the module blue were chosen for target genes. A total of 530 target genes were screened out based on the information in TargetScan, miRanda, and miRwalk. These target genes were

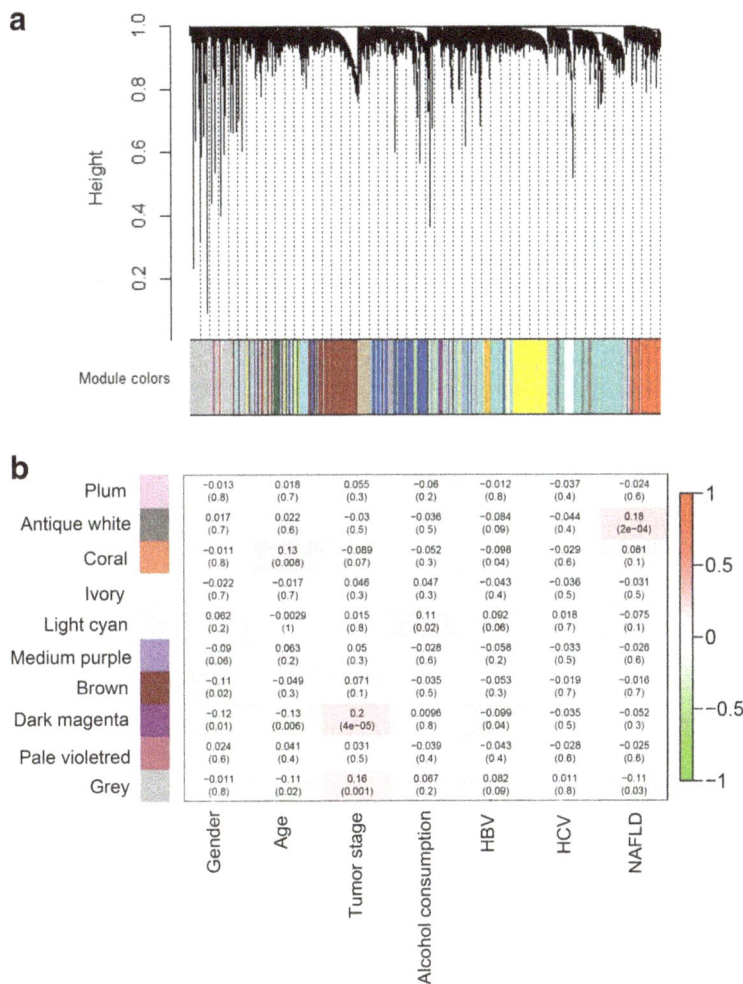

Fig. 2 The color display of co-expression network modules for mRNAs (**a**) and the correlation of mRNA co-expression network modules with clinical prognostic factors of hepatocellular carcinoma (**b**). HBV, hepatitis B virus; HCV, hepatitis C virus; NAFLD, non-alcoholic fatty liver disease

Table 1 Gene Ontology enrichment analysis of genes in the ten network modules

Module	Gene number	Functional Ontology (top)	p value	Discription
Plum	52	keratinization	1.50E-25	Protein involved in keratinization, the process in which the cytoplasm of the outermost cells of the vertebrate epidermis is replaced by keratin. Keratinization occurs in the stratum corneum, feathers, hair, claws, nails, hooves, and horns.
Antique white	122	erythrocyte	1.20E-09	Protein involved in the maturation of erythrocytes, the predominant type of cells present in vertebrate blood and which contain the gas-transporting protein, hemoglobin.
Coral	1488	oxidoreductase	4.20E-49	Enzyme that catalyzes the oxidation of one compound with the reduction of another.
Ivory	124	Secreted	6.20E-11	Protein secreted into the cell surroundings.
Light cyan	3299	acetylation	4.90E-92	Protein which is posttranslationally modified by the attachment of at least one acetyl group; generally at the N-terminus.
Medium purple	35	cell membrane	6.20E-03	Protein found in or associated with the cytoplasmic membrane, a selectively permeable membrane which separates the cytoplasm from its surroundings. Known as the cell inner membrane in prokaryotes with 2 membranes.
Brown	99	glycoprotein	3.90E-04	Protein containing one or more covalently linked carbohydrates of various types, i.e. from monosaccharides to branched polysaccharides, including glycosylphosphatidylinositol (GPI), glycosaminoglycans (GAG).
Dark magenta	8695	alternative splicing	3.20E-39	Protein for which at least two isoforms exist due to distinct pre-mRNA splicing events.
Pale violetred	46	chromosomal protein	1.00E-08	Protein which is associated with chromosomal DNA, including histones, protamines and high mobility group proteins.
Grey	6199	sensory transduction	3.40E-13	Protein involved in sensory transduction, the process by which a cell converts an extracellular signal, such as light, taste, sound, touch or smell, into electric signals.

significantly related to GO functions like alternative splicing, phosphotransferase and immune response (Table 3).

Associations of miRNA target genes and gene network modules

To investigate whether miRNA targets in module blue were genes in the gene network modules, distribution of miRNA targets in the 10 gene network modules was analyzed. More than 200 miRNA targets were distributed in the gene module dark magenta (Fig. 4). Among them, the number of target genes of hsa-miR-363-5p in module dark magenta reached 22, including APOBEC3F, ASB16, GAPVD1, IL6R, MRPL44, MTFMT, MYEF2, PPM1D, RASSF2, RELL1, RGPD5, RGPD6, RHOF, RRP15, SHOX, SLC9A7, SPC24, ST8SIA4, WHSC1, ZNF445, ZNF780B, and ZYG11A.

Table 2 Top 5 Gene Ontology functional terms of genes in module dark magenta associated with the clinical prognostic data

Genes numbers	Functional Ontology (top5)	p value	Discription
3576	alternative splicing	3.5E-39	Protein for which at least two isoforms exist due to distinct pre-mRNA splicing events.
1038	dna-binding	7.6E-36	Protein which binds to DNA, typically to pack or modify the DNA, or to regulate gene expression.
1091	transcription regulation	2.2E-30	Protein involved in the regulation of the transcription process.
1107	Transcription	3.3E-29	Protein involved in the transfer of genetic information from DNA to messenger RNA (mRNA) by DNA-directed RNA polymerase
2102	nucleus	3.8E-27	Protein located in the nucleus of a cell.

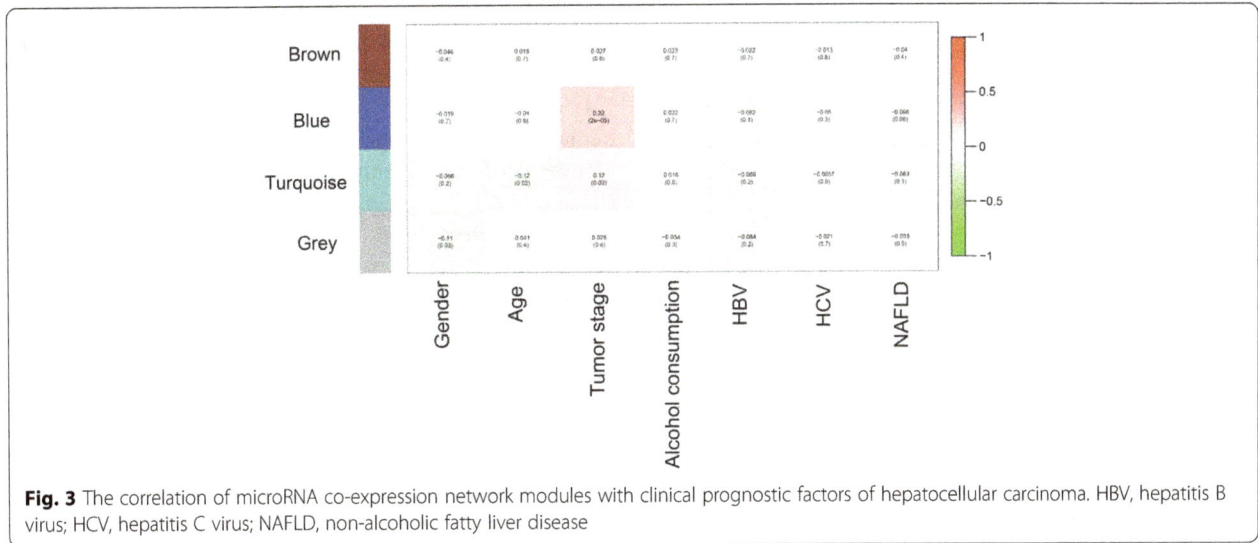

Fig. 3 The correlation of microRNA co-expression network modules with clinical prognostic factors of hepatocellular carcinoma. HBV, hepatitis B virus; HCV, hepatitis C virus; NAFLD, non-alcoholic fatty liver disease

Correlation of hsa-miR-363-5p and prognosis of HCC

To further reveal the correlation of hsa-miR-363-5p and prognosis of HCC, survival curve was analyzed by Kaplan–Meier test. The median value of hsa-miR-363-5p expression (RPKM = 4.61) was set as the cut-off criteria for high- and low-expression groups of HCC patient samples in TCGA. The 5-year survival curve proved the survival difference between the high- and low-expression groups started at 2 years after surgery, and the difference reached 51.4% 5 years (p = 0.012) (Fig. 5) after surgery. The results indicated that hsa-miR-363-5p expression was closely related to the prognosis of HCC.

Discussion

In the present study, 10 mRNA network modules were identified based on the WGCNA of sequencing data of HCC samples, of which three modules were significantly related to tumor stage, NAFLD and patient age. Meanwhile, four miRNA network modules were identified, of which one module was associated with tumor stage of HCC. Target genes of the miRNAs in this miRNA network module were markedly related to alternative splicing.

Alternative splicing is one of the most significant components of the functional complexity of the human genome, and various splicing alterations have been involved

Table 3 The results of Gene Ontology enrichment analysis of target genes of microRNAs in module blue

Function ontology	p value	Description
Alternative splicing	2.90E-05	Protein for which at least two isoforms exist due to distinct pre-mRNA splicing events.
Phosphotransferase	3.90E-03	Protein involved in the phosphotransferase system, the major carbohydrate transport system in bacteria. This phosphotransferase system catalyzes the transfer of the phosphoryl group from phosphoenolpyruvate to incoming sugar substrates concomitant with their translocation across the cell membrane.
Coiled coil	5.30E-03	Protein which contains at least one coiled coil domain, a type of secondary structure composed of two or more alpha helices which entwine to form a cable structure. In proteins, the helical cables serve a mechanical role in forming stiff bundles of fibres.
Immune response	9.00E-03	Protein involved in immunity, any immune system process that functions in the response of an organism to a potential internal or invasive threat. The vertebrate immune system is formed by the innate immune system (composed of phagocytes, complement, antimicrobial peptides, etc) and by the adaptive immune system which consists of T- and B-lymphocytes.
Transferase	1.40E-02	Enzyme that transfers a chemical group, e.g. a methyl group or a glycosyl group from one compound (donor) to another compound (acceptor).

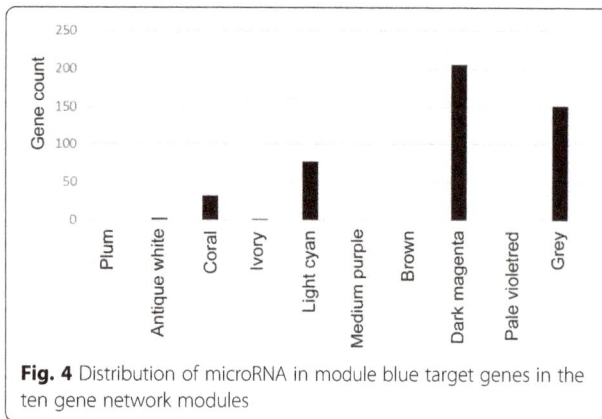

Fig. 4 Distribution of microRNA in module blue target genes in the ten gene network modules

in different steps and aspects of cancer initiation and progression [22]. In HCC, alternative splicing of multiple molecules have been detected. For instance, two alternative splicing isoforms of the cell fate determinant Numb, PRR^L and PRR^S, correlated with the prognosis of patients with HCC [23]. Alternative splicing of A-Raf is regulated by the upregulation of hnRNP A2 in HCC, which activates the Ras-MAPK-ERK pathway [24]. Another study reported that the splicing regulator SLU7 is an essential factor for the preservation of HCC cell viability via oncogenic miR-17-92 cluster expression [25]. Therefore, alternative splicing of some genes plays a critical role in the progression and prognosis of HCC.

Furthermore, a set of target genes of miRNAs were the genes in the gene network modules. Among them, 22 targets of hsa-miR-363-5p were distributed in the gene network modules, such as RGPD5, RGPD6, ZNF445, and ZNF780B. Kaplan–Meier test revealed that

low expression of hsa-miR-363-5p was closely related to better overall survival of HCC patients. miR-363-5p belongs to the miR-363 family, and it modulates endothelial cell properties and their communication with hematopoietic precursor cells [25]. Inhibition of miR-363-5p affect angiogenic properties (e.g. the response to stimulation by angiogenic factors) of endothelial cells and the interaction between endothelial cells and hematopoietic precursors [26]. miR-363-5p has been previously predicted to be down-regulated in HCC tumor endothelial cells compared to normal hepatic sinusoidal endothelial cells [27]. Besides, miR-363-5p also exhibits decreased expression in other tumors, such as human oral squamous carcinoma and triple-negative breast cancer [28, 29]. These studies indicated that miR-363-5p is usually downregulated in cancer. However, low expression of hsa-miR-363-5p was found to be closely associated with the better overall survival of HCC patients. There is no report about the association of miR-363-5p with survival of HCC patients to date. We speculate that low expression of miR-363-5p might has effect on angiogenic properties and interactions with hematopoietic precursors, and thus inhibits the angiogenesis in HCC, weakens the invasion ability of tumor and results in a better overall survival of patients. However, this inference is required to be further validated by experiments, which will be conducted in our future study.

A set of genes, such as RGPD5, RGPD6, ZNF445, and ZNF780B were predicted to be regulated by miR-363-5p in this study. Both RGPD5 and RGPD6 share a high degree of sequence identity with RANBP2, a large RAN-binding protein [30]. Currently, there are limited studies

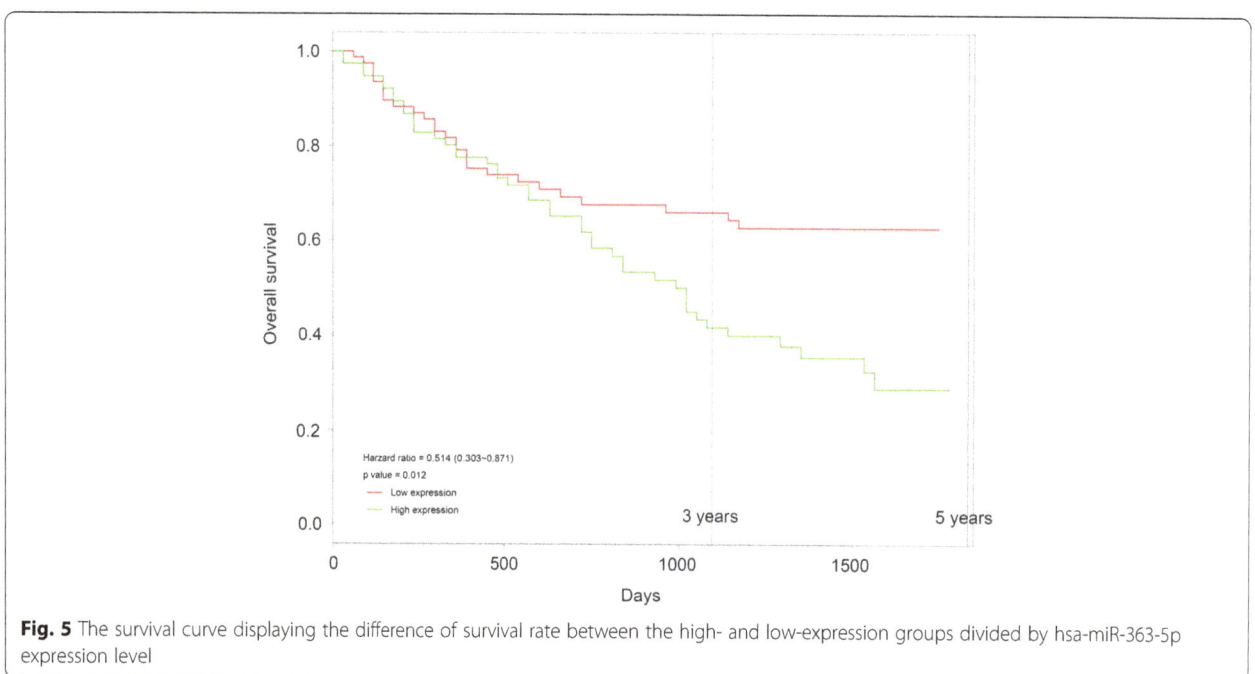

Fig. 5 The survival curve displaying the difference of survival rate between the high- and low-expression groups divided by hsa-miR-363-5p expression level

miR-363-5p as potential prognostic marker for hepatocellular carcinoma indicated by weighted...

77

about the relations between RGPD5/ RGPD6 and cancer. Both ZNF445 (also known as ZNF168) and ZNF780B (also known as ZNF779) encode zinc finger proteins that may be associated with transcriptional regulation [31]. No evidence is now available to show their connection with HCC. However, a previous study has demonstrated that another member of the ZNF family, ZNF165 mRNA and its protein are expressed in HCC, indicating that ZNF family may be involved in tumor biology of HCC [32]. Besides, a recent study has found that zinc finger protein ZBTB20 promotes tumor growth of HCC via transcriptionally repressing FoxO1 [33]. In our further study, we will confirm the regulatory relationships between miR-363-5p and its target genes (e.g. RGPD5, RGPD6, ZNF445 and ZNF780B), and the associations of these genes with HCC.

Conclusion

In conclusion, we found that several gene networks and one miRNA network might be important clinical prognostic factors (e.g. tumor stage, NAFLD or age) for HCC based on the WGCNA of sequencing data. Low expression of hsa-miR-363-5p was closely related to the better overall survival of HCC, and it may be a potential prognostic marker for HCC.

Abbreviations

DAVID: the Database for Annotation, Visualization and Integrated Discovery; FDR: False discovery rate; GO: Gene Ontology; GS: Gene significance; HBV: Chronic hepatitis B virus; HCC: Hepatocellular carcinoma; HCV: Hepatitis C virus; miRNA: microRNA; MS: Module significance; NAFLD: Non-alcoholic fatty liver disease; RPKM: Reads per kilobase of exon per million reads mapped; TCGA: The Cancer Genome Atlas, TOM: Topological overlap matrix; WGCNA: Weighted gene co-expression network analysis

Acknowledgements
None.

Funding
None.

Authors' contributions
JZ and JF participated in the design of this study, and they both performed the statistical analysis. CMZ and JZ carried out the study and collected important background information. YYQ collected the dataset, drafted the manuscript and provided some important intellectual content. All authors read and approved the final manuscript.

Competing interests
The authors declare that they have no competing interests.

Consent for publication
Not applicable.

References

1. Arzumanyan A, Reis HM, Feitelson MA. Pathogenic mechanisms in HBV-and HCV-associated hepatocellular carcinoma. Nat Rev Cancer. 2013;13(2):123–35.
2. Morgan TR, Mandayam S, Jamal MM. Alcohol and hepatocellular carcinoma. Gastroenterology. 2004;127(5):S87–96.
3. Xu J, Wu C, Che X, Wang L, Yu D, Zhang T, et al. Circulating MicroRNAs, miR-21, miR-122, and miR-223, in patients with hepatocellular carcinoma or chronic hepatitis. Mol Carcinog. 2011;50(2):136–42.
4. Tomimaru Y, Eguchi H, Nagano H, Wada H, Kobayashi S, Marubashi S, et al. Circulating microRNA-21 as a novel biomarker for hepatocellular carcinoma. J Hepatol. 2012;56(1):167–75.
5. Zhang J, Yang Y, Yang T, Liu Y, Li A, Fu S, et al. microRNA-22, downregulated in hepatocellular carcinoma and correlated with prognosis, suppresses cell proliferation and tumourigenicity. Br J Cancer. 2010;103(8):1215–20.
6. Huang J, Wang Y, Guo Y, Sun S. Down-regulated microRNA-152 induces aberrant DNA methylation in hepatitis B virus–related hepatocellular carcinoma by targeting DNA methyltransferase 1. Hepatology. 2010;52(1):60–70.
7. Gramantieri L, Ferracin M, Fornari F, Veronese A, Sabbioni S, Liu CG, et al. Cyclin G1 is a target of miR-122a, a microRNA frequently down-regulated in human hepatocellular carcinoma. Cancer Res. 2007;67(13):6092–9.
8. Zheng F, Liao Y-J, Cai M-Y, Liu Y-H, Liu T-H, Chen S-P, et al. The putative tumour suppressor microRNA-124 modulates hepatocellular carcinoma cell aggressiveness by repressing ROCK2 and EZH2. Gut. 2012;61(2):278–89.
9. Yang X, Liang L, Zhang XF, Jia HL, Qin Y, Zhu XC, et al. MicroRNA-26a suppresses tumor growth and metastasis of human hepatocellular carcinoma by targeting interleukin-6-Stat3 pathway. Hepatology. 2013;58(1):158–70.
10. Zheng F, Liao Y-J, Cai M-Y, Liu T-H, Chen S-P, Wu P-H, et al. Systemic delivery of microRNA-101 potently inhibits hepatocellular carcinoma in vivo by repressing multiple targets. PLoS Genet. 2015;11(2):e1004873.
11. Vaira V, Roncalli M, Carnaghi C, Faversani A, Maggioni M, Augello C, et al. MicroRNA-425-3p predicts response to sorafenib therapy in patients with hepatocellular carcinoma. Liver Int. 2015;35(3):1077–86.
12. Chuang KH, Whitney-Miller CL, Chu CY, Zhou Z, Dokus MK, Schmit S, et al. MicroRNA-494 is a master epigenetic regulator of multiple invasion-suppressor microRNAs by targeting ten eleven translocation 1 in invasive human hepatocellular carcinoma tumors. Hepatology. 2015;62(2):466–80.
13. Zhang B, Horvath S. A general framework for weighted gene co-expression network analysis. Stat Appl Genet Mol Biol. 2005;4(1):1128.
14. Langfelder P, Horvath S. WGCNA: an R package for weighted correlation network analysis. BMC Bioinformatics. 2008;9(1):559.
15. Storey JD, Tibshirani R. Statistical significance for genomewide studies. Proc Natl Acad Sci U S A. 2003;100(16):9440–5. doi:10.1073/pnas.1530509100.
16. Yip AM, Horvath S. Gene network interconnectedness and the generalized topological overlap measure. BMC Bioinformatics. 2007;8:22. doi:1471-2105-8-22 [pii] 1186/1471-2105-8-22
17. Langfelder P, Zhang B, Horvath S. Defining clusters from a hierarchical cluster tree: the dynamic tree cut package for R. Bioinformatics. 2008;24(5):719–20.
18. Sedgwick P. Pearson's correlation coefficient. BMJ. 2012;345:e4483.
19. Huang DW, Sherman BT, Lempicki RA. Systematic and integrative analysis of large gene lists using DAVID bioinformatics resources. Nat Protocols. 2008; 4(1):44–57. http://www.nature.com/nprot/journal/v4/n1/suppinfo/nprot. 2008.211_S1.html.
20. Huang DW, Sherman BT, Lempicki RA. Bioinformatics enrichment tools: paths toward the comprehensive functional analysis of large gene lists. Nucleic Acids Res. 2009;37(1):1–13. doi:10.1093/nar/gkn923.
21. Routledge R. Fisher's exact test. Encycl Biostat. 2005.
22. Kroll J, Fonseca A, de Souza S. Alternative splicing and cancer. In: Post-genomic Approaches in Cancer and Nano Medicine, vol. 4; 2015. p. 1.
23. Lu Y, Xu W, Ji J, Feng D, Sourbier C, Yang Y, et al. Alternative splicing of the cell fate determinant numb in hepatocellular carcinoma. Hepatology. 2015; 62(4):1122–31.
24. Shilo A, Hur VB, Denichenko P, Stein I, Pikarsky E, Rauch J, et al. Splicing factor hnRNP A2 activates the Ras-MAPK-ERK pathway by controlling a-Raf splicing in hepatocellular carcinoma development. RNA. 2014;20(4):505–15.
25. Urtasun R, Elizalde M, Azkona M, Latasa M, García-Irigoyen O, Uriarte I, et al. Splicing regulator SLU7 preserves survival of hepatocellular carcinoma cells and other solid tumors via oncogenic miR-17-92 cluster expression. Oncogene. 2016.

26. Costa A, Afonso J, Osório C, Gomes AL, Caiado F, Valente J, et al. miR-363-5p regulates endothelial cell properties and their communication with hematopoietic precursor cells. J Hematol Oncol. 2013;6:87.

27. Z-h C, Shen S-Q, Chen Z-b HC. Growth inhibition of hepatocellular carcinoma tumor endothelial cells by miR-204-3p and underlying mechanism. World J Gastroenterol. 2014;20(18):5493–504.

28. Khuu C, Jevnaker AM, Bryne M, Osmundsen H. An investigation into anti-proliferative effects of microRNAs encoded by the miR-106a-363 cluster on human carcinoma cells and keratinocytes using microarray profiling of miRNA transcriptomes. Front Gen. 2014;5:246.

29. Yang F, Zhang W, Shen Y, Guan X. Identification of dysregulated microRNAs in triple-negative breast cancer (review). Int J Oncol. 2015;46(3):927–32.

30. Neilson DE, Adams MD, Orr CM, Schelling DK, Eiben RM, Kerr DS, et al. Infection-triggered familial or recurrent cases of acute necrotizing encephalopathy caused by mutations in a component of the nuclear pore, RANBP2. Am J Hum Genet. 2009;84(1):44–51.

31. Calabrò V, Pengue G, Bartoli PC, Pagliuca A, Featherstone T, Lania L. Positional cloning of cDNAs from the human chromosome 3p21–22 region identifies a clustered organization of zinc-finger genes. Hum Genet. 1995; 95(1):18–21.

32. Dong X, Yang X, Wang Y, Chen W. Zinc-finger protein ZNF165 is a novel cancer-testis antigen capable of eliciting antibody response in hepatocellular carcinoma patients. Br J Cancer. 2004;91(8):1566–70.

33. Kan H, Huang Y, Li X, Liu D, Chen J, Shu M. Zinc finger protein ZBTB20 is an independent prognostic marker and promotes tumor growth of human hepatocellular carcinoma by repressing FoxO1. Oncotarget. 2016.

11

Efficacy of glutathione for the treatment of nonalcoholic fatty liver disease

Yasushi Honda[1†], Takaomi Kessoku[1†], Yoshio Sumida[2], Takashi Kobayashi[1], Takayuki Kato[1], Yuji Ogawa[1], Wataru Tomeno[1], Kento Imajo[1], Koji Fujita[1], Masato Yoneda[1], Koshi Kataoka[3], Masataka Taguri[3], Takeharu Yamanaka[3], Yuya Seko[4], Saiyu Tanaka[5], Satoru Saito[1], Masafumi Ono[6], Satoshi Oeda[7], Yuichiro Eguchi[7], Wataru Aoi[8], Kenji Sato[9], Yoshito Itoh[4] and Atsushi Nakajima[1*]

Abstract

Background: Glutathione plays crucial roles in the detoxification and antioxidant systems of cells and has been used to treat acute poisoning and chronic liver diseases by intravenous injection. This is a first study examining the therapeutic effects of oral administration of glutathione in patients with nonalcoholic fatty liver disease (NAFLD).

Methods: The study was an open label, single arm, multicenter, pilot trial. Thirty-four NAFLD patients diagnosed using ultrasonography were prospectively evaluated. All patients first underwent intervention to improve their lifestyle habits (diet and exercise) for 3 months, followed by treatment with glutathione (300 mg/day) for 4 months. We evaluated their clinical parameters before and after glutathione treatment. We also quantified liver fat and fibrosis using vibration-controlled transient elastography. The primary outcome of the study was the change in alanine aminotransferase (ALT) levels.

Results: Twenty-nine patients finished the protocol. ALT levels significantly decreased following treatment with glutathione for 4 months. In addition, triglycerides, non-esterified fatty acids, and ferritin levels also decreased with glutathione treatment. Following dichotomization of ALT responders based on a median 12.9% decrease from baseline, we found that ALT responders were younger in age and did not have severe diabetes compared with ALT non-responders. The controlled attenuation parameter also decreased in ALT responders.

Conclusions: This pilot study demonstrates the potential therapeutic effects of oral administration of glutathione in practical dose for patients with NAFLD. Large-scale clinical trials are needed to verify its efficacy.

Keywords: Nonalcoholic fatty liver disease, Glutathione, Controlled attenuation parameter

* Correspondence: nakajima-tky@umin.ac.jp
†Equal contributors
[1]Department of Gastroenterology and Hepatology, Yokohama City University Graduate School of Medicine, Yokohama, Japan
Full list of author information is available at the end of the article

Background

Nonalcoholic fatty liver disease (NAFLD) is an important cause of chronic liver injury worldwide [1, 2]. The spectrum of NAFLD ranges from nonalcoholic fatty liver to nonalcoholic steatohepatitis (NASH), cirrhosis, and hepatocellular carcinoma [3]. NAFLD is associated with metabolic syndromes and the incidence of NAFLD has increased over time [4, 5]. First-line treatment for NAFLD is lifestyle modification to achieve weight reduction, particularly through diet and exercise [6]. However, weight reduction is very difficult to accomplish and maintain. Effective therapy for NAFLD has not yet been established.

Glutathione, γ-L-glutamyl-L-cysteinyl-glycine, is a tripeptide present in every cell of the human body [7]. Although its functions are complex and remain the subject of current research, glutathione is thought to play crucial roles in the detoxification and antioxidant systems in cells. Because a reduction of glutathione levels in cells has been found to increase the risks for diseases and poisoning, direct intravenous injection of glutathione has been used to treat patients with chronic liver diseases and poisoning [8, 9].

Glutathione is synthesized in cells from glutamic acid, cysteine, and glycine. Cysteine and glycine are generated from methionine and serine, respectively, and glutamic acid is synthesized from α-ketoglutarate, a metabolite of glucose. These amino acids are generally supplied from food. It has been reported that oral administration of glutathione did not change the levels of glutathione and glutathione disulfide in the deproteinized fraction of blood [10], and it has been suggested that orally administered glutathione is degraded into constituting amino acids and does not exert specific activity beyond the amino acid source. However, it has been reported that glutathione can pass through the mono layer of Caco-2 cells without degradation [11]. In addition, Park et al. reported an increase in the protein-bound form of glutathione in human blood after oral administration, while glutathione in the deproteinized fraction did not change [12]. These studies suggest that orally administered glutathione is absorbed into the blood and might have effects on the redox status in the human body. Such findings have encouraged us to examine the therapeutic effects of oral administration of glutathione on NAFLD.

The objective of the current study was to demonstrate the therapeutic potential of oral administration of glutathione in an open-label, single-arm, multicenter, pilot study prior to subsequent large-scale clinical trials. In this study, we compared clinical parameters before and after treatment with glutathione. We also evaluated controlled attenuation parameter (CAP) and liver stiffness measurement (LSM), as determined by vibration-controlled transient elastography (VCTE).

Methods

Patients and study design

The study protocol was conducted in accordance with the guidelines contained within the Declaration of Helsinki and was approved by the ethics committees of Yokohama City University and Kyoto Prefectural University of Medicine. Written informed consent was obtained from all participants before entry into the study. The trial is registered with the University Hospital Medical Information Network (UMIN) Clinical Trials Registry (UMIN000011118).

Patient enrollment began in January 2014 and ended when the target sample size was reached in September 2014. Follow-up of participants ended in December 2014. We prospectively evaluated 34 NAFLD patients with liver dysfunction. NAFLD was diagnosed based on ultrasonography. All 34 patients provided a detailed medical history and underwent a physical examination. Patients were excluded if they had infectious hepatitis (hepatitis B or C or Epstein–Barr virus infection), autoimmune hepatitis, primary biliary cirrhosis, sclerosing cholangitis, hemochromatosis, α1-antitrypsin deficiency, Wilson's disease, drug-induced hepatitis, alcoholic hepatitis, or excessive alcohol consumption (present or past consumption of >20 g alcohol/day). No NAFLD patient had clinical evidence of hepatic decompensation, such as hepatic encephalopathy, ascites, variceal bleeding, or a serum bilirubin level greater than twice the upper limit of normal. All patients were started on a standard diet (30 kcal/kg/day, consisting of 50–60% carbohydrate, 20–30% fat, and 15–20% protein) and received exercise counseling beginning 3 months before glutathione treatment. Exercise consisted of 5–6 metabolic equivalents for 30 min daily. Patients taking medication for lifestyle-related comorbid diseases, such as hypertension, dyslipidemia, and diabetes, were included; however, no change in medication or dose was allowed.

Because serum alanine aminotransferase (ALT) levels have been reported to predict the histological course of NASH and because strict control of ALT is required to prevent the progression of NASH [13], the primary outcome of this study was a change in ALT levels.

Anthropometric and laboratory evaluations

Patient weight and height were measured using a calibrated scale after patients removed their shoes and any heavy clothing. Venous blood samples were obtained after patients had fasted overnight (12 h). Platelet counts and concentrations of fasting blood sugar (FBS), hemoglobin A1c (HbA1c), immunoreactive insulin (IRI), high-density lipoprotein (HDL) cholesterol, low-density lipoprotein (LDL) cholesterol, triglycerides, non-esterified fatty acids (NEFA), aspartate aminotransferase (AST), ALT, γ-glutamyl transpeptidase, ferritin, and type

IV collagen 7 were measured using standard laboratory techniques before and after glutathione treatment. Patients with FBS ≥126 mg/dL, HbA1c ≥6.5%, and/or currently using antidiabetic medication were defined as having diabetes according to the criteria of the Japan Diabetes Society [14].

Glutathione in the deproteinized fraction and protein-bound fraction of plasma were determined using the method described by Park et al. [12]. Briefly, 100 μL of plasma was mixed with three parts ethanol. The supernatant was used as the deproteinized fraction. The precipitate was extracted using 100 μL of 5% trichloroacetic containing 2% 2-mercaptoethanol. The supernatant was used as the protein-bound fraction. Glutathione in these fractions were alkalized and derivatized with 6-aminoquinolyl-N hydroxy succinimidyl carbamate as described previously. The derivatives were resolved and detected using liquid chromatography/electron spray ionization/tandem mass spectrometry in multi-reaction monitoring mode.

Vibration-controlled transient elastography
VCTE was performed using an M-probe device (Fibroscan; EchoSens, Paris, France). Details of the technique and the examination procedure for LSM have been described previously [15, 16]. CAP was measured using VCTE to stage steatosis. The technique is a proprietary algorithm based on the ultrasonic attenuation coefficient of the shear wave of VCTE, an estimate of the total ultrasonic attenuation at 3.5 MHz. CAP uses the same radiofrequency data as LSM and is only appraised if the acquisition is valid. It is expressed in decibels per meter. Measurements were obtained from the right lobe of the liver through the intercostal spaces, with a patient lying in the dorsal decubitus position and the right arm in maximal abduction. Only VCTE measurements based on at least 10 valid shots and success rates ≥60% were considered reliable and were used for statistical analysis.

Statistical analysis
Data are expressed as mean ± standard deviation, unless indicated otherwise. The sample size was determined by reference to a previous report [17]. We estimated that with this sample size, the study would have 80% power to detect an absolute difference in the rate of improvement in ALT of 30 percentage points, with a two-sided type 1 error of 0.05. All statistical analyses were performed using JMP ver. 11.2.0 software (SAS Institute, Cary, NC, USA). Univariate comparisons between patient groups were analyzed using the Student's t-test or the Mann–Whitney's U-test, as appropriate. A p-value <0.05 was considered statistically significant.

Results
Biochemical response after 4 months of glutathione treatment
The study flowchart is shown in Fig. 1. Of the 34 patients enrolled, two withdrew before the start of treatment. The remaining 32 were treated with L-glutathione (300 mg/day; KOHJIN Life Sciences, Tokyo, Japan, US FDA GRAS #GRN000293) for 4 months by oral administration. Twenty-nine patients (14 men, 15 women, mean age 56.0 ± 13.3 years) finished the study protocol.

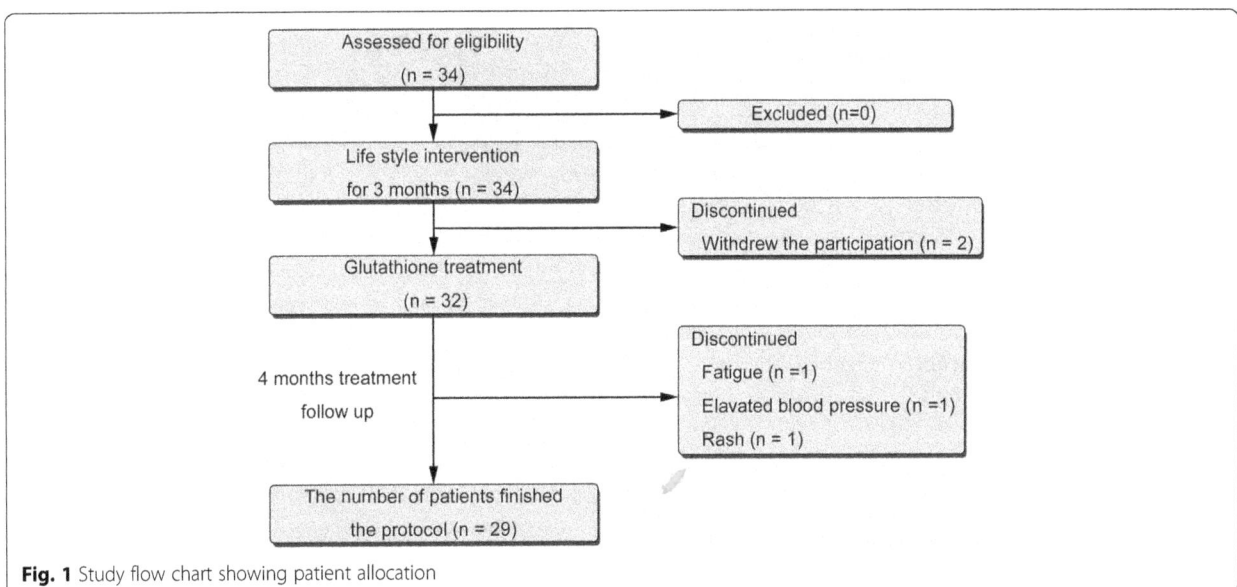

Fig. 1 Study flow chart showing patient allocation

Table 1 Characteristics of patients before and after glutathione treatment ($n = 29$)

	Before treatment	After treatment	P-value
Age (year)	56.0 ± 13.3		-
Male/female (n)	14/15		
Dyslipidemia (%)	24 (82.8)		-
Statin (%)	12 (41.4)		-
Diabetes (%)	14 (48.3)		-
BMI (kg/m^2)	26.5 ± 3.9	26.5 ± 3.9	0.32
FBS (mg/dL)	118.4 ± 34.3	120.0 ± 27.8	0.24
IRI (μU/mL)	23.1 ± 29.8	23.4 ± 33.8	0.38
HbA$_{1c}$ (%)	6.37 ± 1.18	6.46 ± 1.23	0.016
HDL cholesterol (mg/dL)	55.2 ± 16.3	55.0 ± 15.4	0.32
LDL cholesterol (mg/dL)	114.0 ± 28.8	111.3 ± 28.0	0.08
Triglycerides (mg/dL)	195.2 ± 135.9	163.6 ± 121.9	0.007
NEFA (μEq/L)	651.2 ± 242.5	533.5 ± 209.7	0.013
AST (IU/L)	46.7 ± 17.2	47.6 ± 21.2	0.39
ALT (IU/L)	68.9 ± 36.1	58.1 ± 33.5	0.014
GGT (IU/L)	70.4 ± 46.5	66.6 ± 47.5	0.29
Ferritin (ng/mL)	219.8 ± 150.8	194.4 ± 139.2	0.015
Platelet count (×10^4 /μL)	20.8 ± 5.7	20.9 ± 5.3	0.30
Type IV collagen 7 s	5.08 ± 1.95	4.84 ± 1.34	0.40
Glutathione in protein fraction (μM)	1.42 ± 0.87	0.93 ± 0.63	0.010
Glutathione in deproteinized fraction (μM)	0.025 ± 0.040	0.019 ± 0.024	0.27
CAP (db/m)	295.7 ± 44.9	285.4 ± 48.8	0.07
LSM (kPa)	9.94 ± 4.93	9.24 ± 4.48	0.16

Data are expressed as mean ± standard deviation. *BMI* body mass index, *FBS* fasting blood sugar, *IRI* immunoreactive insulin, *HBA1c*, hemoglobin A1c, *HDL cholesterol* high-density lipoprotein cholesterol, *LDL cholesterol* low-density lipoprotein cholesterol, *NEFA* non-esterified fatty acid, *AST* aspartate aminotransferase, *ALT* alanine aminotransferase, *GGT* γ-glutamyl transpeptidase, *CAP* controlled attenuation parameter, *LSM* liver stiffness measurement

Three patients dropped out, one each owing to fatigue, elevated blood pressure, and rash.

The clinical and laboratory characteristics of the study participants are shown in Table 1. Twenty-four patients (82.8%) had dyslipidemia and 12 (41.4%) were taking statins. Fourteen patients (48.3%) had diabetes.

After 4 months of glutathione treatment, ALT levels decreased significantly. Glutathione treatment decreased the concentrations of triglycerides, NEFA, and ferritin. HbA1c levels increased after glutathione treatment. Unexpectedly, glutathione in the plasma protein fraction decreased significantly after glutathione treatment. There was no significant difference in glutathione levels in the deproteinized fraction. Although glutathione treatment did not significantly affect CAP and LSM values, both tended to decrease.

Glutathione treatment improved CAP values in ALT responders

The median decrease in ALT level from baseline was 12.9%. The 29 patients were divided into ALT responders ($n = 15$), defined as those with an ALT reduction ≥12.9%, and ALT non-responders ($n = 14$), defined as those with an ALT reduction <12.9%, and the factors associated with responses to glutathione were evaluated (Table 2). ALT responders were significantly younger than ALT non-responders (50.7 ± 12.1 years vs. 61.7 ± 12.4 years, $p = 0.011$). Body mass index (BMI) did not differ between ALT responders and non-responders (26.5 ± 4.1 kg/m^2 vs. 26.6 ± 3.8 kg/m^2, $p = 0.47$). Although the percentages of ALT responders and non-responders with dyslipidemia did not differ (80.0% vs. 85.7%, $p = 0.68$), HDL cholesterol and LDL cholesterol levels were higher in ALT responders. Rates of statin use tended to be lower in ALT responders than in non-responders (26.7% vs. 57.1%, $p = 0.10$). Rates of diabetes also tended to be lower (33.3% vs. 64.3%, $p = 0.10$) and HbA1c levels were significantly lower in ALT responders compared with non-responders. There were no significant differences in glutathione levels in the plasma protein and deproteinized fractions between ALT responders and non-responders before glutathione treatment.

The characteristics of ALT responders and non-responders before and after glutathione treatment are

Table 2 Characteristics of ALT responders and non-responders

	ALT responders (n = 15)	ALT non-responders (n = 14)	P-value
Age (year)	50.7 ± 12.1	61.7 ± 12.4	0.011
Male/female (n)	9 (6)	5 (9)	0.191
Dyslipidemia (%)	12 (80.0)	12 (85.7)	0.68
Statin (%)	4 (26.7)	8 (57.1)	0.10
Diabetes (%)	5 (33.3)	9 (64.3)	0.10
BMI (kg/m^2)	26.5 ± 4.1	26.6 ± 3.8	0.47
FBS (mg/dL)	115.7 ± 37.9	121.4 ± 31.2	0.33
IRI (µU/mL)	23.5 ± 22.7	22.6 ± 38.0	0.47
HbA$_{1c}$ (%)	5.94 ± 1.03	6.9 ± 1.2	0.019
HDL cholesterol (mg/dL)	60.3 ± 18.6	49.7 ± 11.7	0.04
LDL cholesterol (mg/dL)	124.5 ± 33.1	102.9 ± 18.6	0.021
Triglycerides (mg/dL)	202.4 ± 164.1	187.6 ± 103.3	0.39
NEFA (µEq/L)	720.2 ± 285.0	563.3 ± 143.0	0.055
AST (IU/L)	46.3 ± 20.2	47.1 ± 14.1	0.45
ALT (IU/L)	77.1 ± 38.6	60.1 ± 32.2	0.104
GGT (IU/L)	81.9 ± 58.0	58.0 ± 26.6	0.085
Ferritin (ng/mL)	260.2 ± 164.5	176.6 ± 126.1	0.07
Platelet count (×10^4 /µL)	20.3 ± 4.6	21.3 ± 6.8	0.32
Type IV collagen 7 s	4.61 ± 1.13	5.59 ± 2.51	0.09
Glutathione in protein fraction (µM)	1.53 ± 0.92	1.27 ± 0.83	0.230
Glutathione in deprotenized fraction (µM)	0.017 ± 0.020	0.036 ± 0.057	0.116
CAP (db/m)	300.3 ± 41.1	290.4 ± 50.2	0.29
LSM (kPa)	8.71 ± 4.63	11.36 ± 5.05	0.080

Data are expressed as mean ± standard deviation

Abbreviations: BMI body mass index, *FBS* fasting blood sugar, *IRI* immunoreactive insulin, *HBA1c* hemoglobin A1c, *HDL cholesterol* high density lipoprotein cholesterol, *LDL cholesterol* low density lipoprotein cholesterol, *NEFA* non-esterified fatty acid, *AST* asparate aminotransferase, *ALT* alanine aminotransferase, *GGT* γ-glutamyl transpeptidase, *CAP* controlled attenuation parameter, *LSM* liver stiffness measurement

shown in Table 3. Glutathione treatment decreased ALT levels in ALT responders (Fig. 2a) but increased AST and ALT levels in ALT non-responders (Fig. 2b). In ALT responders, glutathione treatment decreased NEFA, ferritin, and HDL cholesterol levels but increased HbA1c levels. In ALT non-responders, glutathione treatment reduced triglyceride levels but increased FBS levels. Glutathione treatment significantly decreased glutathione in the plasma protein-boud fraction in ALT responders; there was no change in ALT non-responders. Surprisingly, CAP values were significantly reduced in ALT responders; there were no differences in ALT non-responders.

Discussion

Glutathione has a long history for the treatment of chronic liver disease by intravenous injection. This study demonstrates a therapeutic effect of glutathione by oral administration in patients with NAFLD. The primary outcome of this study was a change in ALT levels. The 29 patients who were treated with oral administration of glutathione (300 mg/day) for 4 months showed a reduction in ALT levels as well as reductions in triglycerides, NEFA, and ferritin levels. The findings of the current study suggest the beneficial effects of glutathione by oral administration for NAFLD patients. It is thought that glutathione is degraded into amino acids during digestion and absorption processes. Orally administered glutathione is suggested to serve as a source of amino acids in the synthesis of endogenous glutathione. Supplementation of large doses of glycine and serine, precursors of glutathione, can attenuate NAFLD in human and animal models [18, 19]. In the current study, the dose of glutathione was 300 mg/day. The amount of cysteine potentially released from 300 mg of glutathione is less than 120 mg, the amount that can be obtained from 10 to 20 g of meat or 100 mL of milk. It is, therefore, very unlikely that the current dose of orally administered glutathione attenuates the pathogenesis of NAFLD via an amino acid source for glutathione synthesis.

It is reported that the level of the protein-bound form of glutathione increases 1–2 h after ingestion of glutathione, which suggests that orally administered glutathione is

Table 3 Characteristics of ALT responders and non-responders before and after glutathione treatment

	ALT responders (n = 15)			ALT non-responders (n = 14)		
	Before treatment	After treatment	P-value	Before treatment	After treatment	P-value
Age (year)	50.7 ± 12.1		-	61.7 ± 12.4		-
Male/female (n)	9 (6)		-	5 (9)		-
Dyslipidemia (%)	12 (80.0)		-	12 (85.7)		-
Statin (%)	4 (26.7)		-	8 (57.1)		-
Diabetes (%)	5 (33.3)		-	9 (64.3)		-
BMI (kg/m^2)	26.5 ± 4.1	26.5 ± 4.0	0.23	26.6 ± 3.8	26.4 ± 3.9	0.45
FBS (mg/dL)	115.7 ± 37.9	113.0 ± 23.0	0.38	121.4 ± 31.2	128.2 ± 31.4	0.004
IRI (μU/mL)	23.5 ± 22.7	17.9 ± 14.3	0.14	22.6 ± 38.0	30.5 ± 31.4	0.11
HbA$_{1c}$ (%)	5.94 ± 1.03	6.08 ± 1.10	0.017	6.9 ± 1.2	6.89 ± 1.28	0.14
HDL cholesterol (mg/dL)	60.3 ± 18.6	57.4 ± 16.7	0.001	49.7 ± 11.7	52.2 ± 13.8	0.08
LDL cholesterol (mg/dL)	124.5 ± 33.1	117.1 ± 34.8	0.06	102.9 ± 18.6	104.1 ± 14.5	0.41
Triglycerides (mg/dL)	202.4 ± 164.1	178.8 ± 157.6	0.15	187.6 ± 103.3	146.2 ± 62.1	0.003
NEFA (μEq/L)	720.2 ± 285.0	576.0 ± 230.1	0.032	563.3 ± 143.0	473.9 ± 170.7	0.13
AST (IU/L)	46.3 ± 20.2	40.0 ± 20.7	0.11	47.1 ± 14.1	55.8 ± 19.3	0.003
ALT (IU/L)	77.1 ± 38.6	47.9 ± 28.1	<0.0001	60.1 ± 32.2	68.9 ± 36.3	0.005
GGT (IU/L)	81.9 ± 58.0	64.8 ± 48.4	0.07	58.0 ± 26.6	68.5 ± 48.3	0.06
Ferritin (ng/mL)	260.2 ± 164.5	217.7 ± 162.3	0.015	176.6 ± 126.1	169.5 ± 109.9	0.28
Platelet count (×10^4 /μL)	20.3 ± 4.6	20.2 ± 4.7	0.45	21.3 ± 6.8	21.8 ± 6.0	0.25
Type IV collagen 7 s	4.61 ± 1.13	4.39 ± 1.06	0.10	5.59 ± 2.51	5.42 ± 1.49	0.13
Glutathione in protein fraction (μM)	1.53 ± 0.92	0.88 ± 0.53	0.004	1.27 ± 0.83	1.00 ± 0.77	0.24
Glutathione in deprotenized fraction (μM)	0.017 ± 0.020	0.019 ± 0.029	0.60	0.036 ± 0.057	0.018 ± 0.017	0.19
CAP (db/m)	300.3 ± 41.1	285.1 ± 53.2	0.049	290.4 ± 50.2	285.8 ± 44.9	0.31
LSM (kPa)	8.71 ± 4.63	7.91 ± 4.22	0.19	11.36 ± 5.05	10.9 ± 4.38	0.32

Data are expressed as mean ± standard deviation

Abbreviations: BMI body mass index, *FBS* fasting blood sugar, *IRI* immunoreactive insulin, *HBA1c* hemoglobin A1c, *HDL cholesterol* high density lipoprotein cholesterol, *LDL cholesterol* low density lipoprotein cholesterol, *NEFA* non-esterified fatty acid, *AST* aspartate aminotransferase, *ALT* alanine aminotransferase, *GGT* γ-glutamyl transpeptidase, *CAP* controlled attenuation parameter, *LSM* liver stiffness measurement

absorbed into the blood [12]. This protein-bound glutathione may be deposited in the liver, attenuating hepatitis.

The levels of protein-bound glutathione were reported to return to baseline levels after an overnight fast [12]. In the current study, we found that the baseline level of the protein-bound form of glutathione significantly decreased after an overnight fast following 4 months of glutathione administration, especially in ALT responders. The levels of protein-bound glutathione in patients in the current study were considerably higher than those of healthy

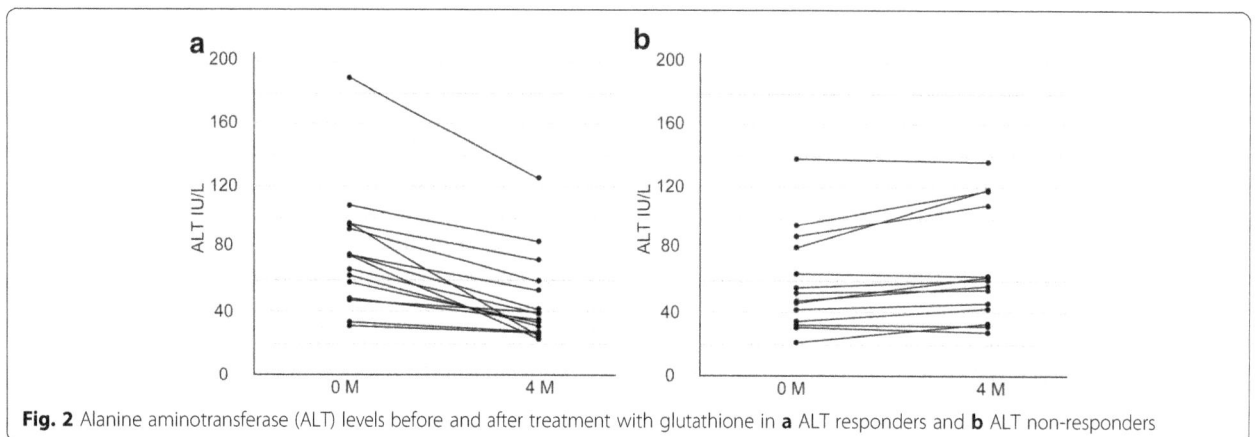

Fig. 2 Alanine aminotransferase (ALT) levels before and after treatment with glutathione in **a** ALT responders and **b** ALT non-responders

volunteers in previous studies [12] estimated using the same method. Glutathione treatment also decreased protein-bound glutathione to normal baseline levels. These findings suggest that oral administration of glutathione may increase the incorporation of protein-bound glutathione into the liver or decrease the pathological excretion of glutathione from the liver.

NAFLD is a complex disease. Its pathogenesis is thought to involve various factors, including insulin resistance, lipotoxicity, gut/nutrient-derived signals, adipocytokines, oxidative stress, and genetic factors. Dyslipidemia has been reported in 20–80% of patients with NAFLD [20]. Our previously study revealed that orally administered glutathione accelerates fatty acid utilization by upregulating levels of the protein peroxisome proliferator-activated receptor-γ coactivator-1α and mitochondrial DNA with reduced plasma NEFA levels [21]. The current study also revealed that 24 (82.8%) of our patients had dyslipidemia, and glutathione treatment reduced triglyceride and NEFA levels significantly.

Increases in ferritin and body iron stores have been detected frequently in NAFLD patients [22, 23]. Ferritin and iron can promote the development of NAFLD through oxidative stress [24]. Results from the PIVENS trial showed that oral administration of the anti-oxidant vitamin E improved liver dysfunction and the pathological conditions of NASH [17]. However, long-term treatment with vitamin E has been associated with increases in all-cause mortality and the risk for prostate cancer [25–27], suggesting the need to evaluate the efficacy and safety of this agent. In the current study, glutathione treatment significantly decreased ferritin levels, but the mechanism behind the decrease remains unclear. Glutathione is thought to ameliorate hyperferritinemia and oxidative stress, and to have therapeutic effects in patients with NAFLD.

Liver fat was non-invasively assessed using VCTE with CAP. A meta-analysis found that CAP has good sensitivity and specificity for detecting liver fat [28]. CAP values in our study tended to decrease in all patients and significantly decreased in ALT responders following 4 months of glutathione treatment. Although the relationship between histologic improvement of hepatic steatosis and the reduction of CAP values has not yet been determined, glutathione may reduce hepatic steatosis.

We also investigated the patient factors associated with the therapeutic effects of glutathione. We found that HDL cholesterol and LDL cholesterol levels were higher and HbA1c levels lower in ALT responders than in non-responders. Although the percentage of patients using statins did not differ significantly between the two groups, the percentage tended to be lower in ALT responders than in ALT non-responders. While it can be nothing more than speculation because of the small sample size, patients who showed therapeutic effects following glutathione treatment appeared to be younger and did not have diabetes or had mild diabetes.

Three patients withdrew from the study because of fatigue, elevated blood pressure, and a rash. In ALT responders, HbA1c levels increased and HDL cholesterol levels decreased after glutathione treatment. A study of 6522 patients found that 24 (0.4%) had experienced adverse reactions, the most frequent being anorexia, nausea, vomiting, and rash [29]. Although administration of glutathione may have been associated with a rash in one patient in the current study, the causal associations between glutathione and other adverse effects are unclear.

This study had some limitations. First, our study was a single-arm study without a control group. Second, the study was limited by the small sample size and the short treatment period (4 months). Third, as the pathological conditions of the patients were not evaluated by liver biopsy, incorporation of orally administered glutathione in the liver was not confirmed. Fourth, a number of patients withdrew from the study but no causal association can be determined.

Conclusions

Treatment with glutathione significantly improved ALT levels. In addition, CAP values were significantly reduced in ALT responders. Our pilot study suggests that oral administration of glutathione supports hepatic metabolism and improves NAFLD. To elucidate the mechanism behind the beneficial effects of glutathione, further studies that examine the incorporation of orally administered glutathione into the liver and the effects on the host redox system using stable isotope-labeled glutathione and animal models are required. Large-scale clinical trials are necessary to confirm the therapeutic effects of glutathione.

Abbreviations

ALT: Alanine aminotransferase; AST: Aspartate aminotransferase; BMI: Body mass index; CAP: Controlled attenuation parameter; FBS: Fasting blood sugar; HbA1c: hemoglobin A1c; HDL: High-density lipoprotein; IRI: Immunoreactive insulin; LDL: Low-density lipoprotein; LSM: Liver stiffness measurement; NAFLD: Nonalcoholic fatty liver disease; NASH: Nonalcoholic steatohepatitis; NEFA: Non-esterified fatty acid; UMIN: University Hospital Medical Information Network; VCTE: Vibration-controlled transient elastography

Acknowledgments

This work was supported in part by the Japan Study Group of NAFLD (JSG-NAFLD, Kyoto, Japan).

Funding

KOHJIN Life Sciences (Tokyo, Japan). a subsidiary of Mitsubishi Corp. Life Sciences, provided glutathione and partial financial support for this work. KOHJIN Life Sciences was not involved in data analysis or manuscript preparation.

Authors' contributions

Designed and coordinated the study: TK, YH, YS, and AN. Performed the experiments: TK, YH, YS, TK, TK, YO, WT, KI, KF, MY, YS, ST, SS, MO, SO, YE, YI, WA, KS, and AN. Performed the statistical analyses: TK, YH, and AN. Collected the data and critically reviewed the manuscript: TK, YH, YS, KK, MT, TY, WA, KS, and AN. Wrote the manuscript: TK, YH, YS, WA, KS, and AN. All authors approved the final version of the manuscript.

Consent for publication

Not applicable.

Competing interests

The authors declare that they have no competing interests.

Author details

[1]Department of Gastroenterology and Hepatology, Yokohama City University Graduate School of Medicine, Yokohama, Japan. [2]Division of Hepatology and Pancreatology, Department of Internal Medicine, Aichi Medical University, Aichi, Japan. [3]Department of Biostatistics, Yokohama City University Graduate School of Medicine, Yokohama, Japan. [4]Department of Gastroenterology and Hepatology, Kyoto Prefectural University of Medicine, Kyoto, Japan. [5]Center for Digestive and Liver Diseases, Nara City Hospital, Nara, Japan. [6]Department of Gastroenterology and Hepatology, Kochi Medical School, Kochi, Japan. [7]Liver Center, Saga University Hospital, Saga, Japan. [8]Division of Applied Life Sciences, Graduate School of Life and Environmental Sciences, Kyoto Prefectural University, Kyoto, Japan. [9]Division of Applied Biosciences, Graduate School of Agriculture, Kyoto University, Kyoto, Japan.

References

1. Day CP. Non-alcoholic steatohepatitis (NASH): where are we now and where are we going? Gut. 2002;50:585–8.
2. Lazo M, Clark JM. The epidemiology of nonalcoholic fatty liver disease: a global perspective. Semin Liver Dis. 2008;28:339–50.
3. Neuschwander-Tetri BA, Caldwell SH. Nonalcoholic steatohepatitis: summary of an AASLD single topic conference. Hepatology. 2003;37:1202–19.
4. Marchesini G, Bugianesi E, Forlani G, et al. Nonalcoholic fatty liver, steatohepatitis, and the metabolic syndrome. Hepatology. 2003;37:917–23.
5. Yilmaz Y, Younossi ZM. Obesity-associated nonalcoholic fatty liver disease. Clin Liver Dis. 2014;18:19–31.
6. Promrat K, Kleiner DE, Niemeier HM, et al. Randomized controlled trial testing the effects of weight loss on nonalcoholic steatohepatitis. Hepatology. 2010;51:121–9.
7. Anderson ME. Glutathione: an overview of biosynthesis and modulation. Chem Biol Interact. 1998;111-112:1–14.
8. Dentico P, Volpe A, Buongiorno R, et al. Glutathione in the treatment of chronic fatty liver diseases. Recenti Prog Med. 1995;86:290–3. [in Italian]
9. Altomare E, Colonna P, D'Agostino C, et al. High-dose antioxidant therapy during thrombolysis in patients with acute myocardial infarction. Curr Ther Res Clin Exp. 1996;57:131–41.
10. Allen J, Bradley RD. Effects of oral glutathione supplementation on systemic oxidative stress biomarkers in human volunteers. J Altern Complement Med. 2011;17:827–33.
11. Kovacs-Nolan J, Rupa P, Matsui T, et al. In vitro and ex vivo uptake of glutathione (GSH) across the intestinal epithelium and fate of oral GSH after in vivo supplementation. J Agric Food Chem. 2014;62:9499–506.
12. Park EY, Shimura N, Konishi T, et al. Increase in the protein-bound form of glutathione in human blood after the oral administration of glutathione. J Agric Food Chem. 2014;62:6183–9.
13. Seko Y, Sumida Y, Tanaka S, et al. Serum alanine aminotransferase predicts the histological course of non-alcoholic steatohepatitis in Japanese patients. Hepatol Res. 2015;45:E53–61.
14. Committee of the Japan Diabetes Society on the Diagnostic Criteria of Diabetes Mellitus, Seino Y, Nanjo K, Tajima, et al. Report of the committee on the classification and diagnostic criteria of diabetes mellitus. J Diabetes Investig. 2010;1:212–28.
15. Sandrin L, Tanter M, Gennisson JL, et al. Shear elasticity probe for soft tissues with 1-D transient elastography. IEEE Trans Ultrason Ferroelectr Freq Control. 2002;49:436–46.
16. Sandrin L, Fourquet B, Hasquenoph JM, et al. Transient elastography: a new noninvasive method for assessment of hepatic fibrosis. Ultrasound Med Biol. 2003;29:1705–13.
17. Sanyal AJ, Chalasani N, Kowdley KV, et al. NASH CRN. Pioglitazone, vitamin E, or placebo for nonalcoholic steatohepatitis. N Engl J Med. 2010;362:1675–85.
18. Zhou X, Han D, Xu R, et al. Glycine protects against high sucrose and high fat-induced non-alcoholic steatohepatitis in rats. Oncotarget. 2016;7:80223–37.
19. Mardinoglu A, Bjornson E, Zhang C, et al. Personal model-assisted identification of NAD+ and glutathione metabolism as intervention target in NAFLD. Mol Syst Biol. 2017;13:916.
20. Souza MR, Diniz Mde F, Medeiros-Filho JE, et al. Metabolic syndrome and risk factors for non-alcoholic fatty liver disease. Arq Gastroenterol. 2012;49:89–96.
21. Aoi W, Ogaya Y, Takami M, et al. Glutathione supplementation suppresses muscle fatigue induced by prolonged exercise via improved aerobic metabolism. J Int Soc Sports Nutr. 2015;12:7.
22. Valenti L, Fracanzani AL, Dongiovanni P, et al. Iron depletion by phlebotomy improves insulin resistance in patients with nonalcoholic fatty liver disease and hyperferritinemia: evidence from a case-control study. Am J Gastroenterol. 2007;102:1251–8.
23. Lapenna D, Pierdomenico SD, Ciofani G, et al. Association of body iron stores with low molecular weight iron and oxidant damage of human atherosclerotic plaques. Free Radic Biol Med. 2007;42:492–8.
24. Dongiovanni P, Valenti L, Ludovica Fracanzani A, et al. Iron depletion by deferoxamine up-regulates glucose uptake and insulin signaling in hepatoma cells and in rat liver. Am J Pathol. 2008;172:738–47.
25. Miller ER 3rd, Pastor-Barriuso R, Dalal D, et al. Meta-analysis: high-dosage vitamin E supplementation may increase all-cause mortality. Ann Intern Med. 2005;142:37–46.
26. Bjelakovic G, Nikolova D, Gluud LL, et al. Mortality in randomized trials of antioxidant supplements for primary and secondary prevention: systematic review and meta-analysis. JAMA. 2007;297:842–57.
27. Klein EA, Thompson IM Jr, Tangen CM, et al. Vitamin E and the risk of prostate cancer: the selenium and vitamin E cancer prevention trial (SELECT). JAMA. 2011;306:1549–56.
28. Shi KQ, Tang JZ, Zhu XL, et al. Controlled attenuation parameter for the detection of steatosis severity in chronic liver disease: a meta-analysis of diagnostic accuracy. J Gastroenterol Hepatol. 2014;29:1149–58.
29. Pharmaceutical Interview Form, Japan Standard Commodity No. 873922, 2014.

12

Portal vein thrombosis in liver cirrhosis: incidence, management, and outcome

Shunichiro Fujiyama[*] ⓘ, Satoshi Saitoh, Yusuke Kawamura, Hitomi Sezaki, Tetsuya Hosaka, Norio Akuta, Masahiro Kobayashi, Yoshiyuki Suzuki, Fumitaka Suzuki, Yasuji Arase, Kenji Ikeda and Hiromitsu Kumada

Abstract

Background: Portal vein thrombosis (PVT) is a serious complication in liver cirrhosis with portal hypertension. We examined the treatment, recurrence and prognosis of PVT in cirrhotic patients.

Methods: The study subjects were all 90 cirrhotic patients with PVT treated with danaparoid sodium (DS) at our department between July 2007 and September 2016. The mean age was 68 years and mean Child-Pugh score was 7. All patients received 2500 U/day of DS for 2 weeks, and repeated in those who developed PVT recurrence after the initial therapy.

Results: Complete response was noted in 49% ($n = 44$), partial response (shrinkage ≥70%) in 33% ($n = 30$), and no change (shrinkage <70%) in 18% ($n = 16$) of the patients after the initial course of treatment. DS treatment neither caused adverse events, particularly bleeding or thrombocytopenia, nor induced significant changes in serum albumin, total bilirubin, prothrombin time, and residual liver function. Re-treatment was required in 44 patients who showed PVT recurrence and 61% of these responded to the treatment. The cumulative recurrence rates at 1 and 2 posttreatment years were 26 and 30%, respectively. The recurrence rates were significantly lower in patients with acute type, compared to the chronic type ($p = 0.0141$). The cumulative survival rates at 1 and 3 years after treatment (including maintenance therapy with warfarin) were 83 and 60%, respectively, and were significantly higher in patients with acute type than chronic type ($p = 0.0053$).

Conclusion: We can expect prognostic improvement of liver cirrhosis by warfarin following two-week DS therapy for the treatment of PVT in patients with liver cirrhosis safety and effectiveness. An early diagnosis of PVT along with the evaluation of the volume of PVT on CT and an early intervention would contribute to the higher efficacy of the treatment.

Keywords: Portal vein thrombosis, Danaparoid sodium, Liver cirrhosis

Background

Liver cirrhosis represents the end stage of chronic diseases of the liver and is associated with life-threatening complications [1, 2]. The natural course of cirrhosis is largely affected by various pathologies, such as variceal bleeding, ascites, and infection [3, 4]. The major predictors of survival of patients with liver cirrhosis are Child-Pugh score; model for end-stage liver disease score; and various biochemical parameters, such as serum bilirubin, albumin, prothrombin time or international normalized ratio, creatinine, as well as encephalopathy and ascites [4, 5].

Recent evidence suggests the association between portal vein thrombosis (PVT) and survival of patients with liver cirrhosis [6], although the data are inconclusive.

Based on the increase in the use of technically-advanced noninvasive liver imaging modalities, PVT has been increasingly identified in patients with cirrhosis, with the estimated current prevalence of PVT in patients with cirrhosis of 0.6 to 26% [3, 7, 8].

The value of anticoagulation in the treatment of PVT in patients with cirrhosis remains controversial [9]. Cirrhosis is associated with bleeding diathesis based on the following factors: prolonged bleeding time, thrombocytopenia associated with hypersplenism, increased prothrombin time/international normalized ratio, reduced synthesis of

* Correspondence: shunichiro-fujiyama@toranomon.gr.jp
Department of Hepatology, Toranomon Hospital, Toranomon 2-2-2, Minato-ku, Tokyo 105-8470, Japan

coagulation factors, and secondary hyperfibrinolysis [10, 11]. More importantly, nearly half of patients with cirrhosis are diagnosed with gastroesophageal varices that can result in life-threatening bleeding events [12]. Taken together, these detrimental conditions greatly limit the use of anticoagulants for patients with cirrhosis. However, recent evidence indicates that both pro- and anticoagulation factors are concomitantly reduced in patients with cirrhosis [13], thereby maintaining a balance in the coagulation system [13–15]. Unfortunately, bleeding risk cannot be accurately assessed in patients with chronic liver disease by globally used coagulation tests [16, 17]. In addition, the occurrence of bleeding in patients with cirrhosis is not primarily dependent on hemostatic abnormalities, but on the severity of portal pressure, endothelial dysfunction, and bacterial infection [14]. Accordingly, the use of anticoagulants for patients with cirrhosis and PVT may be theoretically justified. However, convincing clinicians to prescribe anticoagulants to cirrhotic patients, especially those with decompensated cirrhosis, remains difficult.

Danaparoid sodium (DS) is a glycosaminoglucoronan derived from the same starting material, porcine intestinal mucosa, as unfractured heparin and low-molecular-weight heparins (LMWHs), but its extraction procedure excludes heparin and heparin fragments [18]. Danaparoid is a low-molecular-weight heparinoid consisting of heparin sulfate (84%), dermatan sulfate (12%), and chondroitin sulfate (4%). The mean mass of its components is approximately 6000 Da [18]. Its antithrombotic activity has been well established. Danaparoid catalyzes inactivation of factors Xa (FXa) and thrombin. Like most LMWHs, danaparoid exerts a stronger catalytic effect on inactivation of FXa by antithrombin (AT)-III, than on inactivation of thrombin by AT-III [19].

Anticoagulation therapy is definitely the most effective way to achieve recanalization of the portal vein, thereby improving the prognosis of patients with PVT. To our knowledge, the optimal management of PVT in individuals with cirrhosis has not yet been addressed by any consensus publication or practice guideline. In this study, we examined the response to treatment, recurrence rate and prognosis of PVT in a group of Japanese cirrhotic patients.

Methods
Patients
In the past 9 years, 23,150 contrast-enhanced computed tomography (CECT) was performed at our hospital, among which 3685 were for patients with liver disease. Of these, 1264 patients had portal vein tumor thrombosis. Of the remaining 2421 patients with liver cirrhosis, 1666 patients were diagnosed with liver cirrhosis and portal hypertension. Among these, 101 patient had portal vein thrombosis. In other words, PVT was recognized in 4.2% of patients with cirrhosis of the liver and 6.1% of patients with portal hypertension (Fig. 1). Of the latter group, 90 patients were enrolled in the present study; they represented consecutive cirrhotic patients with PVT who were treated at our hospital with DS between July 2007 and September 2016. We divided the patients into two groups; 27 patients developed PVT within 1 month after hepatectomy (16 cases) or splenectomy (11 cases). We defined this group as an "Acute type". Because CECT is often taken early postoperatively. And 63 patients developed PVT without particular cause. We defined this group as an "Chronic type". Table 1 summarizes the clinical characteristics of the study patients as recorded before treatment, including patients of the two groups. For the entire group, the mean age was 68 years, 55% of the patients were males, 61 (72%) patients had hepatitis C virus-related cirrhosis, and the mean Child-Pugh score was 7. Hepatocellular carcinoma (HCC)

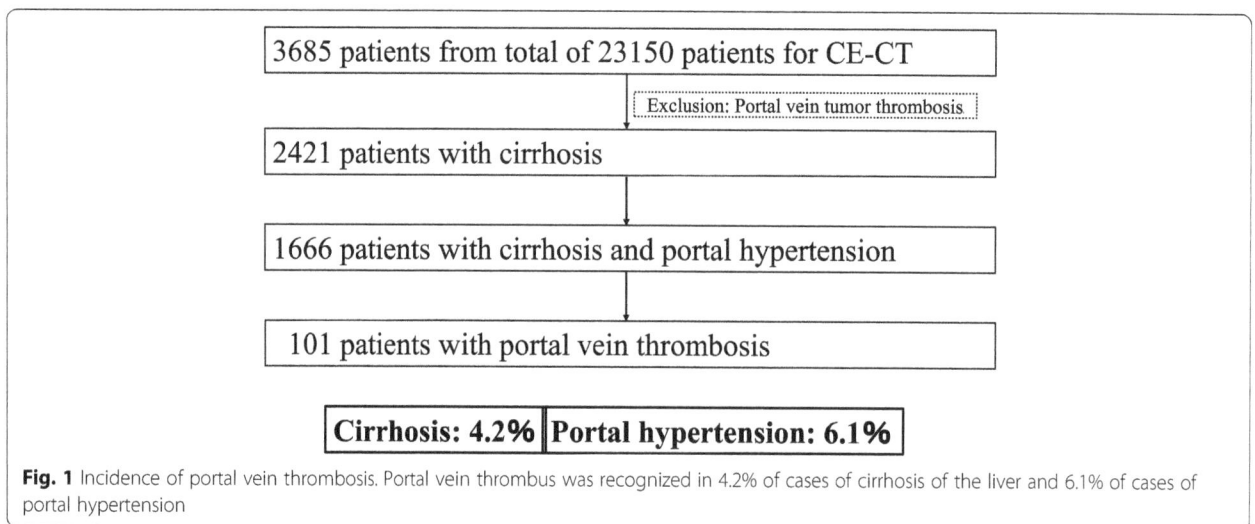

Fig. 1 Incidence of portal vein thrombosis. Portal vein thrombus was recognized in 4.2% of cases of cirrhosis of the liver and 6.1% of cases of portal hypertension

Table 1 Clinical characteristics of cirrhotic patients with PVT

	Total	Acute type	Chronic type	p
Number of patients	90	27	63	
Age (years)[a]	68 (37–84)	62 (37–77)	70 (45–84)	0.0034
Male sex	47	16	31	0.1885
BMI (kg/cm²)[a]	23.0 (16.2–36.5)	23.9 (16.2–31.5)	22.9 (18.1–36.5)	0.1253
Etiology (hepatitis C viral infection)	61	19	42	0.3445
Clinical findings				
Hepatic encephalopathy (+)	5	2	3	0.7748
Ascites (+)	39	11	28	0.9955
Esophagogastric varices (+)	70	13	57	0.0000
HCC (+)	40	1	39	0.0000
Duration of DS treatment (14/28 days)	61/24	18/6	43/18	0.6042
Child-Pugh score	7 (5–12)	7 (5–10)	8 (5–12)	0.0143
Platelet count (μl)	8.0 (1.7–65.5)	20.0 (3.9–65.5)	7.1 (1.7–21.7)	0.0000
Serum albumin (g/dL)	3.1 (2.1–4.5)	3.1 (2.7–4.5)	3.2 (2.1–4.4)	0.5181
Total bilirubin (mg/dL)	1.3 (0.4–5.4)	0.9 (0.4–3.9)	1.5 (0.5–5.4)	0.0000
Aspartate aminotransferase (IU/L)	39 (15–177)	36 (17–103)	41 (15–177)	0.0427
Alanine aminotransferase (IU/L)	23 (0–119)	22 (11–78)	23 (0–119)	0.9222
NH₃ (μg/dL)	70 (21–185)	44 (22–136)	78 (21–185)	0.0064
Prothrombin time (%)	68.3 (27.8–95.3)	73.8 (50.0–85.6)	65.0 (27.8–95.3)	0.1010
Prothrombin time -INR	1.23 (1.02–2.03)	1.19 (1.08–1.38)	1.24 (1.02–2.03)	0.1059
Indocyanine green (%)	38 (2–78)	25 (2–56)	41 (22–78)	0.0024

Data are number of patients, except those denoted by [a], which represent the median (range) values
INR international normalized ratio

without invasion of the bile duct, hepatic vein, or portal vein was diagnosed in 40 (47%) patients at the time of study enrolment.

All patients underwent plain and contrast-enhanced computed tomography (CECT) examination with a multidetector CT scanner (Aquilion-16 or Aquilion-64; Toshiba Medical Systems, Tokyo, Japan), set at 5.0-mm slice thickness at 35, 60, and 180 s to obtain hepatic arterial, portal venous, and equilibrium phase images after the injection of contrast medium (1.5 mL/kg body-weight; Iomeron™ 350 mg I/mL; Eisai, Tokyo) at a rate of 3.0 mL/s. Other parameters of the abdominal CT scan included tube voltage of 120 kVp, tube current of 240 mA, rotation time of 0.6 s, helical pitch of 1.375, field of view of 35–40 cm, and matrix of 512 × 512. Patients with iodine allergy underwent magnetic resonance imaging (MRI).

Protocol for treatment of portal vein thrombosis

The treatment protocol is shown in Fig. 2. Cirrhotic patients with PVT were treated with DS (Orgaran; MSD, Tokyo), 2500 units/day (IV drip) for 2 weeks. The same treatment was repeated for 2 weeks in patients who showed no or partial response to the initial course of treatment. All patients received warfarin as maintenance

therapy. AT-III and other thrombolytic agents were not used during the administration of DS.

Esophageal and gastric varices were assessed endoscopically. Endoscopic injection sclerotherapy or endoscopic variceal ligation was used for treatment of varices assessed as F2 or F3 and/or RC1 or RC2/3 before anticoagulation therapy. Imaging studies, laboratory tests (hepatic reserve test, platelet count, and tests of the coagulation/fibrinolytic system) and complications were assessed before and after treatment.

Evaluation of PVT

CECT was performed in all patients to determine the maximum extent of stenosis and presence of PVT. Multislice CT image data were reconstructed and transferred to a computer workstation (Ziostation; Ziosoft, Tokyo) for postprocessing. The response to treatment was categorized as complete response (CR, complete disappearance of thrombus), partial response (PR, ≥70% reduction in size of thrombus), and no change (no-change, <70% reduction in size of thrombus), compared with the pretreatment thrombus volume.

The study was approved by the institutional review board of the participating clinical sites, the Ethical Committee for Epidemiology of Toranomon Hospital, all

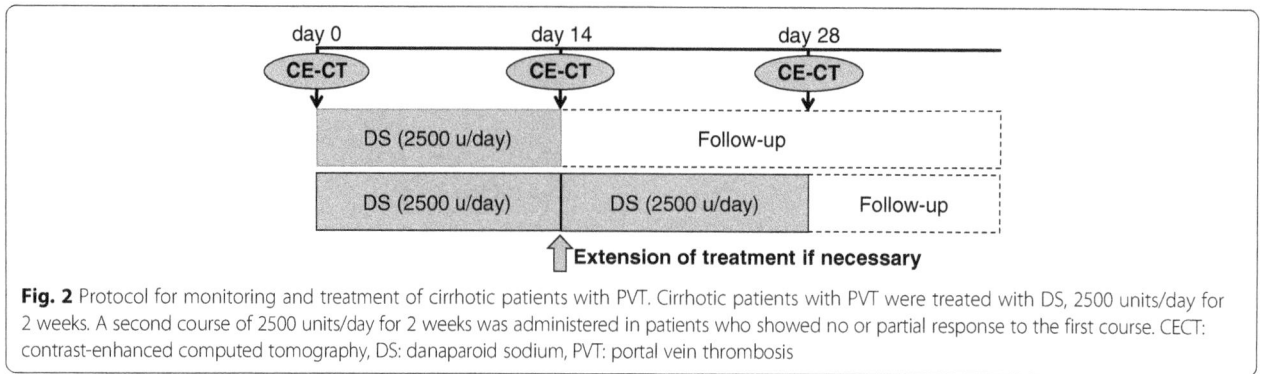

Fig. 2 Protocol for monitoring and treatment of cirrhotic patients with PVT. Cirrhotic patients with PVT were treated with DS, 2500 units/day for 2 weeks. A second course of 2500 units/day for 2 weeks was administered in patients who showed no or partial response to the first course. CECT: contrast-enhanced computed tomography, DS: danaparoid sodium, PVT: portal vein thrombosis

protocols and amendments were approved by the ethics committee (#1096) and conform to the ethics guidelines of the 1975 Declaration of Helsinki. All participating patients provided written informed consent.

Statistical analysis

The maximum extent of stenosis of PVT and differences in tumor response rate among the groups were analyzed by the chi-square test. Recurrence and survival rates were analyzed using the Kaplan-Meier technique with the log-rank test. A P value <0.05 was considered significant. Data were analyzed using IBM SPSS Statistics software (version 19).

Results

Effects of danaparoid sodium treatment on PVT

Figure 3 illustrates the sites of PVT. Most thrombi (71% of 90 patients) were located completely or partially within the main trunk of the PV: in the proximal PV plus the intrahepatic branch in 32 (38%), in the proximal

PV in 18 (21%), proximal PV plus splenic vein in 9 (11%) and proximal PV plus superior mesenteric vein in 1 (1%) patient.

Table 2 shows the response rates to DS after the initial course of 2-week treatment. The median values of the maximum extent of portal vein stenosis before and after treatment were 70% (range, 30–100%) and 20% (range 0–100%), respectively, and the median difference in the extent of stenosis before and after treatment was significant ($p < 0.001$). CR was noted in 44 (49%) patients, PR in 30 (33%), and NC in 16 (18%) patients.

Forty-four patients who developed recurrence required a repeat course of 2-week DS treatment. Table 2 shows the rates of response to DS after the second treatment. CR was obtained in 10 (22%), PR in 17 (39%), and NC in 17 (39%) patients. Retreatment was effective in 54% of the patients who required another course of DS treatment.

The radiological findings in a representative case of CR are presented in Fig. 4. This patient presented with PVT in the main branch of the PV, with maximum stenosis of 80% before and 0% after treatment. Recurrence was noted 7 months after the initial treatment with DS.

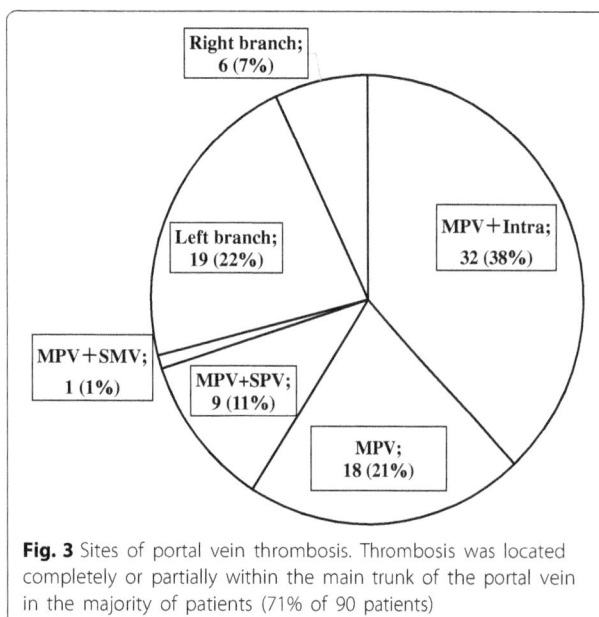

Fig. 3 Sites of portal vein thrombosis. Thrombosis was located completely or partially within the main trunk of the portal vein in the majority of patients (71% of 90 patients)

Table 2 Therapeutic effects of the initial and repeat treatment with danaparoid sodium

Outcome	All patients (n = 90)	Acute type (n = 27)	Chronic type (n = 63)
Initial treatment			
Complete response	44 (49%)	23 (51%)	21 (33%)
Partial response	30 (33%)	2 (35%)	28 (45%)
No change	16 (18%)	2 (14%)	14 (22%)*
Repeat treatment	(n = 44)		
Complete response	10 (22%)		
Partial response	17 (39%)		
No change	17 (39%)		

*$p = 0.001$, compared with the complete and partial response groups, by chi-square test

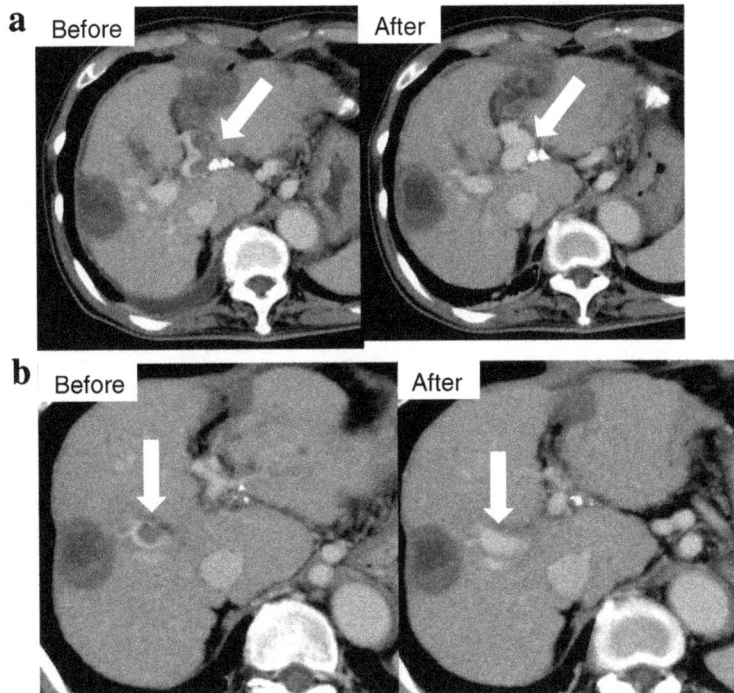

Fig. 4 Representative case of complete response (CR) [Acute type]. **a** The patients was a 66-year-old man with type C cirrhosis, Child-Pugh B. PVT of the main branch of the portal vein disappeared after 2 weeks of treatment. **b** Recurrence in the right branch of the intrahepatic portal vein at 7 months after treatment. The patient was treated again for 2 weeks with DS. Maintenance therapy using warfarin maintained CR. *DS: danaparoid sodium, PVT: portal vein thrombosis, CR: complete response*

DS was administered again for 2 weeks. This was followed by administration of warfarin as maintenance therapy. CR was maintained up to the time of writing of this report. No major or minor bleeding events, episodes of thrombocytopenia, or evidence of liver dysfunction were encountered during the 2 weeks of DS treatment.

Changes in blood parameters
Serum albumin, total bilirubin (T-Bil), prothrombin time (PT), platelet count did not change after therapy in both the acute and chronic categories (Fig. 5). These results indicated that DS does not affect liver residual function. AT-III activity at the start of therapy was significantly higher in patients who achieved CR or PR than in those of the NC group ($P = 0.009$). AT-III can be used for the treatment of patients with low AT-III activity. Serum D-dimer levels were significantly lower after DS therapy in both groups ($P < 0.001$).

Cumulative PVT recurrence rate after the initial course of DS therapy
The recurrence rates at 1 and 3 years after treatment were 26 and 30%, respectively (Fig. 6a). Patients with Acute type had significantly fewer recurrences than patients with Chronic type ($P = 0.0141$) (Fig. 6b).

PVT-related cumulative survival rate after initial DS treatment
The cumulative survival rates at 1 and 3 years after the initial treatment were 83% and 60%, respectively (Fig. 7a). The survival rate was significantly higher in patients with acute cirrhosis than those with chronic cirrhosis ($P = 0.0053$) (Fig. 7b). The survival rate also varied according to the response to DS therapy and was higher in the order of CR, PR, and NC ($P = 0.0053$) (Fig. 7c). The cumulative survival rate was significantly higher for patients without HCC at initial treatment compared to patients with HCC ($P = 0.0000$) (Fig. 7d).

Discussion
The results of this study showed that anticoagulation with DS is safe and effective treatment, significantly reducing the risk of progression of PVT and liver decompensation. In our study, the response rate (CR + PR) was higher than 75% in all the groups of patients tested in this study. These results are to a large extent similar to those reported by Naeshiro et al. [20], who reported response rate of 77% (CR 15%, PR 62%) after 2-week treatment with DS. Interestingly, the treatment was not associated with severe adverse events, such as gastrointestinal bleeding, thrombocytopenia, or worsening of liver dysfunction (Fig. 4).

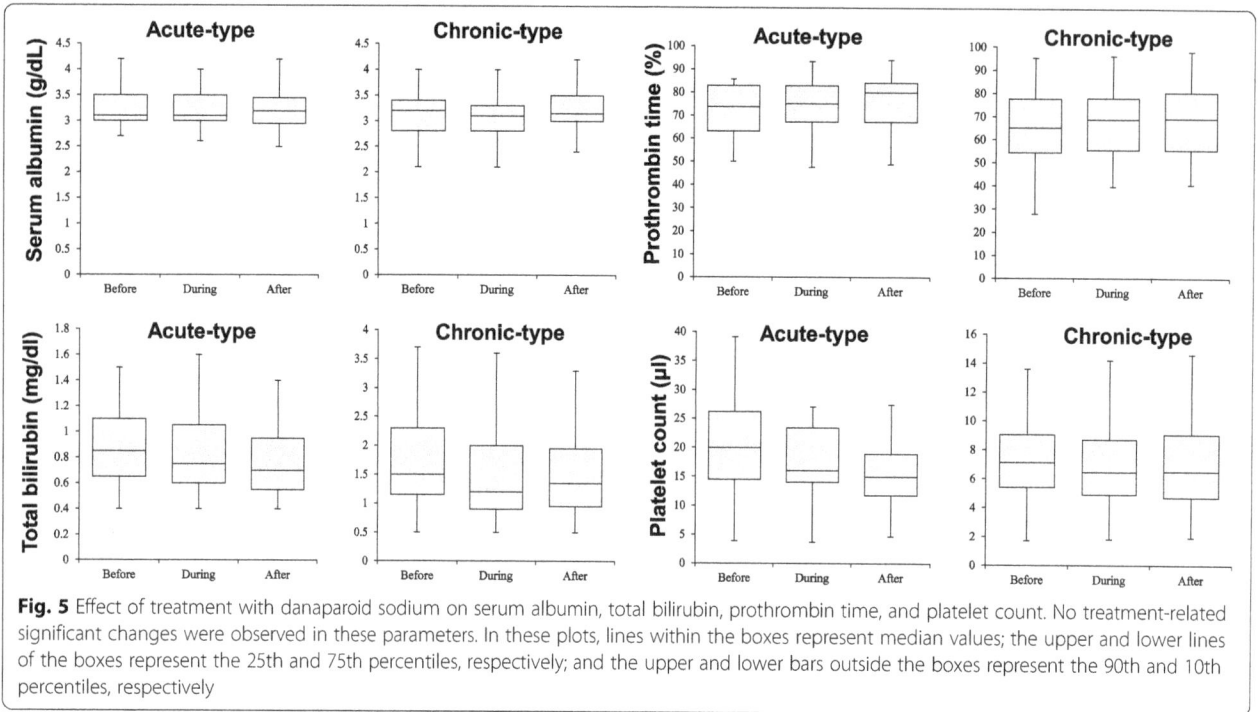

Fig. 5 Effect of treatment with danaparoid sodium on serum albumin, total bilirubin, prothrombin time, and platelet count. No treatment-related significant changes were observed in these parameters. In these plots, lines within the boxes represent median values; the upper and lower lines of the boxes represent the 25th and 75th percentiles, respectively; and the upper and lower bars outside the boxes represent the 90th and 10th percentiles, respectively

Although no side effects were encountered, PVT relapse occurred in about third of the patients, though a second course of DS treatment was efficacious in 54% of the patients. In this regard, the second course of DS treatment was followed by warfarin for maintenance therapy. It is important to keep the international normalized ratio (INR) at less than 2 during warfarin use. The prognosis of patients with unresolved PVT remains poor, including death from hepatic failure.

The treatment goals in PVT include the reversal or prevention of progression of thrombosis in the portal venous system and prevention/treatment of complications. Management decisions must be tailored to the individual patient and should be based on the experience of the attending specialist, since there are only a few randomized controlled trials and no standardized treatment protocols are currently available. The current guidelines of the American Association for the Study of Liver Disease [9] recommend that all patients with acute PVT be anticoagulated for at least 3 months, starting with low-molecular-weight heparin (LMWH), followed by an oral anticoagulant. Long-term anticoagulation is recommended for patients with permanent risk factors or with distal extension of the thrombus into the mesenteric veins. In the setting of chronic PVT, patients should be screened for varices and receive appropriate

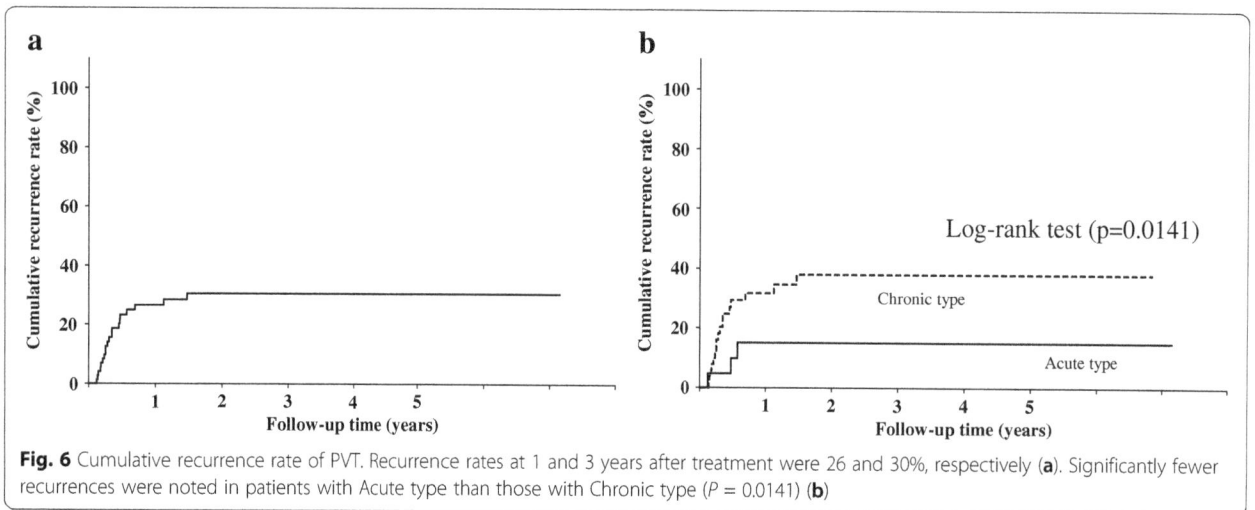

Fig. 6 Cumulative recurrence rate of PVT. Recurrence rates at 1 and 3 years after treatment were 26 and 30%, respectively (**a**). Significantly fewer recurrences were noted in patients with Acute type than those with Chronic type (*P* = 0.0141) (**b**)

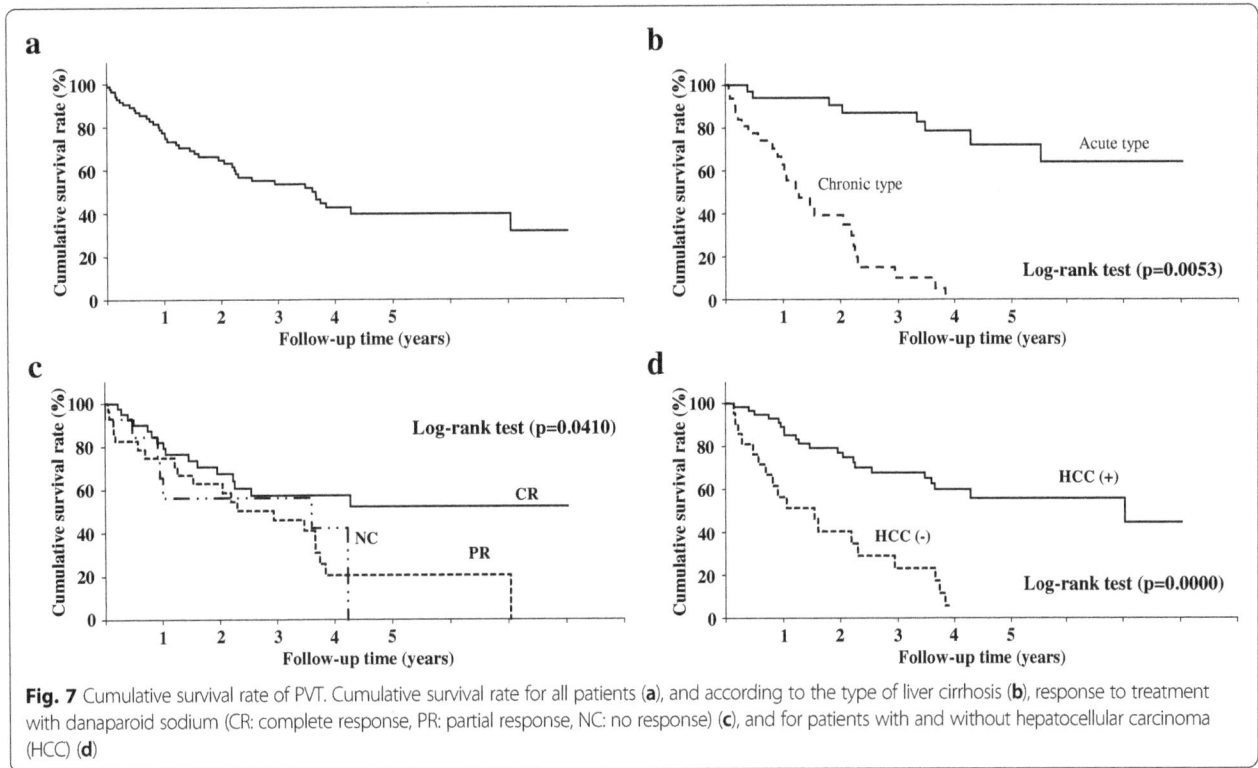

Fig. 7 Cumulative survival rate of PVT. Cumulative survival rate for all patients (**a**), and according to the type of liver cirrhosis (**b**), response to treatment with danaparoid sodium (CR: complete response, PR: partial response, NC: no response) (**c**), and for patients with and without hepatocellular carcinoma (HCC) (**d**)

prophylaxis, with long-term anticoagulation therapy being one consideration for patients with risk factors for thrombosis. At present, no standard recommendations exist for patients with cirrhosis.

DS is devoid of heparin or heparin fragments. Its antithrombotic activity has been well established. The exact antithrombotic mechanism of DS is unclear, but is thought to involve a complex interaction between its two major components. Laboratory monitoring is usually not necessary and bleeding enhancement by DS is minimal. However, patients with serum creatinine above 2 mg/dL should be monitored carefully. There is no antidote for DS, and protamine does not reverse its anticoagulant effect. DS is contraindicated in patients with severe hemorrhagic diathesis; active major bleeding; hypersensitivity to danaparoid, sulfates, or pork products; and those with positive in vitro test for antiplatelet antibodies in the presence of danaparoid.

Several studies have investigated the clinical value of warfarin (a vitamin K antagonist) in the treatment of PVT in cirrhotic patients. The rate of PV recanalization in warfarin-treated patients with cirrhosis is about 40% [21]. Orally administered warfarin is more acceptable to patients; however, treatment with warfarin is particularly difficult in patients with cirrhosis, primarily because monitoring of anticoagulation is complex in this particular situation. Notably, the results of assessments based on the INR in patients with liver disease often overestimate bleeding risk, because this index is determined in

plasma samples from patients taking warfarin [22]. The INR has only been validated in individuals with normal liver function on stable anticoagulation. In this regard, 29% variation in mean INR values was reported in a study of patients with cirrhosis treated with one of three different thromboplastin reagents [23]. Further studies are needed to determine whether the target INR value ranging between 2 and 3 is adequate in individuals with abnormal INR values before anticoagulation therapy.

Administration of AT-III to patients with cirrhosis might be efficacious in the prevention of PVT. Kawanaka et al. [24] demonstrated that low and decreasing AT-III activity was associated with the development of PVT in patients with cirrhosis who have undergone splenectomy, and that treatment with AT-III concentrate would probably prevent the development of PVT in these patients.

Previous studies showed that the rate of portal vein recanalization was significantly higher while the rate of thrombus progression was significantly lower in the anticoagulation group compared with the non-anticoagulation group. These results suggest that anticoagulation, rather than "wait-and-see" strategy, should be actively employed to maximize the recanalization of thrombosed portal veins in liver cirrhosis. However, this recommendation should be cautiously applied for the following reasons. First, only a small number of studies were included in the two comparative analyses, and none of them was nonrandomized. Second, the role of spontaneous portal vein recanalization should be considered always [9, 21]. To avoid overtreatment, future studies of cirrhotic patients with PVT who benefit most from anticoagulation are warranted.

The timing and duration of follow-up are also controversial. We tend to see patients either in the surgical or specialized coagulation outpatient clinics every 3 months for at least 1 year. Depending on the location and the extent of thrombosis, CECT should be used regularly to assess the vessel patency.

The strength of our study relative to previous studies is that we used DS for 4 weeks rather than for only 2 weeks. However, our study has three important limitations. First, we used DS to treat PVT in patients with >70% stenosis. Treatment adaptation depends on the institution. Second, the study included only a small number of patients who received warfarin as maintenance therapy. We hesitate to use warfarin in patients with cirrhosis. Many novel oral anticoagulants have been approved for such patients, but since warfarin is an antagonist, it can be used relatively safely. Third, we did not examine the long-term outcome of patients after treatment and identified the factors that affect survival.

Conclusions

Warfarin following danaparoid sodium for the treatment of PVT in patients with liver cirrhosis was safe and effective. An early diagnosis of PVT along with the evaluation of the volume of PVT on CT and an early intervention would contribute to the higher efficacy of the treatment. Thus, we recommend anticoagulation for the management of PVT in liver cirrhosis. Prevention of PVT or successful recanalization of a previously thrombosed portal vein can potentially improve survival of such patients.

Abbreviations
AT: Antithrombin; CECT: Contrast-enhanced computed tomography; DS: Danaparoid sodium; HCC: Hepatocellular carcinoma (HCC); LMWHs: Low-molecular-weight heparins; MRI: Magnetic resonance imaging; PVT: Portal vein thrombosis

Acknowledgements
Not applicable.

Funding
The authors received no specific funding for this work.

Disclaimers
This paper has not been published or presented elsewhere in part or in entirety, and is not under consideration by another journal.

Authors' contributions
SF participated in the study design, data collection, data analysis, and manuscript drafting and revision processes. YK, HS, TH, NA, MK, YS, FS, YA and KI participated in the data collection process. SS participated in manuscript drafting and revision process. HK gave final approval of the manuscript to be published. All authors read and approved the final manuscript.

Consent for publication
Not applicable. No details, images, or videos relating to individual participants are included in the manuscript.

Competing interests
Hiromitsu Kumada received honorarium from MSD K.K., Bristol-Myers Squibb, Gilead Sciences., AbbVie Inc., GlaxoSmithKline K.K., and Dainippon Sumitomo Pharma. Fumitaka Suzuki received honorarium from Bristol-Myers Squibb. Yoshiyuki Suzuki received honorarium from Bristol-Myers Squibb. Yasuji Arase received honorarium from MSD K.KKenji Ikeda received honorarium from Dainippon. Sumitomo Pharma, Eisai Co., Ltd. All other authors declare that they have no competing interest.

References
1. Tsochatzis EA, Bosch J, Burroughs AK. Liver cirrhosis. Lancet. 2014;383:1749–61.
2. Schuppan D, Afdhal NH. Liver cirrhosis. Lancet. 2008;371:838–51.
3. Tripodi A, Anstee QM, Sogaard KK, Primignani M, Valla DC. Hypercoagulability in cirrhosis: causes and consequences. J Thromb Haemost. 2011;9:1713–23.
4. D'Amico G, Garcia-Tsao G, Pagliaro L. Natural history and prognostic indicators of survival in cirrhosis: a systematic review of 118 studies. J Hepatol. 2006;44:217–31.
5. Kamath PS, Kim WR. The model for end-stage liver disease (MELD). Hepatology. 2007;45:797–805.
6. Qi X, Han G, Fan D. Management of portal vein thrombosis in liver cirrhosis. Nature Rev Gastroenterol Hepatol. 2014;11:435–46.
7. Zocco MA, Di Stasio E, De Cristofaro R, Novi M, Ainora ME, Ponziani F, et al. Thrombotic risk factors in patients with liver cirrhosis: correlation with MELD scoring system and portal vein thrombosis development. J Hepatol. 2009; 51:682–9.
8. Zironi G, Gaiani S, Fenyves D, Rigamonti A, Bolondi L, Barbara L. Value of measurement of mean portal flow velocity by Doppler flowmetry in the diagnosis of portal hypertension. J Hepatol. 1992;16:298–303.
9. De Leve LD, Valla DC, Garcia-Tsao G. Vascular disorders of the liver. Hepatology. 2009;49:1729–64.
10. Reverter JC. Abnormal hemostasis tests and bleeding in chronic liver disease: are they related? Yes. J Thromb Haemost. 2006;4:717–20.
11. Basili S, Raparelli V, Violi F. The coagulopathy of chronic liver disease: is there a causal relationship with bleeding? Yes. Eur J Intern Med. 2010;21:62–4.
12. Garcia-Tsao G, Bosch J. Management of varices and variceal hemorrhage in cirrhosis. N Engl J Med. 2010;362:823–32.
13. Tripodi A, Primignani M, Chantarangkul V, Dell'Era A, Clerici M, de Franchis R, et al. An imbalance of pro- vs anti-coagulation factors in plasma from patients with cirrhosis. Gastroenterology. 2009;137:2105–11.
14. Tripodi A. The coagulopathy of chronic liver disease: is there a causal relationship with bleeding? No. Eur J Intern Med. 2010;21:65–9.
15. Tripodi A, Mannucci PM. The coagulopathy of chronic liver disease. N Engl J Med. 2011;365:147–56.
16. Mannucci PM. Abnormal hemostasis tests and bleeding in chronic liver disease: are they related? No. J Thromb Haemost. 2006;4:721–3.
17. Matsushita T, Saito H. Abnormal hemostasis tests and bleeding in chronic liver disease:are they related? No, but they need a careful look. J Thromb Haemost. 2006;4:2066–7.
18. Meuleman DG. Orgaran (org 10172): its pharmacological profile in experimental models. Haemostasis. 1992;22(2):58–65.
19. Meuleman DG, Hobbelen PM, Van Dedem G, et al. A novel anti-thrombotic heparonoid (org 10172) devoid of bleeding inducing capacity: a survey of its pharmacological properties in experimental animal models. Thromb Res. 1982;27:353–63.
20. Naeshiro N. Efficacy and safety of the anticoagulant drug, danaparoid sodium, in the treatment of portal vein thrombosis in patients with liver cirrhosis. Hepatol Res. 2015;45:656–62.

21. Qi X, Yang Z, Fan D. Spontaneous resolution of portal vein thrombosis in liver cirrhosis: where do we stand, and where will we do? Saudi J Gastroenterol. 2014;20:265–6.
22. Qi X, Wang J, Chen H, Han G, Fan D. Nonmalignant partial portal vein thrombosis in liver cirrhosis: to treat or not to treat? Radiology. 2013;266:994–5.
23. Francoz C, Belghiti J, Vilgrain V, Sommacale D, Paradis V, Condat B, Denninger MH, Sauvanet A, Valla D, Durand F. Splanchnic vein thrombosis in candidates for liver transplantation: usefulness of screening and anticoagulation. Gut. 2005;54:691–7.
24. Kawanaka H, Akahoshi T, Kinjo N, Konishi K, Yoshida D, Anegawa G, Yamaguchi S, Uehara H, Hashimoto N, Tsutsumi N, Tomikawa M, Maehara Y. Impact of antithrombin III concentrates on portal vein thrombosis after splenectomy in patients with liver cirrhosis and hypersplenism. Ann Surg. 2010;251:76–83.

13

Pre-treatment alphafeto protein in hepatocellular carcinoma with non-viral aetiology

Siriwardana Rohan Chaminda[1*], Thilakarathne Suchintha[1], Niriella Madunil Anuk[2], Dassanayake Anuradha Supun[3], Gunathilake Mahen Bhagya[1], Liyanage Chandika Anuruddha Habarakada[1] and De Silva Hithadurage Janaka[2]

Abstract

Background: Alpha-fetoprotein (AFP) is a biomarker for hepatocellular carcinoma (HCC). The significance of pre-treatment AFP (pt-AFP) in non-viral HCC (nvHCC) is not clear.

Methods: Patients with nvHCC, referred to a Hepatobiliary Clinic from September 2011–2015 were screened. HCC was diagnosed using American Association for the Study of Liver Disease guidelines, and TNM staged. nvHCC was diagnosed when HBsAg and anti-HCVAb was negative. Child-Turcotte-Pugh (CTP) and Model for End-stage Liver Disease (MELD) scores were calculated. AFP level was evaluated against patient characteristics, tumour characteristics and survival.

Results: Three hundred eighty-nine patients with nvHCC [age 64(12–88) years; 344(88.4%) males] were screened. Median AFP was 25.46 ng/ml (1.16–100,000). 41.2% ($n = 160$) Of patients had normal AFP level. 22.9% ($n = 89$) had AFP over 400 ng/ml. Female gender ($P < 0.05$), vascular invasion ($P < 0.001$), tumours over 5 cm ($P < 0.05$), late TNM stage ($P < 0.001$) and non-surgical candidates had higher AFP levels. Diffuse type ($P < 0.001$), macro vascular invasion ($P < 0.001$) and late stage tumours ($P < 0.001$) had AFP over 400 ng/ml. Having AFP below 400 ng/ml was associated with longer survival (16 vs. 7 months, $P < 0.001$).

Conclusion: Pre treatment AFP has a limited value In diagnosing nvHCC, Having a AFP value over 400 ng/ml was associated with aggressive tumour behaviour and poor prognosis.

Keywords: Carcinoma hepatocellular/diagnosis, Carcinoma hepatocellular/aetiology, Alpha-fetoproteins/analysis, Prognosis

Background

Hepatocellular carcinoma (HCC) is the second leading cause of cancer death worldwide [1]. Half of all cases of HCC are associated with hepatitis B virus infection and 25% associate with hepatitis C virus [2]. In absence of viral aetiology other factors such as alcoholic liver disease, non - alcoholic steato - hepatitis (NASH), intake of aflatoxin contaminated food, diabetes, and obesity [3, 4] are secondary risk factors. In Sri Lanka, great majority of patients with HCC are not associated with viral aetiology [5] in keeping with the low prevalence of Hepatitis B

and C [6, 7] in the country. Non-alcoholic fatty liver disease (NAFLD) and non-alcoholic steato-hepatitis (NASH) are becoming increasingly prevalent in the Asian continent and are already a leading cause of chronic liver disease in the region [8–10].

Serum alpha-fetoprotein (AFP) is a commonly used screening biomarker in patients at risk for HCC. Use of AFP in diagnosing HCC has been debated due to its variability in sensitivity and specificity [11]. It has been recognized as a poor prognostic factor in patients with HCC. Hence serum AFP level is included in some HCC staging systems [12]. It has also found to vary with the etiology of liver disease [13]. There is paucity of data on the significance of pre treatment alpha–fetoprotein in HCC patients of non-viral aetiology. This study analyse

* Correspondence: rohansiriwardana@yahoo.com
[1]Department of surgery, Faculty of Medicine, University of Kelaniya Sri Lanka, Kelaniya, Sri Lanka
Full list of author information is available at the end of the article

the significance of pre treatment alpha-fetoprotein in a cohort of patients with non-viral HCC.

Methods

Three hundred and ninety patients with hepatocellular carcinoma (HCC) were referred from all around the country from 2011 September to 2015 September. One patient was infected with both hepatitis B and C viruses and excluded from the study. Rest of the patients (n = 389) with hepatocellular carcinoma of non-viral aetiology were selected for the study. Work up of patients included detailed history and examination, haematological investigations including pre-treatment serum alpha - feto protein (AFP) level and imaging with contrast enhanced CT scans of the abdomen. HCC was diagnosed according to the American Association for the Study of Liver Diseases (AASLD) guidelines [14].

Biopsy from the lesion was done only in 4 patients with atypical imaging. A detailed history was taken to assess the degree of alcohol consumption. Patients who had a history of consuming alcohol above the accepted safe limits (Asian standards: <14 units of alcohol per week in men and <7 units per week in women) prior to the diagnosis of cirrhosis were considered as having alcoholic cirrhosis. Patients who did not drink alcohol above the safe limit, had no history of contributing drug or herbal product, who were hepatitis B surface antigen and C antibody was negative, absence of auto immune disease, normal serum ferritin levels and having a normal serum copper levels were taken as cryptogenic cirrhotics.

Staging of the cancer was done according to TNM classification developed jointly by the American Joint Committee on Cancer (AJCC) and the International Union for Cancer Control (UICC). Child-Turcotte-Pugh (CTP) and Model for end stage liver disease (MELD) scores were calculated for further prognostication. Non-viral aetiology of the HCC was confirmed by Hepatitis B surface antigen testing and Hepatitis C antibody testing.

Decisions regarding liver transplantation, surgical resection, ablation, trans-arterial chemoembolization or Sorafenib therapy were made according to tumor morphology, background liver status and functional index. Management decisions were taken at a multi-disciplinary meeting. A team of dedicated hepato biliary surgeons performed surgery. The patients were followed up in a special combined medical and surgical clinic at three monthly intervals. CECT abdomen was performed three monthly in the first year and six monthly in the next two years. All the data were entered in to a database prospectively.

Data are presented as mean with standard deviation (SD), median with interquartile range (IQR) and frequencies with percentages (%). The differences between groups were evaluated using Pearson's Chi-square test, Mann Whitney U, Kruskal-Wallis Test as appropriate. Initially single variable analysis was done to screen the variables and subsequently multiple variable analysis were carried out to determine association between variables. Cumulative survival and recurrence rates were calculated using the Kaplan - Meier method and the difference between survivals was evaluated using the log - rank test. A P value of less than 0.05 was considered statistically significant. IBM SPSS Statistics V22.0 was used for statistical analysis.

Results

The median age of the study population was 64 (range 12–88) years and 88.5% were males. Sixty per cent were diagnosed patients with diabetes mellitus. 48% Were regular alcohol consumers while 20.4% were social drinkers and 31.6% were non-alcohol consumers. Background cirrhosis was noted in 84.5% of the patients. The Child - Pugh class A, B and C had 57.3%, 32.4% and 10.3% patients respectively. The median Child - Pugh score was 6 (range1–14). The median MELD score was 11 (range 5–28). Majority (45.5%) had stage III HCC. The median total tumour diameter was 6 cm (0.9–26.5). Sixty three per cent of the patients had no signs of vascular or visceral invasion. The median INR was 1.23 (0.97–98).

The median alpha feto protein level was 25.46 ng/ml (range 1.16–100,000). Only 41.2% patients had an AFP level above the reference range (0–10 ng/ml) (Fig. 1). Twenty three percent of the patients had AFP level above 400 ng/ml.

The median AFP level was compared in different sub groups (Table 1). In regular alcohol consumers, median AFP level was 38.5 ng/ml while in others median AFP was 18.57 ng/ml showing no statistical difference (P = 0.197). Female gender was associated with statistically significant higher median AFP level (P = 0.049). Tumours with vascular invasion had a higher median AFP value (P = 0.002). HCC with total tumour diameter more than 5 cm (P = 0.013) and diffuse type tumours (P = 0.002) had higher AFP levels. Late tumour stage (stage 3 and 4) was associated with a higher median AFP value compared to early stage tumours (P = 0.001).

21% (n = 81) of patients underwent curative resection, three patients were offered liver transplantation. Radiofrequancy and alcohol ablation was performed in 10% (n = 38). Trans arterial chemo embolization was done in 34% (n = 131). 35% (n = 136) of the patients were offered Sorafinib or palliative care. Patients who were candidates for surgical treatment had lower median AFP level compared to the patients who underwent nonsurgical treatment (P = 0.001). Factors such as cirrhosis, diagnosis of diabetes mellitus, Childs class, state of non-tumour liver, bile duct invasion, recurrence of tumour after treatment, metastatic tumour at presentation and number of tumour nodules were not associated with significantly elevated median AFP values.

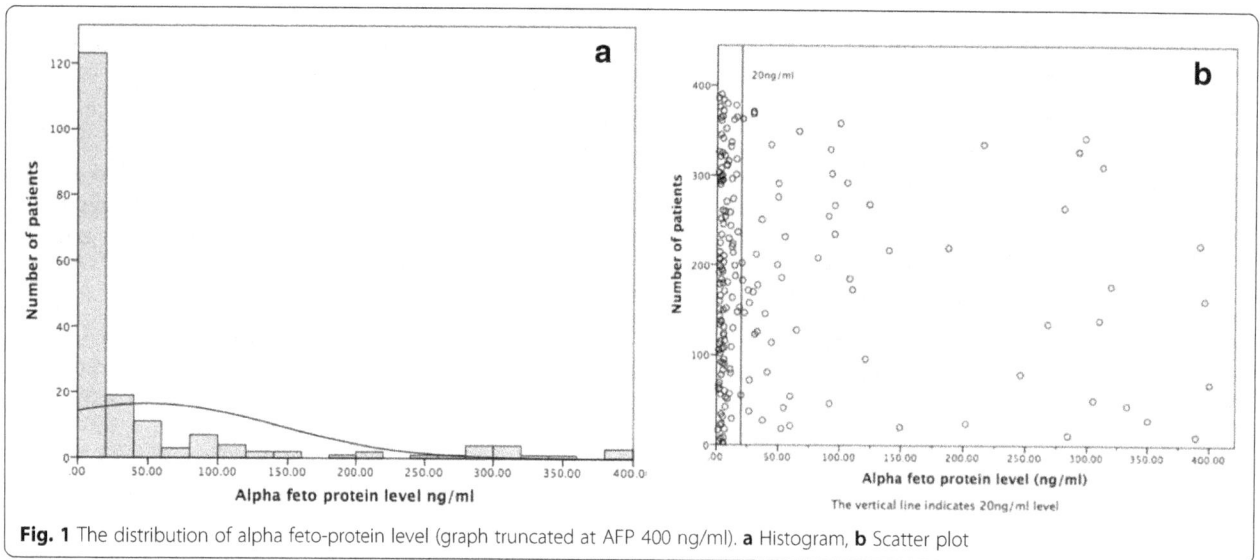

Fig. 1 The distribution of alpha feto-protein level (graph truncated at AFP 400 ng/ml). **a** Histogram, **b** Scatter plot

Patients who had AFP less than 400 ng/ml and more than 400 ng/ml were compared in different sub groups. Diffuse tumours ($P = 0.001$), invasive tumours ($P = 0.002$) and late stage tumours ($P = 0.004$) had statistically significant association of having an AFP level above 400 ng/ml. However multi nodular tumours ($P = 0.992$), large tumour diameter ($P = 0.155$) and presence of background cirrhosis ($P = 0.694$), history of alcohol consumption did not have a significant association of having an AFP level above 400 ng/ml.

Patient survival was compared taking AFP of 400 ng/ml level as the cut off point. Patients with AFP value less than 400 ng/ml had a median overall survival of sixteen months and AFP more than 400 ng/ml had only a median survival of seven months (Fig. 2a). There was a statistically significant increased survival in the patient group with an AFP value less than 400 ng/ml ($P = 0.002$). On multivariate Cox regression analysis presence of macro vascular invasion ($P = 0.940$), Child Turcotte-Pugh class ($P = 0.171$), tumour size below or above 5 cm ($P = 0.068$) were not individual predictors. Tumour nodularity ($P = 0.026$), AFP

level ($P = 0.008$), and early stage ($P = 0.042$) were individual predictors of survival.

When patients who underwent surgery as the primary treatment modality (Fig. 2b) were analysed, patients who had AFP values less than 400 ng/ml had statistically significant better survival compared to those who had AFP more than 400 ng/ml ($P = 0.013$). How ever there was no difference in survival between two AFP categories among the patients who underwent trans arterial chemo embolization as the primary treatment modality ($P = 0.545$) and the patients who did not undergo any form of treatment ($P = 0.263$).

Discussion

In this cohort of patients with non-viral aetiology, 41% patients had AFP above the reference range while 23% had AFP over 400 ng/ml. higher percentage of larger, vascular invading and advanced stage tumours had AFP level over 400 ng/ml. Surgical candidates had a lower AFP levels. Having AFP over 400 ng/ml predicted poor outcome after surgery.

Table 1 Comparison of median AFP among groups of patient

Factor (number within brackets)	AFP level (ng/ml) median and range		P value
Gender (Males 343, 88.2%)	Male 20 (1.16–100,000)	Female 268 (3–26,172)	0.049
Macro vascular invasion (Present 110, 28.3%)	Present 908 (1.16–100,000)	Absent 12.6 (1.48–92,120)	0.002
Tumour diameter (<5 cm 176, 45.2%)	<5 cm 11.5 (1.84–50,000)	>5 cm 32 (1.16–94,120)	0.013
Stage (Early 196, 50.4%)	Early 10.54 (1.48–50,000) (Stage I/II)	Late 202 (1.16–100,000) (Sage III/IV)	0.001
Macroscopic tumour (Nodular 269, 69.1%)	Nodular 9.6 (1.16–50,000)	Diffuse 2308.5 (1.84–100,000)	0.002
Cirrhotic state (Cirrhotics 301, 77.4%)	Cirrhotic 20.4 (1.48–10,000)	Non cirrhotic 65 (1.16–94,120)	0.150
Alcohol consumption (Alcoholics −266, 68.4%)	Alcoholic 26.6 (1.48–94,120)	Non alcoholic 21 (1.16–100,000)	0.197
Diabetes mellitus (Diabetics 234, 60.1%)	Diabetics 26.6 (1.48–100,000)	Non diabetics 22 (1.16–94,120)	0.808
Child-Pugh (Class A - 223, 57.3%)	Class A 12.33(1.66–94,120)	Class B/C 26.03 (1.76–100,000)	0.179
Tumour nodularity (Single 199, 51.2%)	Single 9.6 (1.16–50,000)	Multiple 17.36 (1.85–94,120)	0.119

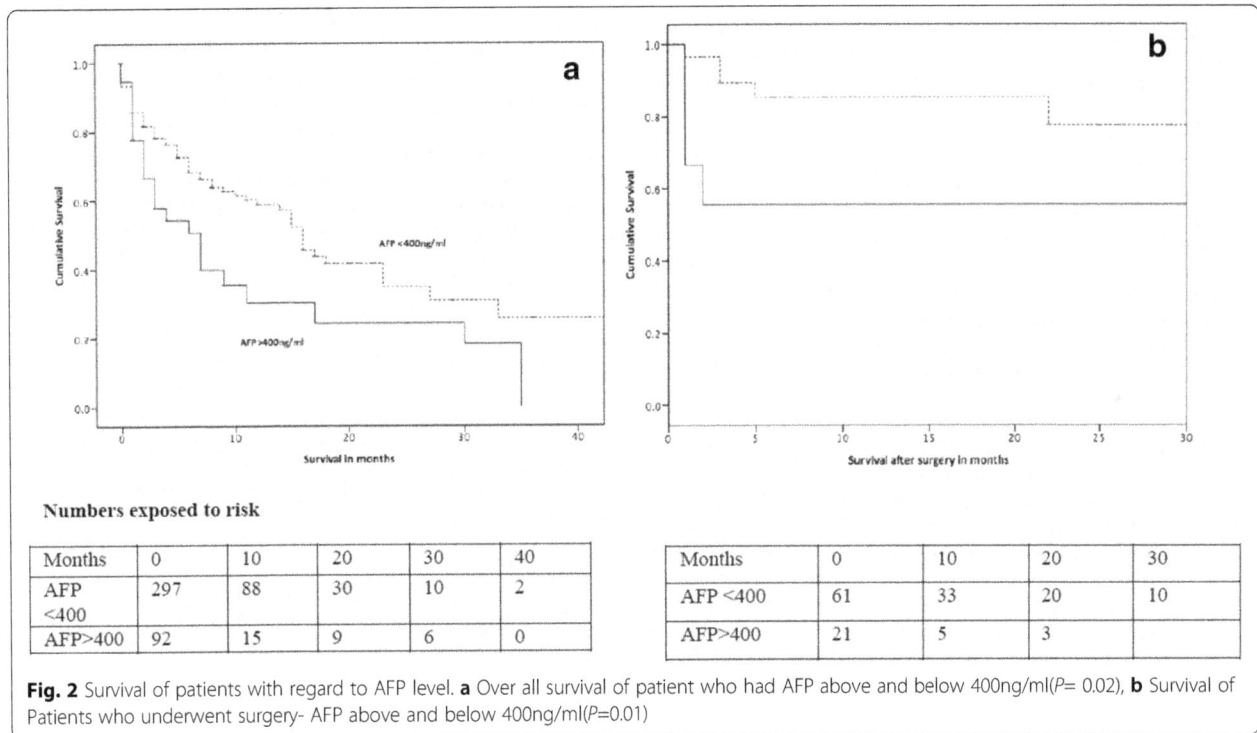

Numbers exposed to risk

Months	0	10	20	30	40
AFP <400	297	88	30	10	2
AFP>400	92	15	9	6	0

Months	0	10	20	30
AFP <400	61	33	20	10
AFP>400	21	5	3	

Fig. 2 Survival of patients with regard to AFP level. **a** Over all survival of patient who had AFP above and below 400ng/ml(P= 0.02), **b** Survival of Patients who underwent surgery- AFP above and below 400ng/ml(P=0.01)

Worldwide pattern of aetiology of HCC seem to be changing. Previously dominated hepatitis B and C are falling in incidence due to vaccination and effective treatment [15]. Non-viral HCC is becoming the predominant variety. With this change in pattern of disease, it is worth re-evaluating the previously used criteria in managing HCC.

Serum alpha-fetoprotein is a traditional tumour maker used in HCC screening and surveillance. Sensitivity and specificity of AFP in diagnosing HCC varies widely and depends on the cut off level [16, 17]. Variations in the AFP levels depending on the etiology have been observed before. In a cohort of patients with hepatitis B related HCC, AFP at 200 ng/ml and 400 ng/ml showed a sensitivity of 79.8% and 91.5% respectively. In another study specificity was 50% in HBV-positive patients compared to 78% in HBV-negative patients [18].

Limited number of researchers has looked in to the value of AFP in HCC of non-viral aetiology. In our study population of non-viral aetiology, 58.8% had normal AFP levels (<10 ng/ml). Low levels of AFP positivity was also seen in a study done by Murugavel et al. where they studies a group of HCC patients with mixed aetiology [13]. In their study AFP positivity was 20.5% (negative in 79.5%) when the patients were of non viral aetiology. This is comparable with our findings. Patients with non-viral aetiology seem to have a lower AFP levels. Thomson et al. in a systematic review on screening a cohort of mixed aetiology HCC came to the conclusion that screening ultrasound is cost effective when it is offered to patients with an AFP value more than 20 ng/ml [19]. With This criterion applied to our study it

would miss 48% of the patients with HCC. Using AFP as a screening or diagnostic investigation seem to be unreliable in them. Block et al. in their study of molecular pathology of viral HCC indicated high hepatocyte turnover in these patients [2]. Relatively lower AFP in non-viral HCC could be related to low rate of hepatocyte turn over.

In this analysis, having a higher AFP level (more than 400 ng/ml) was associated with a significant reduction in overall survival. This was also apparent when survival was analysed in subgroup of patients who underwent surgery. A similar impact of AFP on survival was noted in patients with HCC having viral aetiology [20]. Similarly, AFP is a well-known marker that predicts the outcome after liver transplantation [15] for HCC.

Conclusion

AFP level at presentation is a poor indicator for screening and diagnosing HCC in patients with non-viral aetiology. Like in other types of HCC, markedly elevated AFP levels seem to predict prognosis in these patients as well.

Abbreviations
AASLD: American Association for the Study of Liver Diseases; AFP: alpha-fetoprotein; AJCC: American Joint Committee on Cancer; CECT: contrast enhanced computed tomogram; CTP: Child-Turcotte-Pugh; HBsAg: hepatitis B surface antigen; HCC: hepato cellular carcinoma; HCVAb: hepatitis C viral antibody; INR: international normalised ratio; MELD: model for end stage liver disease; NAFLD: non alcoholic fatty liver disease; NASH: non - alcoholic steato - hepatitis; nv- HCC: non vital hepato cellular carcinoma; pt.-AFP: pre treatment alpha feto protein; SD: standard deviation; TNM: tumour node metastasis; UICC: international Union for Cancer Control

Acknowledgements
Not applicable

Funding
The project was not supported by any funding source.

Authors' contributions
RCS – concept, planning, clinical management, analysis and manuscript writing, ST- analysis and manuscript writing, MAN, ASD, MBG and CAHL – planning clinical management and manuscript writing, HJdeS – manuscript writing and final approval. All authors read and approved the final manuscript.

Consent for publication
Not applicable

Competing interests
All authors declare that there are no competing interest.

Author details
[1]Department of surgery, Faculty of Medicine, University of Kelaniya Sri Lanka, Kelaniya, Sri Lanka. [2]Department of medicine, Faculty of Medicine, University of Kelaniya Sri Lanka, Kelaniya, Sri Lanka. [3]Department of pharmacology, Faculty of Medicine, University of Kelaniya Sri Lanka, Kelaniya, Sri Lanka.

References
1. Ferlay J, Soerjomataram I, Dikshit R, Eser S, Mathers C, Rebelo M, et al. Cancer incidence and mortality worldwide: sources, methods and major patterns in GLOBOCAN 2012. Int J Cancer. 2015;136(5):E359–86.
2. Block TM, Mehta AS, Fimmel CJ, Jordan R. Molecular viral oncology of hepatocellular carcinoma. Oncogene. 2003;22(33):5093–107.
3. Sanyal AJ, Yoon SK, Lencioni R. The etiology of hepatocellular carcinoma and consequences for treatment. Oncologist. 2010;15(Suppl 4):14–22.
4. Blum HE, Moradpour D. Viral pathogenesis of hepatocellular carcinoma. J Gastroenterol Hepatol. 2002;17(Suppl 3):S413–20.
5. Siriwardana RCLCAH, Gunethileke MB. Hepatocellular carcinoma in Sri Lanka - where do we stand? The Sri Lanka journal of. Surgery. 2013;31(2)
6. Senevirathna D, Amuduwage S, Weerasingam S, Jayasinghe S, Fernandopulle N, Hepatitis C. Virus in healthy blood donors in Sri Lanka. Asian J Transfus Sci. 2011;5(1):23–5.
7. Vitarana T. Viral hepatitis in Sri Lanka. Ceylon Med J 1989;34(4):163–177.
8. Siriwardana RN, Niriella MA, Liyanage CA, Wijesuriya SR, Gunathilaka B, Dassanayake AS. Cryptogenic cirrhosis is the leading cause for listing for liver transplantation in Sri Lanka. Indian J Gastroenterol. 2013;32:397–9.
9. Dassanayake AS, AK S, Rajindrajith U, Kalubowila S, Chakrawarthi AP. De Silva. Prevalence and risk factors for non-alcoholic fatty liver disease among adults in an urban Sri Lankan population. J Gastroenterol Hepatol. 2009;24:1284–8.
10. Chitturi SFG, George J. Non-alcoholic steatohepatitis in the Asia-Paci c region: future shock? J Gastroenterol Hepatol. 2004;19:368–74.
11. Lok AS, Sterling RK, Everhart JE, Wright EC, Hoefs JC, Di Bisceglie AM, et al. Des-gamma-carboxy prothrombin and alpha-fetoprotein as biomarkers for the early detection of hepatocellular carcinoma. Gastroenterology. 2010;138(2):493–502.
12. Subramaniam S, Kelley RK, Venook APA. Review of hepatocellular carcinoma (HCC) staging systems. Chin Clin Oncol. 2013;2(4):33.
13. Murugavel KG, Mathews S, Jayanthi V, Shankar EM, Hari R, Surendran R, et al. Alpha-fetoprotein as a tumor marker in hepatocellular carcinoma: investigations in south Indian subjects with hepatotropic virus and aflatoxin etiologies. Int J Infect Dis. 2008;12(6):e71–6.
14. Bruix J, Sherman M. American Association for the Study of liver D. Management of hepatocellular carcinoma: an update. Hepatology. 2011;53(3):1020–2.
15. Kaplan DE, Reddy KR. Rising incidence of hepatocellular carcinoma: the role of hepatitis B and C; the impact on transplantation and outcomes. Clin Liver Dis. 2003;7(3):683–714.
16. Sherman M, Peltekian KM, Lee C. Screening for hepatocellular carcinoma in chronic carriers of hepatitis B virus: incidence and prevalence of hepatocellular carcinoma in a north American urban population. Hepatology. 1995;22(2):432–8.
17. Oka H, Tamori A, Kuroki T, Kobayashi K, Yamamoto S. Prospective study of alpha-fetoprotein in cirrhotic patients monitored for development of hepatocellular carcinoma. Hepatology. 1994;19(1):61–6.
18. Lee HS, Chung YH, Kim CY. Specificities of serum alpha-fetoprotein in HBsAg+ and HBsAg- patients in the diagnosis of hepatocellular carcinoma. Hepatology. 1991;14(1):68–72.
19. Thompson Coon J, Rogers G, Hewson P, Wright D, Anderson R, Cramp M, et al. Surveillance of cirrhosis for hepatocellular carcinoma: systematic review and economic analysis. Health Technol Assess. 2007;11(34):1–206.
20. Huo TI, Huang YH, Lui WY, JC W, Lee PC, Chang FY, et al. Selective prognostic impact of serum alpha-fetoprotein level in patients with hepatocellular carcinoma: analysis of 543 patients in a single center. Oncol Rep. 2004;11(2):543–50.

14

Metabolic syndrome and biochemical changes among non-alcoholic fatty liver disease patients attending a tertiary care hospital of Nepal

Bashu Dev Pardhe[1,2*] [iD], Shreena Shakya[1], Anjeela Bhetwal[1], Jennifer Mathias[2], Puspa Raj Khanal[1], Roshan Pandit[1], Jyotsna Shakya[1], Hari Om Joshi[3] and Sujan Babu Marahatta[4]

Abstract

Background: Non-alcoholic fatty liver disease (NAFLD) is mutually and bidirectionally linked with metabolic syndrome (MetS) of which it is both the cause and the consequences. Worldwide, 6.3 to 33% of the general populations are estimated to suffer from the disease with even higher prevalence in the group sharing metabolic co-morbidities. Hence, this study aims to recognize various risk factors including metabolic components and blood parameters to predict the possible incidence of the disease.

Methods: Total of 429 (219 NAFLD and 210 control) subjects were conveniently selected for study during the period of 9 months. Diagnosis of non-alcoholic fatty liver disease was done by liver imaging and based on liver enzymes. Assessment of metabolic syndrome was done by International Diabetic Federation (IDF) and National Cholesterol Education Program Adult Treatment Panel III (NCEP ATP III) criteria. All biochemical and hematological parameters and liver enzymes were estimated by using standard guideline. Mean comparison of quantitative data in different groups were performed using analysis of variance (one-way ANOVA). Risk estimation of NAFLD associated with each character was verified by Chi-square test.

Results: There was significant high levels of body mass index (BMI), waist circumference (WC) and lipid profiles in NAFLD patients in comparison to control population ($p < 0.001$). Further, according to the NCEP ATP III criteria, 13.6% of NAFLD were present with MetS where risk estimate was significant (OR = 2.15). Whereas, other criteria (IDF) for MetS showed higher frequency (30.1%) with higher risk (OR = 29.75) for the presence of MetS in NAFLD patients. The change in triglycerides (TG) and HDL-C (high density lipoprotein cholesterol) was also statistically significant in different grades of NAFLD. High risk for NAFLD was associated with existing co-morbid conditions like cardiovascular risk patients (3.18 times) followed by obese patients (1.72 times) and Diabetes Mellitus patients (1.68 times) at a significant level.

Conclusion: The result of this study suggests that there is an increased prevalence of all the components of MetS and significant changes in biochemical markers in cases of NAFLD. Timely diagnosis would help in delaying its complications and co-morbidities.

Keywords: Non-alcoholic fatty liver disease, Transaminases, Metabolic syndrome, Biochemical markers

---

* Correspondence: bashudev.pardhe@mmihs.edu.np
[1]Department of Laboratory Medicine, Manmohan Memorial Institute of Health Sciences, Kathmandu, Nepal
[2]Department of Health Science, National Open College, Sanepa, Lalitpur, Nepal
Full list of author information is available at the end of the article

Background

Nonalcoholic fatty liver disease (NAFLD) was described almost 6 decades ago and has emerged as the most common form of the chronic liver disease and its prevalence is likely to continue rising [1, 2]. Worldwide, 6.3 to 33% of the general population are estimated to suffer from the disease with even higher prevalence in the group sharing metabolic co-morbidities [3].

Hepatic steatosis based on either imaging studies or liver biopsy confirms NAFLD in patients with clinical signs and symptoms without the considerable abuse of alcohol (< 20 g ethanol/ day) [4]. The pathological spectrum of this disease ranges from a simple steatosis to steatohepatitis, fibrosis or cirrhosis of the liver [5]. Underlying metabolic risk factors for the disease progression include old age (> 50 years), sex (male> female), central obesity, insulin resistance (IR), Type 2 diabetes mellitus (T2DM), increased ferritin levels and genetic polymorphisms (patatin-like phospholipase domain-containing 3 (PNPLA3) I148M polymorphism) [6].

Previously, NAFLD has been considered as a hepatic component of metabolic syndrome (MetS), [7] but recently an association between NAFLD and MetS in type 2 diabetes mellitus has been described but the phenomenon is very complex. Indeed NAFLD is mutually and bidirectionally linked with MetS of which it is both the cause and the consequences. [2] Tan et al. [8] suggested International Diabetic Federation (IDF) criteria is applicable in an Asian population for risk assessment of MetS while Pokharel et al [9] suggests National Cholesterol Education Program Adult Treatment Panel III (NCEP ATP III) to be specific for MetS in our population but not applicable.

NAFLD progresses as a silent disease which is disclosed only after a routine health check-up following elevated transaminases levels with no any other recognized causes of fatty liver like alcohol, virus, drugs, autoimmunity [10, 11]. Liver biopsy remains the gold standard method for the diagnosis of hepatic steatosis and helps in exclusion from secondary etiology of liver injuries like drug-induced hepatotoxicity, Wilson disease and autoimmune hepatitis [4, 12]. Histological examination also differentiates NAFLD into its sub-stages; non-alcoholic fatty liver (NAFL) and non-alcoholic steatohepatitis [3, 13, 14]. The development of new technology has given the alternatives to screen the patients without much of inconvenience like ultrasonography, computed tomography, magnetic resonance imaging, transient elastography [15]. Furthermore, semiquantitative ultrasound score i.e. ultrasonographic fatty live indicator (US-FLI) is more specific for metabolic/histological variables in NAFLD [16]. Due to cost-effectiveness and availability of ultrasonography, it is widely used to detect and grade NAFLD in our country.

Various changes in the biochemical profile can be observed in the patients with the disease. Elevated serum transaminases level remains the most common or sometimes the only abnormal laboratory finding. Although the prime abnormality, liver enzymes may be normal in greater than 70% of the patients with NAFLD [4]. Serum level of alkaline phosphatase (ALP), γ-glutamyl transferase (GGT) or both is frequently elevated although the level is lower than in alcoholic hepatitis. There is also an increase in the triglyceride (TG) and low-density lipoprotein cholesterol (LDL-C) level posing a cardiovascular risk [17].The mechanisms underlying excess cardiovascular risk in NAFLD patients is much more complex and involves both generic mechanisms associated with the MetS and other specifically associated with NAFLD [2, 18]. The studies from the past decade have projected the increasing morbidity and mortality of the patients with NAFLD, not due to the liver-related complications but primarily because of cardiovascular disease [19].

Early diagnosis is very important in the timely management of the NAFLD. But there is not a single biochemical marker for confirmation of NAFLD. Hence, this study aims to recognize various risk factors including metabolic components and blood parameters to predict the possible incidence of the disease.

Methods

A hospital-based cross-sectional study was conducted in a tertiary care teaching hospital in Nepal during the period of 9 months. A total number of 429 (219 NAFLD and 210 control) subjects were selected conveniently for the study from the patients visiting for their regular medical checkup. Diagnosis of NAFLD was based on imaging (fatty liver) in the absence of competing for the cause of steatosis [12, 20]. Fatty live imaging by ultrasonography was performed by experienced Radiologist by Medison SonoAce R7 ultrasound machine and patient with visual diffused hepatic steatosis were further graded to describe the extent of fatty change in the liver. Grading was done based on the standard criteria accepted by American, Gastroenterological Association [21].

Grade I: Increased hepatic echogenicity with visible periportal and diaphragmatic echogenicity.

Grade II: Increased hepatic echogenicity with imperceptible periportal echogenicity, without obscuration of the diaphragm.

Grade III: Increased hepatic echogenicity with imperceptible periportal echogenicity and obscuration of the diaphragm.

Patients with normal hepatic ultrasonography were categorized as a control. Information regarding the patient demography (age, sex), height, weight, blood pressure, and related drug therapy were collected, measured by standard protocol and recorded in a clinical profile form. About 5 ml of fasting blood specimen was collected from every individual, processed and then analyzed for blood chemistry parameters (lipid profile, liver profile and renal profile) by standard methods as per the guideline provided by the reagent manufacturer (Human Gm Bh, Germany). Fasting blood glucose was estimated to diagnose Diabetes Mellitus. For categorization of DM from the total population, the T2DM diagnostic criteria provided by the International Diabetes Federation (IDF) was used [22]. Further, the study population was categorized as with and without metabolic syndrome based on the cut-offs value provided by National Cholesterol Education Adult Treatment Panel III (NCEP/ATP III) criteria 2001 and International Diabetic Federation (IDF) criteria 2005 [23]. Total cholesterol (TC), TG, and high density lipoprotein cholesterol (HDL-C) were estimated and LDL-C was calculated by using Friedwald equation. Aspartate aminotransferase (AST), alanine aminotransferase (ALT), ALP, total protein, and albumin were estimated in the total population to assess liver function by using standard methods. The normal range for both ALT and AST was considered up to 42 U/L in male and up to 32 U/L in female as provided by reagent manufacturer guideline [24]. All biochemical parameters were analyzed by HumaStar 300 fully automated analyzer following manufacturers' instructions. Hematological parameters were analyzed by automated cell counter (Huma Count 30^{TS} - HUMAN DIAGNOSTICS).

Inclusion and exclusion criteria
Patients above the age of 30 years and below 60 years attending Manmohan Memorial Teaching Hospital (MMTH) during the period of 9 months were included in the study after taking their informed and written consent.

Control- Apparently healthy individuals visiting for their regular health checkup and without any history of elevated liver enzymes during past 6 months and without fatty liver (imaging) on diagnosis were included.

NAFLD- Patients with a history of elevated liver enzymes at least once during past 6 months of their hospital visit were included and evaluated by imaging (fatty liver) for the confirmation of NAFLD. The population with a history of regular alcohol intake in past 6 months, history of steroid intake for > 2 weeks in past 6 months and any evidence of prescribed hepatotoxic drugs (methotrexate) were excluded from the study. In addition Patients with liver cirrhosis, kidney disease, evidence of bone diseases were also excluded from the study. Further, patients with positive Hepatitis B surface antigen and positive hepatitis C antibody on blood test were also barred.

Ethical approval was taken from the Institutional Review Committee (IRC) of Manmohan Memorial Institute of Health Sciences (MMIHS).Written consent was taken from each individual before their participation in the study. Data regarding personal information were coded and kept confidential.

Data analysis
Data were analyzed using SPSS version 20.0 (IBM Corp., Armonk, NY, USA) and Microsoft Excel 2013. Quantitative data recorded with normal distribution were expressed in mean ± SD and were analyzed by Student's t-test. Mean comparison of quantitative data in different groups were performed using analysis of variance (one--way ANOVA). Qualitative data were analyzed by Chi-square test. Risk estimation of NAFLD associated with each character was also verified by Chi-square test. $P < 0.05$ was considered statistically significant.

Results
The study was carried out in Manmohan Memorial Teaching Hospital (MMTH) among 429 study population of which 225 were male and 204 were female. The mean age of study population was 56 ± 10 year. On diagnosis by ultrasonography, 54% were present in grade I, 39% with grade II and 7% were with grade III NAFLD. On average, AST exceeded the upper normal limit in 46% of cases, ALT in 54%, ALP in 9% and GGT in 23%. There were significant high levels of body mass index (BMI), waist circumference (WC), systolic blood pressure (SBP), and diastolic blood pressure (DBP) in NAFLD patients as compared to control population ($p < 0.001$). In addition, lipid profile parameters showed significant statistical elevation among NAFLD patients. (Table 1).

Overall, distributions of metabolic components in NAFLD and control groups are illustrated in Table 2. The varied frequency distribution of metabolic components was reported as, low HDL-C with the highest frequency (69.8%), and followed by high TG (60.27%), overweight (57.5%) and hypertension (56.1%). Further, according to the NCEP ATP III criteria, 13.6% of NAFLD were present with MetS where risk estimate was significant (OR = 2.15). In addition, other criteria (IDF) for MetS showed higher frequency (30.1%) with higher risk (OR = 29.75) for the presence of MetS in NAFLD patients.

When variations in liver enzymes were compared in different grades of NAFLD, it was observed that with an increase in hepatic steatosis, ALP level also increased significantly. Also, changes in ALT were significant between the grades of NAFLD while no significant change in AST was observed. The change in TG and HDL-C was also statistically significant in different grades of NAFLD where TG was found to increase while HDL-C decreased with steatosis. There was no significant change in TC and LDL-C between different grades of NAFLD-(Table 3).

Table 1 Comparisons of biochemical parameters between control and NAFLD populations

	NAFLD	Control	p
Age (years)	44.24 ± 13.45	45.38 ± 14.67	0.985
BMI (kg/m²)	26.41 ± 4.74	23.61 ± 3.51	**< 0.001**
WC (cm)	89.55 ± 9.73	76.34 ± 6.12	**< 0.001**
SBP (mmHg)	133.79 ± 12.72	126.64 ± 10.13	**< 0.001**
DBP (mmHg)	85.82 ± 7.91	80.85 ± 7.01	**< 0.001**
Total Bilirubin (mg/dl)	0.85 ± 0.162	0.85 ± 0.097	0.776
Direct Dilirubin (mg/dl)	0.24 ± 0.081	0.23 ± 0.047	0.619
ALT (U/L)	41.93 ± 23.98	22.86 ± 6.99	**< 0.001**
AST (U/L)	38.66 ± 20.20	25.64 ± 7.27	**< 0.001**
ALP (U/L)	170.74 ± 51.39	143.62 ± 40.79	**< 0.001**
Uric Acid (mg/dl)	5.34 ± 1.18	4.64 ± 1.08	**< 0.001**
FBS (mg/dl)	106.52 ± 37.82	89.23 ± 16.43	**< 0.001**
Total cholesterol (mg/dl)	191.62 ± 40.0	154.51 ± 18.9	**< 0.001**
Triglyceride (mg/dl)	191.30 ± 94.29	113.83 ± 21.56	**< 0.001**
HDL-C (mg/dl)	42.51 ± 3.50	46.18 ± 3.82	**< 0.001**
LDL-C (mg/dl)	110.82 ± 35.79	85.57 ± 18.76	**< 0.001**
Creatinine (mg/dl)	0.93 ± 0.16	0.92 ± 0.16	0.561
Urea (mg/dl)	25.41 ± 5.96	27.014 ± 6.63	0.13
Hemoglobin (g/dl)	14.47 ± 1.83	17.46 ± 2.21	0.25
TLC (cells/µl)	8895.89 ± 1226.22	5931.43 ± 1003.12	0.43
RBC (millions/ µl)	4.98 ± 0.69	4.83 ± 0.52	0.145
Platelet (cells/ µl)	282,000.01 ± 72,872.61	297,442.86 ± 69,208.074	0.196
Total protein (g/dl)	6.49 ± 0.65	7.38 ± 0.65	**< 0.001**
Albumin (g/dl)	3.42 ± 0.41	4.41 ± 0.53	**< 0.001**

Bold represents statistically significant values

BMI body mass index, *WC* waist circumference, *SBP* systolic blood pressure, *DBP* diastolic blood pressure, *ALT* alanine aminotransferase, *AST* aspartate aminotransferase, *ALP* alkaline phosphatase, *FBS* fasting blood sugar, *HDL-C* high density lipoprotein cholesterol, *LDL-C* low density lipoprotein cholesterol, *TLC* total leucocyte count, *RBC* red blood cell count

Table 2 Distribution of metabolic components in study population

Metabolic components	Control	NAFLD	X²	OR (95%CI)
Age: > 50 years	10%	16.4%	1.28	0.56(0.21–1.53)
BMI: ≥25 kg/m²	30%	57.5%	10.99	3.16(1.58–6.31)[a]
WC: > 94 cm (M),> 80 cm (F)	11.4%	56.1%	31.75	0.10(0.04–0.24)[a]
WC: > 102 cm (M),88 cm (F)	1.4%	30.1%	21.821	29.76(3.88–228.03)[a]
Blood Pressure: ≥130/85 mmHg	35.7%	56.1%	6.01	2.30(1.17–4.50)
TG: ≥150 mg/dl	2.9%	60.27%	53.98	51.58(11.71–227.12)[a]
Low HDL: < 40 mg/dl(M),< 50 mg/dl (F)	47.1%	69.8%	7.61	2.59(1.30–5.16)[b]
MetS + (NCEP ATPIII-criteria)	1.4%	13.6%	10.31	2.15(1.70–2.52)[b]
MetS + (IDF-criteria)	1.4%	30.1%	21.82	29.75(3.888–228.03)[a]

[a]-*p* < 0.001, [b]-*p* < 0.005

F female, *M* male, *MetS + (NCEPATPIII)* metabolic syndrome present by National Cholesterol Education Program Adult Treatment Panel III, *MetS + (IDF)* metabolic syndrome present by International Diabetic Federation

Table 3 Comparison of liver markers and lipid profile between different grades of NAFLD

Liver markers	Grade I- NAFLD (n = 120)	Grade II- NAFLD (n = 87)	Grade III- NAFLD (n = 12)	p
ALT (U/L)	33.65 ± 16.51	53.52 ± 29.20	40.75 ± 9.42	**0.002**
AST (U/L)	34.87 ± 20.63	43.86 ± 19.37	38.75 ± 17.53	0.191
ALP (U/L)	160.80 ± 51.28	177.48 ± 44.57	221.25 ± 74.10	**0.049**
TP (g/dl)	6.70 ± 0.57	6.26 ± 0.70	6.20 ± 0.47	**0.014**
Albumin (g/dl)	3.53 ± 0.42	3.31 ± 0.38	3.07 ± 0.13	**0.021**
TB (mg/dl	0.85 ± 0.16	0.82 ± 0.09	1.07 ± 0.36	**0.011**
DB (mg/dl)	0.23 ± 0.06	0.24 ± 0.10	0.27 ± 0.15	0.593
Lipid profile				
TC	184.21 ± 36.67	197.71 ± 41.05	221.51 ± 53.35	0.117
TG	156.97 ± 62.95	227.86 ± 112.32	269.57 ± 85.23	**0.001**
HDL-C	43.62 ± 2.87	41.34 ± 3.99	40.00 ± 2.16	**0.009**
LDL-C	109.18 ± 32.48	110.71 ± 38.44	127.51 ± 53.25	0.627

Bold represents statistically significant values ($p < 0.05$). n- the number of patients

The relative risk of co-morbidity along with NAFLD is demonstrated in Table 4. High risk for NAFLD was associated with existing co-morbid conditions like cardiovascular risk patients (3.18 times) followed by obese patients (1.72 times) and Diabetes Mellitus patients (1.68 times) at a significant level. (Table 4).

Discussion

In our study, the overall incidence of NAFLD was about 51%. The overall prevalence of NAFLD was reported in Western countries, ranging from 15 to 51%. However, Asian countries have reported lowest prevalence of NAFLD, for instance, Japan's prevalence rate ranged from 9 to 14% [25]. Elevated liver enzymes (ALT, GGT, AST) are the sign of liver injury and may be the potent

Table 4 Risk estimation for NAFLD in association with pre-existing co-morbid conditions

	NAFLD (n)	Control (n)	X^2	RR	p
Diabetes (FBS ≥ 126 mg/dl)					
Yes	36	9	5.621	1.68	0.016
No	183	201			
Cardiovascular Risk (TC/HDL-C > 5)					
Yes	135	9	52.721	3.18	**< 0.001**
No	84	201			
Hyperurecemia (UA > 7.5 mg/dl)					
Yes	33	15	2.259	1.41	0.107
No	186	195			
Central Obesity (WC > 94 cm(M),> 80 cm(F))					
Yes	123	24	34.909	2.50	**< 0.001**
No	96	186			

Bold represents statistically significant values ($p < 0.05$). RR- relative risk, n- the number of population

surrogate markers of NAFLD [26]. In the present study, there was a significant rise in the liver enzymes and lipid profiles except for HDL-C, which was significantly less as compared to the controls. Likewise, a study carried out by Agarwal et al. and Uttareshvar et al also reported an increase in TG, TC, VLDL-C, LDL-C and decrease HDL-C levels, indicating possible atherogenic dyslipidaemia [27, 28] . Thus, most of the earlier studies are in concordance with our observation. The influx of high fatty acids in the liver causes liver toxicity and additionally, inflammatory cytokines, TNF-6 also plays a major role in the development of hepatocellular injury causes NAFLD and fatty liver with mild to moderate increase of liver enzymes [29].

Noteworthy, important and well-established clinical association of NAFLD with dyslipidaemia, hypertension, and obesity has been documented in several studies resulting in increased mortality rates in many countries. In our study, low HDL-C and hypertriglyceridaemia are present in 69.8 and 60.27% of NAFLD patients respectively which was in accordance with the study done by Santhoshakumari et al. [30]. Additionally, the prevalence of low HDL-C was about 71.7% and hypertriglyceridaemia was about 42.4% in a study by Rafique et al [31]. The probable reason for the high incidence of dyslipidaemia might be due to unhealthy diet and lack of exercise. Similarly, the present study showed that over-weight was present in 57.5% and hypertension in 56.1% of NAFLD patients which was higher compared to the study of Santhoshakumari et al and Shen et al [30, 32].

The overall prevalence of metabolic syndrome in NAFLD patients varied based on the diagnostic criteria used (IDF, NCEP ATP III). In the present study, the prevalence of MetS was highest (30.1%) with the IDF criteria, showing higher risk (OR = 29.75, 95%CI: 3.88–

228.03). In the study of Chen et al., the prevalence of MetS was 11.11, 8.48 and 5.30% on the basis of diagnostic criteria IDF, NCEP ATP III and Chinese Diabetes Society (CDS) respectively [33]. This difference might be due to the population sample studied and the diagnostic criteria used. The lower prevalence (13.6%) of NCEP ATP III criteria is due to its relatively higher cut off values for waist circumference and this can underestimate the prevalence of MetS and risk of CVD in our population [34].

In this study, the majority of patients (54.8%) had grade I NAFLD. When liver enzymes were compared in different grades of NAFLD, ALP level increased significantly with increase in hepatic steatosis. Further, changes in ALT were also significant between the grades of NAFLD while no significant change in AST was observed. To the flip side, Cordeiro et al reported no significant changes in ALT, AST, and ALP levels among individuals with hepatic steatosis [35]. In the current study, the change in TG and HDL-C was also statistically significant in different grades of NAFLD reflecting increased TG but decreased HDL-C levels with steatosis. No any significant changes in TC and LDL-C were noted between different grades of NAFLD. In contrast to our study, the differences in serum TG and TC were not statistically significant with the increasing grades of NAFLD but statistically significant lower serum HDL-C was observed in the study of Kirovski et al. [36]. Furthermore, in the study of Mahaling et al., the change in TC, HDL-C, LDL-C, and VLDL-C showed statistical significance with increasing grades of NAFLD ($P < 0.05$), yet TG showed no significance change [27].

We also observed the higher risk of developing NAFLD with existing co-morbid conditions like cardiovascular risk, obesity and Diabetes Mellitus. In our study, cardiovascular risk patients had 3.18 times the risk of having NAFLD as compared to the control group. Incongruous, a meta-analysis study conducted in 2011 reported that the patients with NAFLD had a twofold higher risk of CVD than the control population [37]. Likewise, the obese group showed 1.72 times the risk in our setting, whereas, from a study by Khadka B et al., overweight and obese groups had 4.2 and 5.1 times the risk of having fatty liver, respectively, as compared to their normal counterparts [38].

Moreover, insulin resistance in addition to chronic dyslipidaemia appears to be a crucial mechanism of NAFLD. There is evidence that NAFLD is highly prevalent in patients with diabetes mellitus and increasing evidence suggests that diabetic patients are at high risk for developing NAFLD [10]. In addition, T2DM increases the risk of developing liver-related death by up to 22-fold as well as overall death by 2.6–3.3-fold in patients with NAFLD [4].

This study provides insight on the relationship between NAFLD and MetS and risk of co-morbidity in NAFLD patients in a specific geographical area, which could be wothful in monitoring and management of NAFLD. This was time framed cross-sectional study in a small setting with relatively lower sample size. Further, well-designed follow-up studies are needed to elucidate the causative relationship between NAFLD and MetS. The diagnosis of NAFLD was only based on imaging of hepatic steatosis and further fibrosis and cirrhosis were not confirmed by liver biopsy. Diagnosis of MetS was based on broad clinical criteria's proposed by NCEP ATP III and IDF with fulfilling three minimum components, but there may be multiple clinical and biochemical presentation on the different clustering of risk factors. Hence, the optimal defining criteria need to be followed in future studies.

Conclusion

The result of this study suggests that there is an increased prevalence of all the components of MetS and significant changes in biochemical markers in cases of NAFLD. Therefore, whenever metabolic components are encountered in the clinical setting, patients must be evaluated for the diagnosis of NAFLD by imaging (fatty liver). Furthermore, incessant endeavors are essential to study the prevalence of NAFLD within the population to monitor the epidemiology of this disease. Timely diagnosis would help in delaying its complications and also play a major role in preventing cardiac diseases as its association with metabolic syndrome is frequent.

Abbreviations

ALP: Alkaline Phosphatase; ALT: alanine aminotransferase; AST: aspartate aminotransferase; BMI: body mass index; CDS: Chinese Diabetes Society; CVD: cardiovascular disease; FBS: fasting blood sugar; HDL-C: high density lipoprotein cholesterol; IDF: International Diabetic Federation; IR: insulin resistance; LDL-C: low density lipoprotein cholesterol; MetS: metabolic syndrome; NAFLD: non-alcoholic fatty liver disease; NCEP/ATP III: National Cholesterol Education Program Adult Treatment Panel III; PNPLA: patatin-like phospholipase domain-containing 3; T2DM: type 2 Diabetes Mellitus; TC: total cholesterol; TG: triglyceride; TNF: tumor necrosis factor; WC: waist circumference

Acknowledgments

We are deeply thankful to all the patients participating in this study. Our special thanks go to all the laboratory staffs, management and officials of Manmohan Memorial Teaching Hospital Kathmandu for providing the opportunity to carry out this research work.

Authors' contributions

BDP and AB - conceived the design of the study, reviewed literature, performed necessary interventions. SS, PRK, JS, and HOJ- participated in hospital data collection and laboratory investigations. BDP, RP, and JM performed statistical analysis of data. BDP, SS, SBM, and AB - prepared the manuscript. All authors contributed toward drafting and critically revising the paper and agree to be accountable for all aspects of the work. All authors read the final version of the manuscript and approved it for submission.

Consent for publication
Not applicable.

Competing interests
The authors declare that they have no competing interests.

Author details
[1]Department of Laboratory Medicine, Manmohan Memorial Institute of Health Sciences, Kathmandu, Nepal. [2]Department of Health Science, National Open College, Sanepa, Lalitpur, Nepal. [3]Department of Radiology, Bhaktapur District Hospital, Bhaktapur, Nepal. [4]Department of Public Health, Manmohan Memorial Institute of Health Sciences, Kathmandu, Nepal.

References
1. Santoshini A, Swathi P, Babu SR, Nair R. Estimation of lipid profile in various grades of non alcoholic fatty liver disease diagnosed on ultrasonography. Int J Pharm Bio Sci. 2016;7(3):1198–203.
2. Lonardo A, Nascimbeni F, Mantovani A, Targher G. Hypertension, diabetes, atherosclerosis and NASH: cause or consequence? J Hepatol. 2018;68(2):335–52.
3. Chalasani N, Younossi Z, Lavine JE, Diehl AM, Brunt EM, Cusi K, et al. The diagnosis and management of non-alcoholic fatty liver disease: practice guideline by the American Association for the Study of Liver Diseases, American College of Gastroenterology, and the American Gastroenterological Association. Hepatology. 2012;55(6):2005–23.
4. Obika M, Noguchi H. Diagnosis and evaluation of nonalcoholic fatty liver disease. Exp Diabetes Res. 2012;2012(145754):12. https://doi.org/10.1155/2012/145754.
5. Wang S, Zhang C, Zhang G, Yuan Z, Liu Y, Ding L, et al. Association between white blood cell count and non-alcoholic fatty liver disease in urban Han Chinese: a prospective cohort study. BMJ Open. 2016;6(6):e010342.
6. Lonardo A, Bellentani S, Argo CK, Ballestri S, Byrne CD, Caldwell SH, et al. Epidemiological modifiers of non-alcoholic fatty liver disease: focus on high-risk groups. Dig Liver Dis. 2015;47(12):997–1006.
7. Villegas R, Xiang Y-B, Elasy T, Cai Q, Xu W, Li H, et al. Liver enzymes, type 2 diabetes, and metabolic syndrome in middle-aged, urban Chinese men. Metab Syndr Relat Disord. 2011;9(4):305–11.
8. Tan C-E, Ma S, Wai D, Chew S-K, Tai E-S. Can we apply the National Cholesterol Education Program Adult Treatment Panel definition of the metabolic syndrome to Asians? Diabetes Care. 2004;27(5):1182–6.
9. Pokharel DR, Khadka D, Sigdel M, Yadav NK, Acharya S, Kafle RC, et al. Prevalence of metabolic syndrome in Nepalese type 2 diabetic patients according to WHO, NCEP ATP III, IDF and harmonized criteria. J Diabetes Metab Disord. 2014;13(1):104.
10. Oliveira CP, de Lima Sanches P, de Abreu-Silva EO, Marcadenti A. Nutrition and physical activity in nonalcoholic fatty liver disease. J Diabetes Res. 2016;2016:4597246. https://doi.org/10.1155/2016/4597246.
11. Byrne CD, Targher G. NAFLD: a multisystem disease. J Hepatol. 2015;62(1):S47–64.
12. Bugianesi E, Rosso C, Cortez-Pinto H. How to diagnose NAFLD in 2016. J Hepatol. 2016;65(3):643. -4-4
13. Virk A, Steckelberg JM, editors. Clinical aspects of antimicrobial resistance. In: Mayo Clinic Proceedings: Elsevier; 2000.editors
14. Brunt EM. Nonalcoholic fatty liver disease and the ongoing role of liver biopsy evaluation. Hepatology Communications. 2017;1(5):370–8.
15. Nascimbeni F, Ballestri S, Machado MV, Mantovani A, Cortez-Pinto H, Targher G, et al. Clinical relevance of liver histopathology and different histological classifications of NASH in adults. Expert Rev. Gastroenterol. Hepatol. 2018;12(4):351–67. (just-accepted)
16. Ballestri S, Nascimbeni F, Baldelli E, Marrazzo A, Romagnoli D, Targher G, et al. Ultrasonographic fatty liver indicator detects mild steatosis and correlates with metabolic/histological parameters in various liver diseases. Metab Clin Exp. 2017;72:57–65.
17. Siddiqui MS, Fuchs M, Idowu MO, Luketic VA, Boyett S, Sargeant C, et al. Severity of nonalcoholic fatty liver disease and progression to cirrhosis are associated with atherogenic lipoprotein profile. Clin Gastroenterol Hepatol. 2015;13(5):1000–8.
18. Targher G, Lonardo A, Byrne CD. Nonalcoholic fatty liver disease and chronic vascular complications of diabetes mellitus. Nat Rev Endocrinol. 2018;14(2):99–114.
19. Mantovani A, Gisondi P, Lonardo A, Targher G. Relationship between non-alcoholic fatty liver disease and psoriasis: a novel Hepato-dermal Axis? Int J Mol Sci. 2016;17(2):217.
20. Nascimbeni F, Pais R, Bellentani S, Day CP, Ratziu V, Loria P, et al. From NAFLD in clinical practice to answers from guidelines. J Hepatol. 2013;59(4):859–71.
21. Sanyal AJ. AGA technical review on nonalcoholic fatty liver disease. Gastroenterology. 2002;123(5):1705–25.
22. Guideline for Type 2 Diabetes. International diabetes federation. In: Brussels Belgium; 2012.
23. Huang PL. A comprehensive definition for metabolic syndrome. Dis Model Mech. 2009;2(5–6):231–7.
24. Schumann G, Klauke R. New IFCC reference procedures for the determination of catalytic activity concentrations of five enzymes in serum: preliminary upper reference limits obtained in hospitalized subjects. Clin Chim Acta. 2003;327(1–2):69–79.
25. Chen C-H, Huang M-H, Yang J-C, Nien C-K, Yang C-C, Yeh Y-H, et al. Prevalence and risk factors of nonalcoholic fatty liver disease in an adult population of Taiwan: metabolic significance of nonalcoholic fatty liver disease in nonobese adults. J Clin Gastroenterol. 2006;40(8):745–52.
26. Sanyal D, Mukherjee P, Raychaudhuri M, Ghosh S, Mukherjee S, Chowdhury S. Profile of liver enzymes in non-alcoholic fatty liver disease in patients with impaired glucose tolerance and newly detected untreated type 2 diabetes. Indian J Endocrinol Metab. 2015;19(5):597.
27. Mahaling DU, Basavaraj MM, Bika AJ. Comparison of lipid profile in different grades of non-alcoholic fatty liver disease diagnosed on ultrasound. Asian Pac J Trop Biomed. 2013;3(11):907–12.
28. Agarwal A, Jain V, Singla S, Baruah B, Arya V, Yadav R, et al. Prevalence of non-alcoholic fatty liver disease and its correlation with coronary risk factors in patients with type 2 diabetes. J Assoc Physicians India. 2011;59:351–4.
29. Esteghamati A, Jamali A, Khalilzadeh O, Noshad S, Khalili M, Zandieh A, et al. Metabolic syndrome is linked to a mild elevation in liver aminotransferases in diabetic patients with undetectable non-alcoholic fatty liver disease by ultrasound. Diabetol Meta. Syndr. 2010;2(1):65.
30. Santhoshakumari T, Radhika G, Kanagavalli P. A Study of Anthropometric And Lipid Profile Parameters in Non-Alcoholic Fatty Liver Disease Patients Attending A Tertiary Care Hospital at Puducherry.
31. Taslima R, Zebunnesa Z, Rahelee Z. Core components of the metabolic syndrome in Nonalcohlic fatty liver disease. J Biochem Biophys. 2015;1(2):21–5.
32. Shen L, Fan J-G, Shao Y, Zeng M-D, Wang J-R, Luo G-H, et al. Prevalence of nonalcoholic fatty liver among administrative officers in shanghai: an epidemiological survey. World J Gastroenterol. 2003;9(5):1106–10.
33. Chen SH, He F, Zhou HL, Wu HR, Xia C, Li YM. Relationship between nonalcoholic fatty liver disease and metabolic syndrome. J Dig Dis. 2011;12(2):125–30.
34. Sharma SK, Ghimire A, Radhakrishnan J, Thapa L, Shrestha NR, Paudel N, et al. Prevalence of hypertension, obesity, diabetes, and metabolic syndrome in Nepal. Int J Hypertens. 2011;2011:821971. https://doi.org/10.4061/2011/821971.

35. Cordeiro A, Pereira SE, Saboya CJ, Ramalho A. Nonalcoholic fatty liver disease relationship with metabolic syndrome in class III obesity individuals. Biomed Res Int. 2015;2015:839253. https://doi.org/10.1155/2015/839253.

36. Kirovski G, Schacherer D, Wobser H, Huber H, Niessen C, Beer C, et al. Prevalence of ultrasound-diagnosed non-alcoholic fatty liver disease in a hospital cohort and its association with anthropometric, biochemical and sonographic characteristics. Int J Clin Exp. 2010;3(3):202.

37. Demirtunc R, Duman D, Basar M, Bilgi M, Teomete M, Garip T. The relationship between glycemic control and platelet activity in type 2 diabetes mellitus. J Diabetes Complicat. 2009;23(2):89–94.

38. Khadka B, Shakya RM, Bista Y. Non-alcoholic fatty liver disease assessment in Nepal. International journal of community medicine and. Public Health. 2017;3(6):1654–9.

15

Transarterial chemoembolization plus sorafenib for the management of unresectable hepatocellular carcinoma

Lin Li[1†], Wenzhuo Zhao[1†], Mengmeng Wang[2†], Jie Hu[3], Enxin Wang[3], Yan Zhao[4*] and Lei Liu[1,5*] (iD)

Abstract

Background: Transarterial chemoembolization (TACE) is the recommended treatment for hepatocellular carcinoma (HCC) patients at Barcelona Clinic Liver Cancer (BCLC) B-stage, whereas sorafenib is an orally administered small molecule target drug for BCLC C-stage. This updated systemic review and meta-analysis focuses on identifying the efficacy of the combination of TACE with sorafenib, which remains controversial despite years of exploration.

Methods: PubMed, EMBASE, Scopus and the Cochrane Library were systematically reviewed to search for studies published from January 1990 to May 2017. Studies focusing on the efficacy of combination therapy for unresectable HCC were eligible. The hazard ratio (HR) with 95% confidence intervals (95% CIs) for time to progression (TTP), overall survival (OS), disease control rate (DCR) and aetiology were collected. The data were then analysed through fixed/random effects meta-analysis models with STATA 13.0. The incidence and severity of treatment-related adverse events (AEs) were also evaluated.

Results: Twenty-seven studies were included. Thirteen non-comparative studies reported median OS (ranging from 18.5 to 20.4 months), median TTP (ranging from 7 to 13.9 months) and DCR (ranging from 18.4 to 95%). Fourteen comparative studies provided median OS (ranging from 7.0 to 29.7 months) and median TTP (ranging from 2.6 to 10.2 months). Five comparative studies provided DCR (ranging from 32 to 97.2%). Forest plots showed that combination therapy significantly improved TTP (HR = 0.66, 95% CI 0.50–0.81, $P = 0.002$) rather than OS (HR = 0.63, 95% CI 0.55–0.71, $P = 0.058$), compared to TACE alone. DCR increased significantly in the combination therapy group (OR = 2.93, 95% CI 1.59–5.41, $P = 0.005$). Additional forest plots were drawn and no significant differences were observed with regard to survival outcome among various aetiologies. Forest plots for separate analysis of regions showed the HR for TTP was 0.62 (95% CI 0.45–0.79, $P = 0.002$) in the Asian countries group, and 0.82 (95% CI 0.59–1.05, $P = 0.504$)) in western countries. The HR for OS was 0.61 (95% CI 0.48–0.75, $P = 0.050$) in the Asian countries group and was 0.88 (95% CI 0.56–1.20, $P = 0.845$) in western countries. These data may indicate positive TTP outcome in Asian patients but not in European patients while no positive findings regarding OS were observed in either region. The most common AEs included fatigue, hand-foot skin reaction, diarrhoea and hypertension.

(Continued on next page)

* Correspondence: yanzhao211@163.com; 18700972783@163.com
†Lin Li, Wenzhuo Zhao and Mengmeng Wang contributed equally to this work.
⁴Department of Gastroenterology, First Affiliated Hospital of Xi'an Jiaotong University, 277 West Yanta Road, Xi'an 710061, China
¹Department of Gastroenterology, Tangdu Hospital, Military Medical University of PLA Airforce (Fourth Military Medical University), 1 Xinsi Road, Xi'an 710038, China
Full list of author information is available at the end of the article

(Continued from previous page)

Conclusions: Combination therapy may benefit unresectable HCC patients in terms of prolonged TTP and DCR. More well-designed studies are needed to investigate its superiority for OS.

Keywords: Hepatocellular carcinoma, Transarterial chemoembolization, Sorafenib, Systemic review, Meta-analysis

Background

Hepatocellular carcinoma (HCC) is the most common liver malignancy. Causing approximate 700,000 deaths per year around the world, it is the third leading cause of cancer death and the fifth most common malignancy globally [1]. Furthermore, Asian countries contribute a large proportion of global HCC, making it a heavy burden in the Asia-Pacific region [2].

Currently, the most widely perceived staging system for HCC is the Barcelona Clinic Liver Cancer (BCLC) system, which integrates prognostic classification and corresponding treatment of HCC. According to the BCLC system, very early and early-stage HCC (BCLC 0 or A) should be treated with curative modalities [3–5], whereas BCLC B and C HCC classified as unresectable HCC should be considered for transarterial chemoembolization (TACE) and sorafenib, respectively [1].

Previous randomized controlled trials (RCTs) have shown that TACE can bring survival benefits to unresectable HCC patients [1]. However, the high recurrence rate after TACE treatment is a major limitation of conventional TACE (c-TACE), possibly resulting from increased expression of vascular endothelial growth factor (VEGF) and vplatelet-derived growth factor (PDGF). Repeated TACE may cause liver function deterioration [6]. Fortunately, as an inhibitor of many kinases, sorafenib can reduce proliferation and angiogenesis of tumour cells, increasing tumour apoptosis by inhibiting VEGF and PDGF receptors [7]. Therefore, combining sorafenib with TACE may be a promising strategy to reduce the recurrence rate of disease and improve the treatment efficacy compared to TACE mono-therapy [2].

Several clinical trials have evaluated survival outcomes in HCC patients who received combination therapy, but the findings differed greatly among studies and thus remain debatable. It remains a pending issue as to whether TACE plus sorafenib enhances TACE efficacy and improves survival. This updated meta-analysis aimed to analyse relevant clinical trials in recent years as much as possible (including comparative and non-comparative trials) to evaluate the efficacy of combination therapy used for unresectable HCC patients and ascertain the benefits of combination therapy.

Methods

Identification and eligibility of relevant studies

To cover as much of the relevant literature as possible, we comprehensively searched PubMed, EMBASE, Scopus and the Cochrane Library for studies published from January 1990 to May 2017. Search terms were as follows: "transarterial chemoembolization" or "chemoembolization" or "TACE" AND "hepatocellular carcinoma" or "hematoma" or "HCC" or "liver cancer" or "liver tumour" AND "sorafenib". The references of retrieved articles were also screened. The search was limited to English articles involving only adult patients.

Inclusion and exclusion criteria
Inclusion criteria
Studies that focused on combination therapy of sorafenib plus TACE in unresectable HCC were included. Studies were limited to English articles and adult patients. Necessary information included overall survival (OS), time to progression (TTP), disease control rate (DCR), adverse events (AEs) and tumour response.

Exclusion criteria
Studies that compared efficacy of combination therapy versus sorafenib alone were excluded. Non-English studies or comments, editorials, letters, case reports, reviews and meta-analyses were not considered. Studies unrelated to our topic or lacking useful information were also excluded.

Definitions and standardization
Two types of TACE were analysed in our meta-analysis, including conventional TACE (c-TACE) and TACE with drug-eluting beads (DEB-TACE). Treatments including TACE before or after sorafenib were both defined as combination therapies. Patients should receive at least one session of TACE during their treatment.

TTP was defined as the time from initial treatment to tumour progression or last follow-up. OS was defined as the time from first TACE to the date of death or last follow-up. DCR was defined as the combination of complete response rate, partial response rate and stable disease rate.

Data extraction
After initial identification of articles from databases, two researchers (Lin Li, Wenzhuo Zhao) screened studies according to the abovementioned criteria by reading titles and abstracts. At each screening step, the number of studies and the reasons for exclusion were recorded. Subsequently, the full-text of articles eligible for inclusion were independently assessed and necessary information was

extracted, including baseline characteristics, treatment strategy, OS, TTP, DCR, AEs, HR and tumour responses. Finally, all available data were pooled and analysed. Disagreements between the two researchers were discussed until consensus was reached.

Statistical analysis

Meta-analysis was performed by STATA 13.0 according to the Cochrane Handbook for Systematic Reviews of Interventions. The quality of included RCT studies was assessed by the Jadad scale [8], while non-RCT studies were assessed by the methodological index for non-randomized studies (MINORS) [9]. HR and 95% CI of TTP, OS, DCR, as well as aetiology of various studies were collected. I^2 analysis was used to assess the heterogeneity among studies. If the I^2 value was less than 50%, a fixed-effects meta-analysis model was conducted, and if the I^2 value was not less than 50% the random-effects meta-analysis model was performed. For all outcomes, a P-value less than 0.05 was considered statistically significant.

Results

Identification of eligible studies

After searching the literature within several databases, a total of 1551 studies were eventually identified for screening. According to titles and abstracts, 1507 studies were excluded, and the full texts of the remaining 44 articles were examined. Finally, 27 studies were included in our analysis, with 14 comparative studies and 13 non-comparative studies. The screening flowchart of the study is shown in Fig. 1.

Study characteristics

The 13 non-comparative studies published from 2009 to 2016 included 8 phase-II studies, 2 phase-I studies and 3 retrospective studies (Table 1). C-TACE was used in 9 studies, and DEB-TACE was used in 4 studies. Seven of the thirteen studies were conducted in Asia. The number of patients per study ranged from 14 to 222. All patients in 13 non-comparative studies were graded as either Child-Pugh (CP) class A or B, among which most patients (65–94%) were at CP A. The proportion of patients at BCLC B stage was 20–100% and there were 1.9–80% at BCLC C stage. The ECOG performance status was reported to be 0 or 1 (94–100%). Eleven studies provided aetiology information about the patients. The total rates of hepatitis viral infection ranged from 24 to 100%. The detailed baseline characteristics of patients, duration of sorafenib and the number of TACE sessions (ranging from 1 to 3) are displayed in Table 1.

Fourteen comparative studies enrolled 1689 patients in total, including 3 RCTs, 4 non-randomized controlled studies and 7 retrospective studies (Table 2). C-TACE was used in 11 studies and DEB-TACE was used in 3 studies. The proportions of patients at BCLC B and C stages were 15–100% and 38–100%, respectively. The

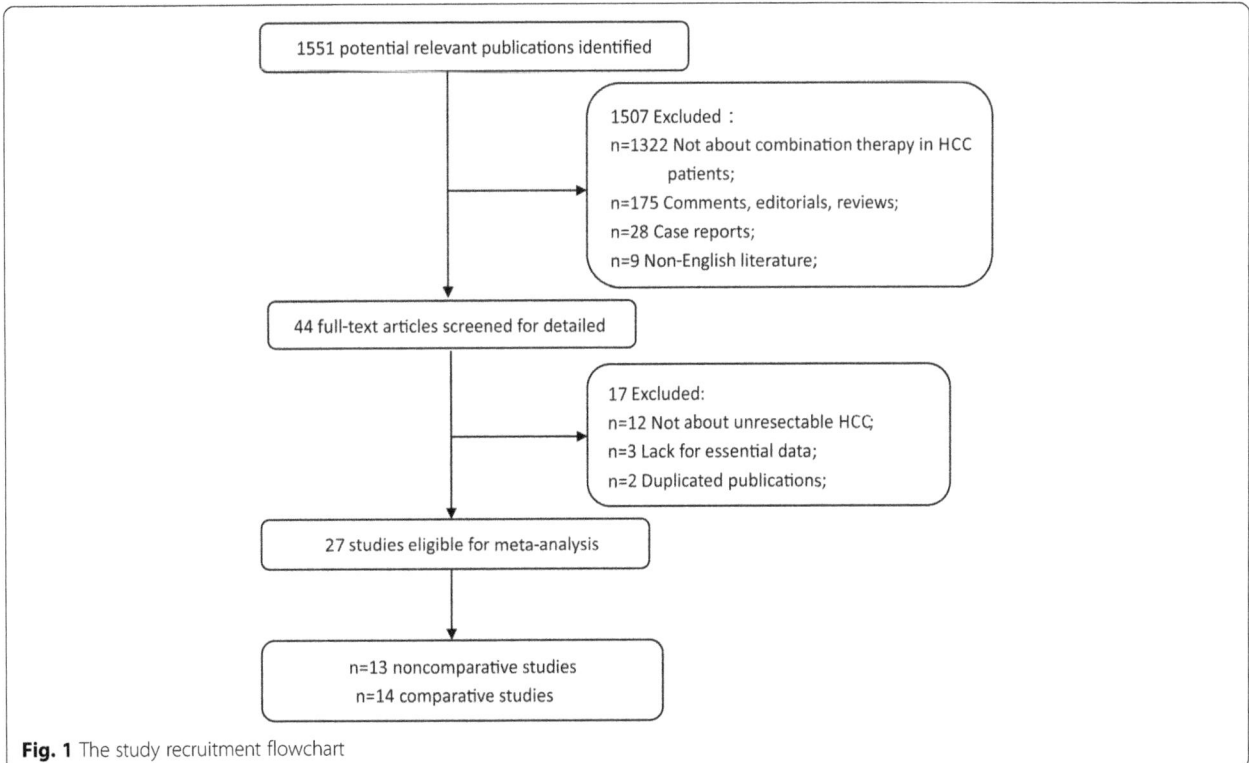

Fig. 1 The study recruitment flowchart

Table 1 Baseline characteristics of 13 non-comparative studies and patients

Authors (year) [Ref]	Study Design	Region	Patients	CPS ≤8scores	BCLC	ECOG	Aetiology	Treatment	No. of TACE	Duration Time of sorafenib
Erhardt et al. (2014) [33]	Phase II	Germany	38	NA	NA	0–2	NA	Continuous sorafenib, interrupted only around TACE	2.0(mean)	NA
Dufour et al. (2010) [34]	Phase I Open-label	Switzerland	14	A = 93% B = 7%	B = 64% C = 36%	0 = 93% 1 = 7%	HCV = 29%	Sorafenib started 1 week prior to TACE without pause for TACE	2.0(median)	NA
Cabrera et al. (2011) [a] [35]	Phase II Prospective	USA	47	A = 72% B = 28%	B = 81% C = 19%	0 = 75% 1 = 25%	HCV = 60%	Continuous sorafenib started 2–4 weeks before DEB-TACE	3.0(median)	NA
Lee et al. (2011) [36]	Phase II Prospective	South Korea	59	A = 93% B = 7%	B = 100%	NA	HBV = 88%	Sorafenib, TACE was performed at every 6–8 weeks	NA	NA
Pawlik et al. (2011) [a] [37]	Phase II Prospective	USA	35	A = 89% B = 11%	B = 34% C = 66%	0 = 46% 1 = 54%	HCV = 37%	Continuous sorafenib started 1 week before DEB-TACE	2.0(median)	NA
Park et al. (2012) [38]	Phase II Prospective	South Korea	50	A = 94% B = 6%	B = 82% C = 18%	0 = 44% 1 = 56%	HBV = 68% HCV = 18%	Sorafenib started 3 days after TACE	1.0(median)	6 month
Sieghart et al. (2012) [39]	Phase I	Austria	15	A = 80% B = 20%	B = 70% C = 30%	0 = 92% 1 = 8%	HBV = 4% HCV = 20%	Sorafenib started 2 weeks before the first TACE	3.0(median)	5.2 month (median)
Chung et al. (2013) [40]	Phase II Prospective	China and South Korea	151	A = 92% B = 8%	A = 16% B = 82% C = 1.9%	0 = 82% 1 = 18%	NA	Sorafenib started 4–7 days after TACE	2.1(mean)	NA
Zhao et al. (2013) [41]	Prospective	China	222	A = 86% B = 14%	B = 20% C = 80%	0 = 44% 1 = 50% 2 = 6%	HBV = 80% HCV = 5%	Continuous sorafenib with no breaks before or after TACE	2.0(median)	NA
Pan et al. (2014) [7]	Retrospective	China	41	A = 85.4% B = 14.6%	NA	0 = 48.8% 1 = 51.2%	HBV = 97.6% HCV = 2.4%	Sorafenib was taken 3 days after the first TACE procedure	2.0(median)	NA
Chao et al. (2014) [2]	Phase II Prospective	Taiwan	192	A = 91.8% B = 7.1%	A = 16.9% B = 81.5% C = 1.6%	0 = 81.8% 1 = 17.7% 3 = 0.5%	NA	Sorafenib on day 4 (to day 7) after the first TACE (day 1) the interrupt on day 4 before the next TACE	3.0(median)	NA
Yao et al. (2015) [32]	Retrospective	China	50	A = 88% B = 12%	B = 52% C = 48%	0 = 46% 1 = 54%	HBV = 84% HCV = 4%	Sorafenib before and after 1 week of TACE	3.0(median)	1.4 month (median)
Cosgrove et al. (2015) [a] [42]	Phase II	USA	50	A = 92% B = 8%	A = 6% B = 32% C = 62%	0 = 52% 1 = 48%	HBV = 8% HCV = 44%	Sorafenib was started 1 week before the first round of DEB-TACE	2.0(median)	1.5 month

Abbreviations: BCLC The Barcelona Clinic Liver Cancer, CPS Child-Pugh classification, ECOG Eastern Cooperative Oncology Group, NO. number, NA not available, HBV hepatitis B virus, HCV hepatitis C virus
[a] TACE with drug-eluting beads (DEB) was performed in the studies. Patients in other studies treated with conventional TACE (c-TACE)

Table 2 Baseline characteristics of 14 comparative studies and patients

Authors (year) [Ref]	Study Design	Region	Patients	CPS	BCLC	ECOG	Aetiology	Treatment	Quality Assessment
Martin et al. (2010)[a][43]	Prospective	several countries	150	ST:B = 31% DT:B = 39%	NA	NA	NA	ST, n = 30; DT, n = 120.	17
Kudo et al. (2011)[15]	Phase III Randomized	Japan South Korea	229	A = 100%	NA	0 = 87% 1 = 13%	HBV = 20% HCV = 60%	Sorafenib was given 1–3 months after TACE till progression	18
Sansonno et al. (2012)[44]	Phase II prospective randomized	Italy	40	A = 100%	B = 100%	0 = 86% 1 = 24%	HCV = 100%	Sorafenib started 1 month after TACE till progression nor unacceptable toxicity	4
Lencioni et al. (2012)[a][10]	Phase II prospective randomized	several countries	307	A = 100%	B = 100%	0 = 100%	NA	Continuous sorafenib 3–7d before TACE	4
Qu et al. (2012)[45]	Retrospective	China	45	A = 65% B = 35%	B = 35% C = 65%	0 = 95% 1 = 5%	HBV = 100%	Sorafenib started after TACE	17
Bai et al. (2013)[46]	Prospective	China	82	A = 77% B = 23%	B = 23% C = 77%	0 = 36.5% 1 = 46.5% 2 = 14.6% 3 = 1.2% 4 = 1.2%	HBV = 87.9% HCV = 4.9%	Continuous sorafenib started within 1d after TACE	19
Muhammad et al. (2013)[a][47]	Retrospective	USA	43	ST:A = 85% DT:A = 77%	A = 46% B = 15% C = 38%	NA	ST:HCV = 69% DT:HCV = 93%	Sorafenib started with 200 mg bid and then increased to 400 mg in the majority of patients	20
Huang et al. (2013)[48]	Prospective	China	155	NA	NA	NA	NA	Sorafenib started within 2 weeks of the first cycle of TACE	14
Hu et al. (2014)[14]	Retrospective	China	280	ST:A = 70.7% T:A = 67.7%	B = 100%	NA	ST:HBV = 82.9% T:HBV = 79.8%	Sorafenib after TACE	20
Ohki et al. (2015)[6]	Retrospective	Japan	95	ST:A = 70.8% T:A = 56.3%	NA	NA	ST:HCV = 75.0% T:HCV = 67.6%	Sorafenib was started within 2 weeks after TACE	17
Yao et al. (2016)[12]	Prospective	China	150	A = 84% B = 16%	B = 42% C = 58%	0 = 42% 1 = 58%	ST:HBV = 84% T:HBV = 83%	Sorafenib therapy was initiated within 1 week before or after the initial TACE treatment	20
Zhang et al. (2016)[49]	Retrospective	China	20	A = 100%	NA	0 = 85% 1 = 15%	HBV = 80%	Sorafenib was given with an interval of 4–7 days before or after TACE session	19
Wan et al. (2016)[50]	Retrospective	China	450	A = 87% B = 13%	NA	0–1 = 91% 2 = 9%	NA	Oral sorafenib was administrated before or after TACE	14
Varghese et al. (2017)[13]	Retrospective	India	124	B:A = 55.9% B = 44.1% C:A = 46.2% B = 53.8%	B = 47.6% C = 52.4%	NA	B:HBV = 37.3% HCV = 18.7% C:HBV = 26.2% HCV = 23%	Sorafenib was introduced 5d after TACE	17

Abbreviations: BCLC The Barcelona Clinic Liver Cancer, *CPS* Child-Pugh classification, *ECOG* Eastern Cooperative Oncology Group, *NA* not available, *ST* sorafenib plus TACE, *DT* DEB –TACE, *HBV* hepatitis B virus, *HCV* hepatitis C virus, *MINORS* methodological index for non-randomized studies
[a] TACE with drug-eluting beads (DEB) was performed in the studies. Patients in other studies treated with conventional TACE (c-TACE). Quality assessment of RCT trial adopted Jadad scale. Scores of non-randomized experimental study were assessed by MINORS

ECOG Performance Status was 0 or 1 (71–100%). For aetiology, HBV (hepatitis B virus)/HCV (hepatitis C virus) infection rates varied greatly. Patients in the Asian-Pacific region were mostly infected with HBV, while Japanese and European countries had more HCV infections. In 13 comparative studies, patients were TACE-responsive before sorafenib administration. Some patients in the study of Ohki et al. were unresponsive to TACE. Detailed procedures in treatment of each study are also provided in Table 2.

Tumour response, DCR, TTP, OS
Non-comparative studies
In terms of the assessment of tumour response, six studies applied the response evaluation in solid tumours (RECIST) and 6 studies applied the modified RECIST (mRECIST). Eleven studies reported DCR ranging from 18.4 to 95%. Six studies reported median TTP ranging from 7 to 13.9 months. Four studies reported median OS ranging from 12 to 20.4 months (Additional file 1: Table S1).

Comparative studies

DCR In 14 comparative studies, five studies reported DCR in combined groups ranging from 32 to 97.2% (Additional file 2: Table S2). For all five studies, DCR in the combination therapy group was substantially higher than those in the TACE alone group. The forest plot showed that the increase of DCR in combination therapy was significant (OR = 2.93, 95% CI 1.59–5.41, $P = 0.005$).

TTP Ten studies provided TTP with a median ranging from 2.6 to 10.2 months. Nine studies provided available HR for TTP (Table 3). The forest plot showed that the overall HR for TTP was 0.66 (95% CI 0.50–0.81, $P = 0.002$), indicating that combination

therapy significantly prolonged TTP. The analysis was performed in a random effect model and the I^2 was 66.4% (Fig. 2). To minimize heterogeneity, TTP in Asia-Pacific and Western studies were separately analysed by the sub-analysis of forest plots. The forest plot showed that the HR for TTP in Asian countries was 0.62 (95% CI 0.45–0.79, $P = 0.002$) and was 0.82 (95% CI 0.59–1.05, $P = 0.504$) in western countries (Fig. 3). These data may indicate positive TTP outcome of statistical significance in Asian countries. Regions may show differences in survival outcome through various factors.

OS Ten studies reported median OS ranging from 7.0 to 29.7 months, while HR of OS was available in 8 studies (Table 4). The forest plot indicated that the overall HR for OS was 0.63 (95% CI 0.55–0.71, $P = 0.058$), suggesting that combination therapy may not significantly improve OS. The analysis was performed in a fixed effect model and the I^2 was 48.7% (Fig. 4). The subgroup analysis according to different region was also performed, and the HR for OS was 0.61 (95% CI 0.48–0.75, $P = 0.050$) in Asian countries and was 0.88 (95% CI 0.56–1.20, $P = 0.845$) in western countries (Fig. 5), without statistical significance across different regions.

Relationship between aetiology and survival outcome
Four studies provided HR of aetiology for OS, and 3 studies provided HR for TTP (Table 5). Using random effect models, the forest plots indicated that the overall HR of aetiology for OS was 1.10 (0.78–1.41, $P = 0.888$) (Additional file 3: Figure S1), and the overall HR for TTP was 0.88 (0.72–1.05, $P = 0.565$) (Additional file 4: Figure S2). We may deduce that the aetiology of HCC might not have significant influence on survival outcome.

Table 3 Median TTP, HR and 95%CIs between combination therapy group and TACE alone group

Authors (year)	Combination group (95% CI)/months	TACE alone group (95% CI)/months	HR (95% CI)
Kudo et al. (2011) [15]	5.4(3.8–7.2)	3.7 (3.5–4.0)	0.87(0.70–1.09)
Sansonno et al.(2012) [44]	9.2	4.9	2.5(1.66–7.56)
Lencioni et al. (2012) [10]	5.6	5.5	0.797 (0.588–1.08)
Bai et al. (2013) [46]	6.3	4.3	0.6 (0.422–0.853)
Muhammad et al. (2013) [47]	NA	NA	0.93 (0.45–1.89)
Huang et al. (2013) [48]	5.4	3.7	0.99 (0.67–1.47)
Hu et al. (2014) [14]	2.6	1.9	0.62 (0.47–0.82)
Ohki et al. (2015) [6]	6.3	3.5	0.38 (0.22–0.63)
Yao et al. (2015) [12]	10.2	6.7	0.403 (0.251–0.646)
Zhang et al. (2016) [49]	4.9 (3.7–6.0)	2.4 (1.3–3.4)	NA

Abbreviations: *TTP* time to progression, *HR* hazard ratio, *95%CIs* 95% confidence intervals, *NA* not available

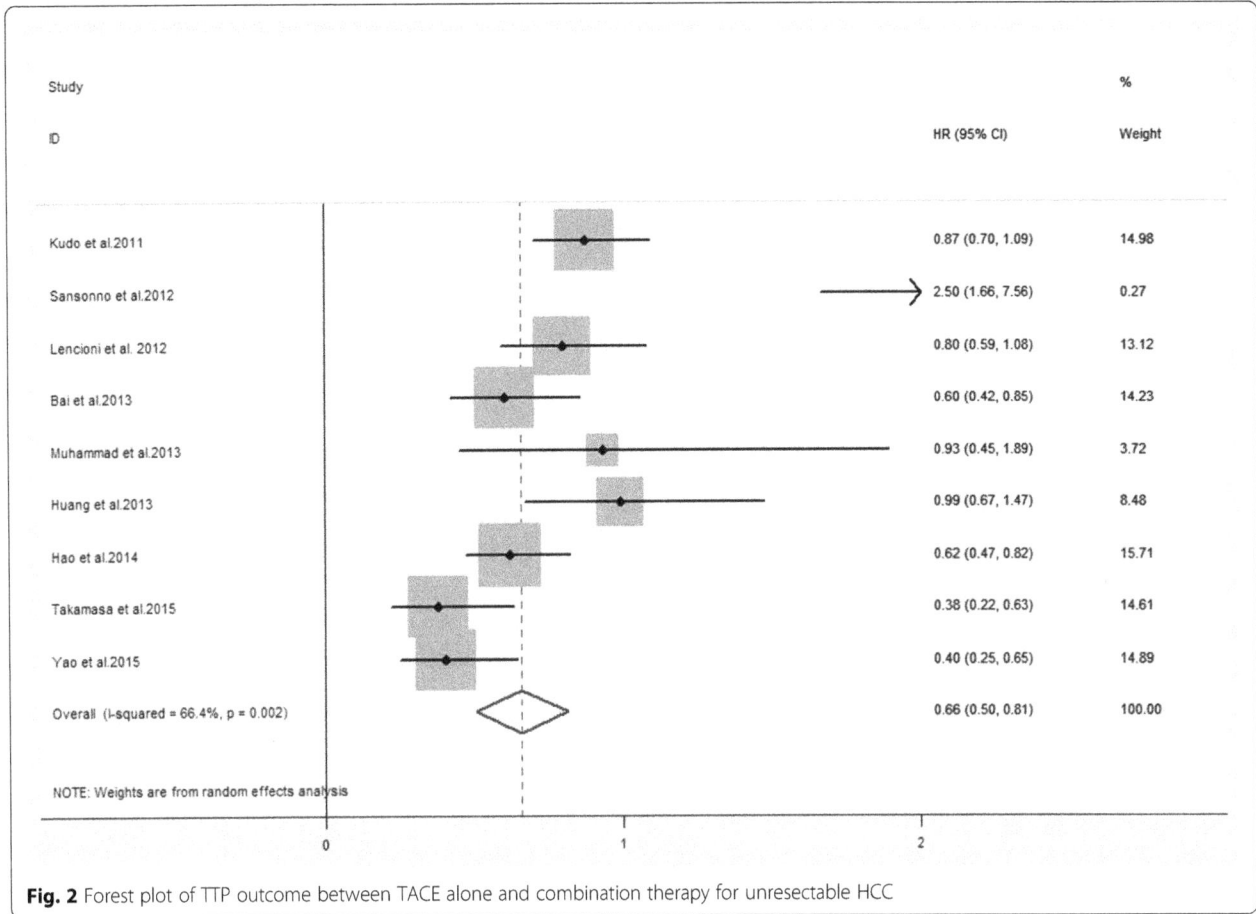

Fig. 2 Forest plot of TTP outcome between TACE alone and combination therapy for unresectable HCC

Adverse events

AEs of combination therapy included fatigue, diarrhoea, nausea, hand-foot skin reaction (HFSR), haematological events, alopecia, hepatotoxicity, hypertension and rash (Additional file 5: Table S3). Among these, the incidence of HFSR was highest. Most patients experienced at least one type of sorafenib-related AE during drug administration. Most AEs were mild to moderate and could be controlled through appropriate management, including temporary dose reduction or another syndrome-relieving treatment. The incidence of severe AEs, such as hepatic failure or gastrointestinal haemorrhage, was very low. No treatment-related deaths and disabilities occurred in these studies.

Discussion

Several clinical trials have been conducted to evaluate the efficacy of combination therapy. Our systematic review and meta-analysis collected the updated studies that evaluated the efficacy of combination therapy for unresectable HCC. The studies were published during the past 8 years, including comparative and non-comparative trials. The comprehensive analysis of 27 studies indicated that combination therapy may

have significant superiority over TACE mono-therapy in terms of TTP but not OS.

As the first globally randomized controlled trial with a relatively large sample size, the SPACE trial (sorafenib or placebo in combination with TACE for intermediate-stage HCC) conducted by Lencioni et al. showed no significant difference of TTP between the combination therapy group and the TACE alone group [10]. Later, many clinical trials conducted in different countries also evaluated the efficacy of combination treatment, and most reported findings that combination therapy was more effective than mono-therapy in terms of TTP. Among 14 comparative studies that we analysed, most studies concluded that, compared with TACE alone, combination treatment with TIPS followed by sorafenib increased the TTP in patients unresponsive to TACE [11–14].

Kudo et al. found the outcomes of clinical trials varied across different races and regions. For Japanese patients, the HR for TTP was 0.94 (95% CI, 0.75–1.19), while for Korean patients it was 0.38 (95% CI, 0.18–0.81), suggesting that the Korean patients may benefit more from combination therapy than Japanese patients [15]. Compared with other Asian countries, Japanese HCC patients

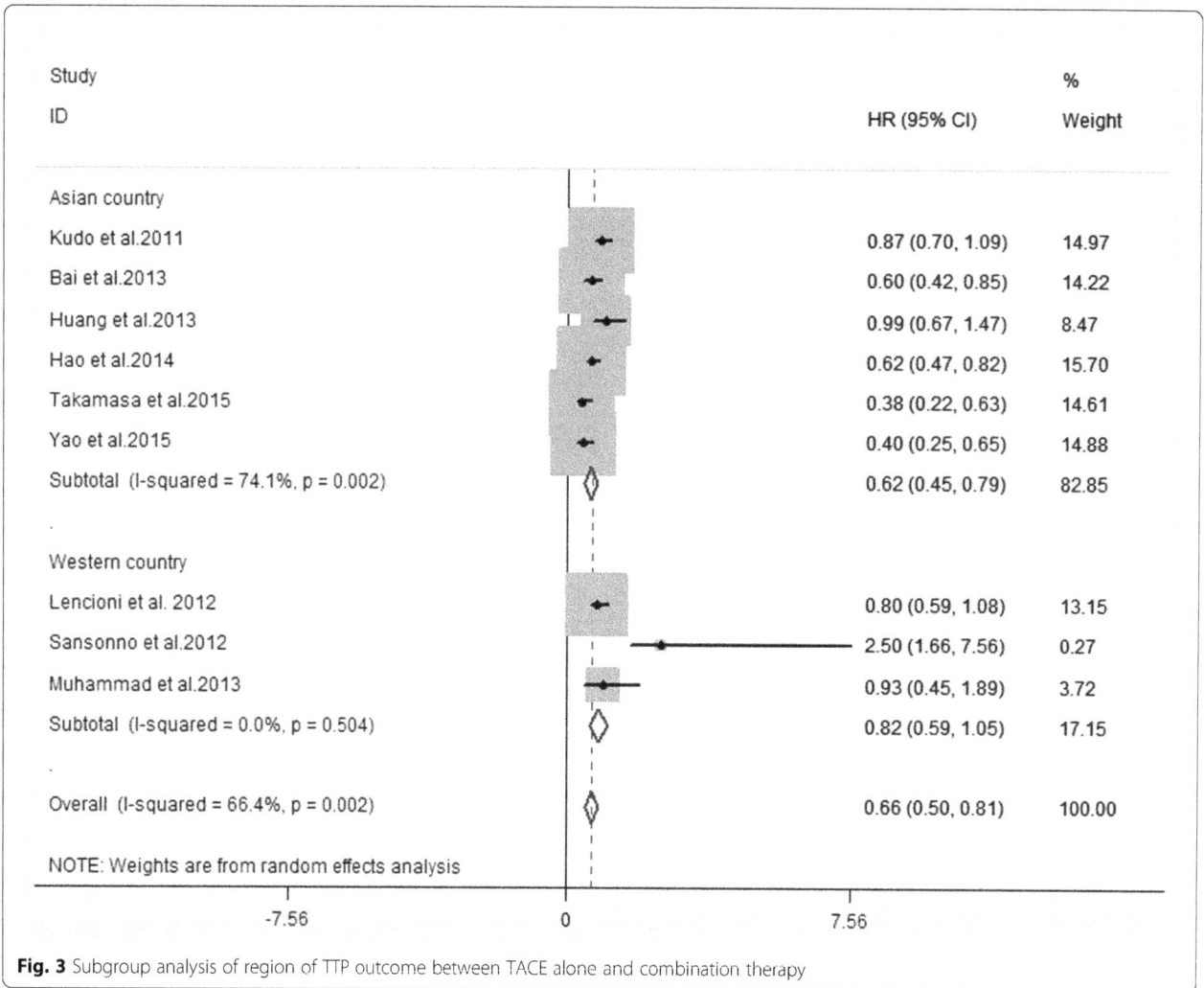

Fig. 3 Subgroup analysis of region of TTP outcome between TACE alone and combination therapy

Table 4 Median OS, HR and 95%CIs between intervention and contrast group

Authors (year)	Combination group (95% CI)/months	TACE alone group (95% CI)/months	HR (95% CI)
Kudo et al. (2011) [15]	29.7 (28.6-NA)	NA	1.06 (0.69–1.64)
Lencioni et al. (2012) [10]	NA	NA	0.898 (0.606–1.33)
Qu et al. (2012) [45]	27 (21.9–32.1)	17 (8.9–25.0)	NA
Bai et al. (2013) [46]	7.5	5.1	0.61 (0.423–0.884)
Muhammad et al. (2013) [47]	20.6 (13.4–38.4)	18.3 (11.8–32.9)	0.82 (0.38–1.77)
Hu et al. (2014) [14]	7.0	4.9	0.63 (0.48–0.84)
Ohki et al. (2015) [6]	28.7	15.6	0.43 (0.24–0.76)
Yao et al. (2015) [12]	21.7	11.5	0.449 (0.302–0.668)
Wan et al.(2016) [50]	20.23	13.97	0.75 (0.61–0.94)
Zhang et al. (2016) [49]	14.9 (6.8–23.0)	6.1 (4.0–8.1)	NA
Varghese et al. (2017) [13]	BCLC-B = 16 (12.9–19.1)	BCLC-B = 9 (6.3–11.7)	BCLC-B:NA
	BCLC-C = 9 (6.8–11.2)	BCLC-C = 4(3–5)	BCLC-C:NA

Abbreviations: OS overall survival, *HR* hazard ratio, *95%CI* 95% confidence intervals, *NA* not available

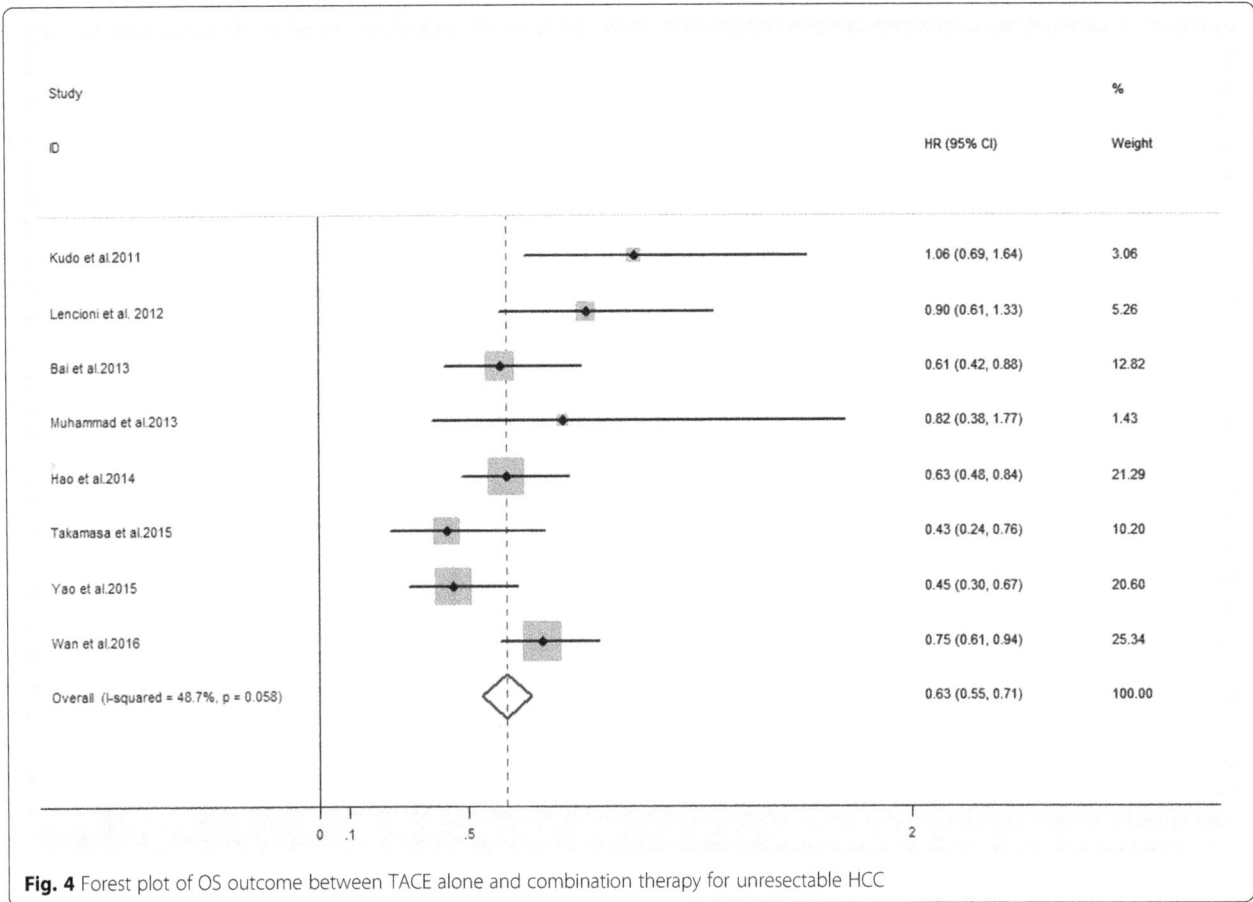

Fig. 4 Forest plot of OS outcome between TACE alone and combination therapy for unresectable HCC

had higher HCV infection rates. However, our analysis between aetiology and survival showed no significant difference. Studies have shown that the mechanism of HCC caused by HBV and HCV is different [16], and pathological manifestations and gene expression differ between HBV- and HCV-related HCC [17, 18]. In terms of tumour survival and prognosis, some studies found significantly better survival and smaller recurrence rates in HCV-related HCC than with HBV-related HCC [19, 20]. In contrast, other studies showed that the prognosis of HCV-related HCC patients was worse than that of HBV-related HCC patients [21]. This might be a potential reason for our negative finding, since the proportion of HCV-related HCC patients in the 27 studies included in this analysis was small.

The survival rate in the Asian-Pacific region was lower than that of European countries. In particular, the mortality rate of Chinese patients was higher than the average value of other regions in the world. Our analysis of regions showed that the TTP outcome in the Asian group was positive, while the European group returned a negative result. In another analysis, both groups showed a negative OS outcome. However, regions show differences through many factors. Take treatment procedure

for example; in SPACE trials, there was a greater improvement in TTP and OS HRs in patients from Asian countries than from non-Asian countries. Because non-Asian patients in the sorafenib arm discontinued TACE treatments earlier and had a shorter duration of sorafenib, both factors may have contributed to the outcome difference and may have caused bias [10]. Well-designed studies, regular drug administration and good control of confounding factors are needed to reflect the real efficacy of combination therapy.

C-TACE is performed by the injection of a mixture of a chemotherapeutic drugs and lipiodol, which block feeding vessels, and thus cause tumour necrosis [22]. DEB-TACE releases chemotherapeutic agents from micro-beads, facilitating further, more effective and more focused embolization [23, 24]. However, compared with C-TACE, it appears that DEB-TACE shows similar clinical outcomes with fewer adverse events. In terms of efficacy, whether DEB-TACE is superior to C-TACE remains debatable [25, 26].

Although there were no positive findings regarding OS in the meta-analysis, this does not necessarily suggest that combination therapy was not futile for improving the survival time of HCC patients. Many

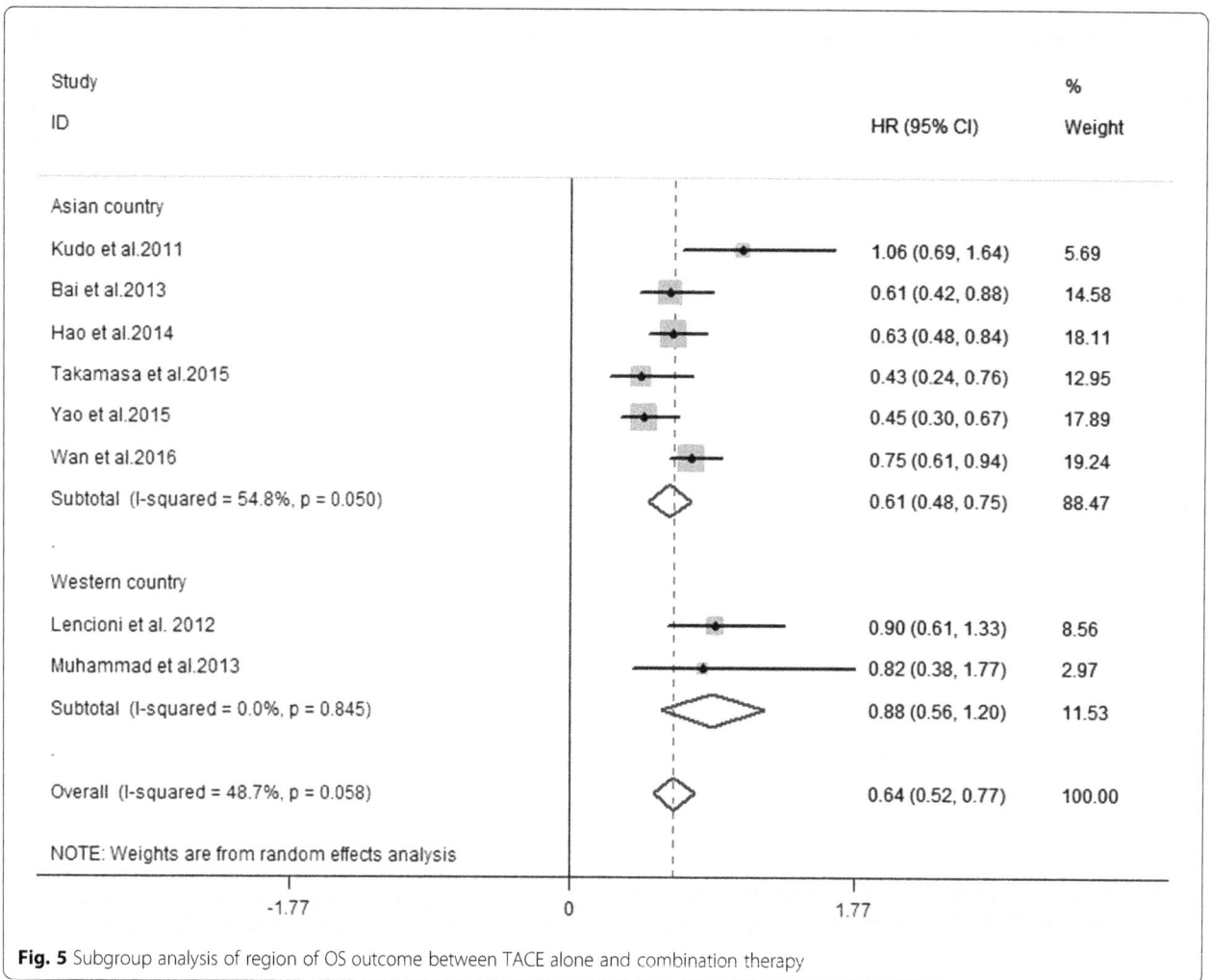

Fig. 5 Subgroup analysis of region of OS outcome between TACE alone and combination therapy

Table 5 The HR of etiology in the studies

Authors (year)	Study design	Aetiology	Endpoint	HR
Kudo et al. (2011) [15]	RCT trial	HBV = 20%	TTP	0.81(0.62–1.07)
		HCV = 60%		
Bai et al. (2013) [46]	Comparative study	HBV = 87.9%	OS	1.01(0.60–1.71)
		HCV = 4.9%		
Muhammad et al. (2013) [47]	Comparative study	ST:HCV = 69%	OS	1.04(0.66–1.63)
		DT:HCV = 93%		
Zhao et al. (2013) [41]	Non-comparative study	HBV = 80%	OS	1.372(0.773–2.437)
		HCV = 5%		
Hu et al. (2014) [14]	Comparative study	ST:B = 82.9%	TTP	1.01(0.76–1.34)
		T:B = 79.8%		
Yao et al. (2016) [12]	Comparative study	ST:HBV = 84%	OS	1.228(0.593–2.540)
		T:HBV = 83%	TTP	0.878(0.494–1.561)

Abbreviations: HR hazard ratio, *OS* overall survival, *TTP* time to progression, *RCT* randomized controlled trials, *ST* sorafenib plus TACE, *DT* DEB –TACE

clinical trials also have shown that combination therapy can prolong OS [4, 6, 11–13]. The heterogeneity of patients' physical conditions may be the primary factor affecting OS, as candidate selection may make a difference. Various study designs, including treatment procedure, number of TACE and duration of sorafenib administration might also have an effect on the outcome. In this case, reasonable study design, including proper candidate selection and appropriate treatment administration, are of great concern [6].

Lead time bias is another factor that may have impact on survival outcome. Lead time means the interval by which the disease was diagnosed by screening in advance [27]. It might create bias in observational studies of screening efficacy and may affect the comparison of overall survival among various studies [28]. However, the BCLC staging system might have made a relatively clear classification for HCC. Currently, most clinical trial designs use inclusion criteria based on BCLC stage, possibly helping to reduce this bias to some degree.

Some studies that included HCC patients with portal vein invasion have shown that combination therapy was more effective than TACE alone in terms of TTP and OS [29, 30]. However, other studies suggested negative efficacy that combination therapy brought for HCC patients with portal vein invasion [7, 14]. The extent of portal vein invasion may make difference to the survival effects. Moreover, promising OS of combined therapy with worse baseline condition may be attributed to incorporate administered systemic therapy and loco-regional treatments [30]. Another study focusing on combination efficacy between elderly and non-elderly patients concluded that age was not a prognostic factor for treatment outcome in advanced HCC patients [11, 31].

In terms of AEs, the study by Yao et al. found that combination therapy induced greater AEs than did TACE mono-therapy [32]. According to the final analysis of the START trials, combination therapy did not appear to lead to worse AEs. Moreover, the presence of some AEs such as HFSR indicated positive correlation with anti-tumour efficacy [15].

The major potential limitations of the present study are as follows: First, the number of studies included in this meta-analysis was relatively large, with half being non-comparative — the heterogeneity of available data from these studies was correspondingly substantial. The funnel plots also showed potential publication bias. Second, only several studies conducted OS and TTP analysis. The detailed information available for meta-analysis was limited. Third, the retrospective nature, small sample size, non-randomized study design and the various treatment procedures may increase the uncertainty of the conclusions.

Conclusions

As a meta-analysis which included a large number of studies, overall results of this systematic review and meta-analysis suggest that the combination of sorafenib plus TACE was superior to TACE alone in terms of TTP but not OS. Nevertheless, combination therapy is still effective and promising. This study not only analysed the relationship between combination therapy and survival efficacy to clarify this controversial issue, but also provided conclusions that aetiological differences may not influence survival outcomes. Separated regions analysis contributed to less heterogeneity while other similar studies currently lack such analysis. In the future, well-designed, randomized-controlled, prospective trials with optimized study designs and large sample sizes are required.

Additional files

Additional file 1: Table S1. Tumor response criteria, DCR, TTP and OS in 13 non-comparative studies.

Additional file 2: Table S2. DCR in 5 comparative studies.

Additional file 3: Figure S1. Forest plot of TTP outcome about the relationship between etiology and treatment outcome. (TIF 1710 kb)

Additional file 4: Figure S2. Forest plot of OS outcome about the relationship between etiology and treatment outcome.

Additional file 5: Table S3. The AEs occurred during combination therapy in 13 non-comparative studies.

Abbreviations
95% CIs: 95% confidence intervals; AEs: Adverse events; BCLC: Barcelona Clinic Liver Cancer; c-TACE: Conventional transarterial chemoembolization; DCR: Disease control rate; DEB-TACE: Transarterial chemoembolization with drug-eluting beads; HBV: Hepatitis B virus; HCC: Hepatocellular carcinoma; HCV: Hepatitis C virus; HFSR: Hand-foot skin reaction; HR: The hazard ratio; MINORS: Methodological index for non-randomized studies; mRECIST: Modified RECIST; OS: Overall survival; PDGF: Platelet-derived growth factor; RECIST: Response Evaluation in Solid Tumors; TACE: Transarterial chemoembolization; TTP: Time to progression; VEGF: Vascular endothelial growth factor

Acknowledgements
The authors are very thankful for JH and EW valuable revision assistance.

Funding
This study was supported by grants from the National Natural Science Foundation of China (81702999, Lei Liu) and the Health and Family Planning commission of Shaanxi province (2017SF-208, Lei Liu). The funding only provided financial support for this study without intervention in any part of the research process.

Authors' contributions
Manuscript writing, LL; Collection and analysis of data, WZ and MW; Revision of the manuscript, JH and EW; Study design, critical revision of the manuscript, YZ; Conceived and designed the study, funds collection, Corresponding Author LL; and all authors approved the final manuscript.

Consent for publication

Not applicable.

Competing interests

The authors declare that they have no competing interests.

Author details

[1]Department of Gastroenterology, Tangdu Hospital, Military Medical University of PLA Airforce (Fourth Military Medical University), 1 Xinsi Road, Xi'an 710038, China. [2]Department of Drug and Equipment, Aeromedicine Identification and Training Centre of Air Force, Lintong District, Xi'an, China. [3]Department of Liver Disease and Digestive Interventional Radiology, Xijing Hospital of Digestive Diseases, Military Medical University of PLA Airforce (Fourth Military Medical University), Xi'an, China. [4]Department of Gastroenterology, First Affiliated Hospital of Xi'an Jiaotong University, 277 West Yanta Road, Xi'an 710061, China. [5]Cell Engineering Research Center and Department of Cell Biology, State Key Laboratory of Cancer Biology, Military Medical University of PLA Airforce), Xi'an, China.

References

1. Bruix J, Reig M, Sherman M. Evidence-Based Diagnosis, Staging, and Treatment of Patients With Hepatocellular Carcinoma. Gastroenterology. 2016;150(4):835–53.
2. Chao Y, Chung Y-H, Han G, Yoon J-H, Yang J, Wang J, Shao G-L, Kim BI, Lee T-Y. The combination of transcatheter arterial chemoembolization and sorafenib is well tolerated and effective in Asian patients with hepatocellular carcinoma: Final results of the START trial. Int J Cancer. 2015; 136(6):1458–67.
3. Bruix J, Sherman M. Management of hepatocellular carcinoma: An update. Hepatology. 2011;53(3):1020–2.
4. EASL-EORTC clinical practice guidelines: management of hepatocellular carcinoma. J Hepatol. 2012;56(4):908–43.
5. Forner A, Llovet JM, Bruix J. Hepatocellular carcinoma. Lancet. 2012; 379(9822):1245–55.
6. Ohki T, Sato K, Yamagami M, Ito D, Yamada T, Kawanishi K, Kojima K, Seki M, Toda N, Tagawa K. Efficacy of Transcatheter Arterial Chemoembolization Followed by Sorafenib for Intermediate/Advanced Hepatocellular Carcinoma in Patients in Japan: A Retrospective Analysis. Clin Drug Investig. 2015; 35(11):751–9.
7. Pan T, Li X-S, Xie Q-K, Wang J-P, Li W, Wu P-H, Zhao M. Safety and efficacy of transarterial chemoembolization plus sorafenib for hepatocellular carcinoma with portal venous tumour thrombus. Clin Radiol. 2014;69(12): e553–61.
8. Jadad AR, Moore RA, Carroll D, Jenkinson C, Reynolds DJM, Gavaghan DJ, McQuay HJ. Assessing the quality of reports of randomized clinical trials: Is blinding necessary? Control Clin Trials. 1996;17(1):1–12.
9. Slim K, Nini E, Forestier D, Kwiatkowski F, Panis Y, Chipponi J. Methodological index for non-randomized studies (MINORS): development and validation of a new instrument. ANZ J Surg. 2003;73(9):712–6.
10. Lencioni R, Llovet JM, Han G, Tak WY, Yang J, Guglielmi A, Paik SW, Reig M, Do YK, Chau G-Y, Luca A, del Arbol LR, Leberre M-A, Niu W, Nicholson K, Meinhardt G, Bruix J. Sorafenib or placebo plus TACE with doxorubicin-eluting beads for intermediate stage HCC: The SPACE trial. J Hepatol. 2016; 64(5):1090–8.
11. Hu H, Duan Z, Long X, Hertzanu Y, Tong X, Xu X, Shi H, Liu S, Yang Z. Comparison of Treatment Safety and Patient Survival in Elderly versus Nonelderly Patients with Advanced Hepatocellular Carcinoma Receiving Sorafenib Combined with Transarterial Chemoembolization: A Propensity Score Matching Study. PLoS One. 2015;10(2):e0117168.
12. Yao X, Yan D, Zeng H, Liu D, Li H. Concurrent sorafenib therapy extends the interval to subsequent TACE for patients with unresectable hepatocellular carcinoma. J Surg Oncol. 2016;113(6):672–7.
13. Varghese J, Kedarisetty C, Venkataraman J, Srinivasan V, Deepashree T, Uthappa M, Ilankumaran K, Govil S, Reddy M, Rela M. Combination of TACE and Sorafenib Improves Outcomes in BCLC Stages B/C of Hepatocellular Carcinoma: A Single Centre Experience. Ann Hepatol. 2017;16(2):0–0.
14. Hu H, Duan Z, Long X, Hertzanu Y, Shi H, Liu S, Yang Z, Woloschak GE. Sorafenib Combined with Transarterial Chemoembolization versus Transarterial Chemoembolization Alone for Advanced-Stage Hepatocellular Carcinoma: A Propensity Score Matching Study. PLoS One. 2014;9(5):e96620.
15. Kudo M, Imanaka K, Chida N, Nakachi K, Tak W-Y, Takayama T, Yoon J-H, Hori T, Kumada H, Hayashi N, Kaneko S, Tsubouchi H, Suh DJ, Furuse J, Okusaka T, Tanaka K, Matsui O, Wada M, Yamaguchi I, Ohya T, Meinhardt G, Okita K. Phase III study of sorafenib after transarterial chemoembolisation in Japanese and Korean patients with unresectable hepatocellular carcinoma. Eur J Cancer. 2011;47(14):2117–27.
16. Guo J-T, Zhou H, Liu C, Aldrich C, Saputelli J, Whitaker T, Barrasa MI, Mason WS, Seeger C. Apoptosis and Regeneration of Hepatocytes during Recovery from Transient Hepadnavirus Infections. J Virol. 2000;74(3):1495–505.
17. Nishikawa H, Arimoto A, Wakasa T, Kita R, Kimura T, Osaki Y. Comparison of clinical characteristics and survival after surgery in patients with non-B and non-C hepatocellular carcinoma and hepatitis virus-related hepatocellular carcinoma. J Cancer. 2013;4(6):502–13.
18. Sinn DH, Gwak GY, Cho J, Paik SW, Yoo BC. Comparison of clinical manifestations and outcomes between hepatitis B virus- and hepatitis C virus-related hepatocellular carcinoma: analysis of a nationwide cohort. PLoS One. 2014;9(11):e112184.
19. Sun H-C, Zhang W, Qin L-X, Zhang B-H, Ye Q-H, Lu W, Ren N, Zhuang P-Y, Zhu X-D, Fan J, Tang Z-Y. Positive serum hepatitis B e antigen is associated with higher risk of early recurrence and poorer survival in patients after curative resection of hepatitis B-related hepatocellular carcinoma. J Hepatol. 2007;47(5):684–90.
20. Hassan MM, Frome A, Patt YZ, El-Serag HB. Rising prevalence of hepatitis C virus infection among patients recently diagnosed with hepatocellular carcinoma in the United States. J Clin Gastroenterol. 2002;35(3):266–9.
21. Peng SY, Mou YP, Liu YB, Ying S, Peng CH, Cai XJ, Wu YL, Zhou LH. Binding pancreaticojejunostomy: 150 consecutive cases without leakage. J Gastrointest Surg. 2003;7(7):898–900.
22. Lencioni R. Loco-regional treatment of hepatocellular carcinoma. Hepatology. 2010;52(2):762–73.
23. Sottani C, Poggi G, Quaretti P, Regazzi M, Montagna B, Quaquarini E, Imbriani M, Leoni E, Di Cesare P, Riccardi A, et al. Serum pharmacokinetics in patients treated with transarterial chemoembolization (TACE) using two types of epirubicin-loaded microspheres. Anticancer Res. 2012;32(5):1769–74.
24. Varela M, Real MI, Burrel M, Forner A, Sala M, Brunet M, Ayuso C, Castells L, Montañá X, Llovet JM, Bruix J. Chemoembolization of hepatocellular carcinoma with drug eluting beads: Efficacy and doxorubicin pharmacokinetics. J Hepatol. 2007;46(3):474–81.
25. Facciorusso A. Drug-eluting beads transarterial chemoembolization for hepatocellular carcinoma: Current state of the art. World J Gastroenterol. 2018;24(2):161–9.
26. Song JE, Kim DY. Conventional drug-eluting beads transarterial chemoembolization for hepatocellular carcinoma. World J Hepatol. 2017; 9(18):808.
27. Jansen RJ, Alexander BH, Anderson KE, Church TR. Quantifying lead-time bias in risk factor studies of cancer through simulation. Ann Epidemiol. 2013;23(11):735–741.e1.
28. Gray S, White J, Peng L, Cannon R, Kilgore W, Redden D, Abdel Aal A, Simpson H, Mcguire B, Eckhoff D, Dubay D. Trans-arterial chemoembolization of hepatocellular carcinoma is efficacious, regardless of hospital characteristics or TACE volume. HPB. 2017;19:S123.
29. Li X. Expression of plasma vascular endothelial growth factor in patients with hepatocellular carcinoma and effect of transcatheter arterial chemoembolization therapy on plasma vascular endothelial growth factor level. World J Gastroenterol. 2004;10(19):2878.
30. Wilhelm SM, Adnane L, Newell P, Villanueva A, Llovet JM, Lynch M. Preclinical overview of sorafenib, a multikinase inhibitor that targets both Raf and VEGF and PDGF receptor tyrosine kinase signaling. Mol Cancer Ther. 2008;7(10):3129–40.
31. El-Serag HB, Mason AC. Rising Incidence of Hepatocellular Carcinoma in the United States. N Engl J Med. 1999;340(10):745–50.
32. Yao X, Yan D, Liu D, Zeng H, Li H. Efficacy and adverse events of transcatheter arterial chemoembolization in combination with sorafenib in the treatment of unresectable hepatocellular carcinoma. Mol Clin Oncol. 2015;3(4):929–35.

33. Erhardt A, Kolligs F, Dollinger M, Schott E, Wege H, Bitzer M, Gog C, Lammert F, Schuchmann M, Walter C, Blondin D, Ohmann C, Häussinger D. TACE plus sorafenib for the treatment of hepatocellular carcinoma: results of the multicenter, phase II SOCRATES trial. Cancer Chemother Pharmacol. 2014;74(5):947–54.

34. Dufour J-F, Hoppe H, Heim MH, Helbling B, Maurhofer O, Szucs-Farkas Z, Kickuth R, Borner M, Candinas D, Saar B. Continuous Administration of Sorafenib in Combination with Transarterial Chemoembolization in Patients with Hepatocellular Carcinoma: Results of a Phase I Study. Oncologist. 2010; 15(11):1198–204.

35. Cabrera R, Pannu DS, Caridi J, Firpi RJ, Soldevila-Pico C, Morelli G, Clark V, Suman A, George TJ Jr, Nelson DR. The combination of sorafenib with transarterial chemoembolisation for hepatocellular carcinoma. Aliment Pharmacol Ther. 2011;34(2):205–13.

36. Lee J-H, Chung Y-H, Kim JA, Shin E-S, Lee D, Shim JH, Lee HC, Yoon JH, Kim BI, Bae SH, Koh KC, Kim G, Park N-H. 639 SINGLE NUCLEOTIDE POLYMORPHISM ASSOCIATED WITH TUMOR RESPONSE TO THE COMBINED THERAPY WITH TRANSARTERIAL CHEMOEMBOLIZATION AND SORAFENIB IN PATIENTS WITH HEPATOCELLULAR CARCINOMA. J Hepatol. 2011;54:S258–9.

37. Reyes D, Azad N, Koteish A, Kamel I, Hamilton J, Pawlik T, Choti M, Bhagat N, Geschwind JF. Abstract No. 4: Phase II trial of sorafenib combined with doxorubicin eluting bead-transarterial chemoembolization for patients with unresectable hepatocellular carcinoma: Interim efficacy analysis. J Vasc Interv Radiol. 2011;22(3):S4–5.

38. Park J-W, Amarapurkar D, Chao Y, Chen P-J, Geschwind J-FH, Goh KL, Han K-H, Kudo M, Lee HC, Lee R-C, Lesmana LA, Ho YL, Paik SW, Poon RT, Tan C-K, Tanwandee T, Teng G, Cheng A-L. Consensus recommendations and review by an International Expert Panel on Interventions in Hepatocellular Carcinoma (EPOIHCC). Liver Int. 2013;33(3):327–37.

39. Sieghart W, Pinter M, Reisegger M, Müller C, Ba-Ssalamah A, Lammer J, Peck-Radosavljevic M. Conventional transarterial chemoembolisation in combination with sorafenib for patients with hepatocellular carcinoma: a pilot study. Eur Radiol. 2012;22(6):1214–23.

40. Chung Y-H, Han G, Yoon J-H, Yang J, Wang J, Shao G-L, Kim BI, Lee T-Y, Chao Y. Interim analysis of START: Study in asia of the combination of TACE (transcatheter arterial chemoembolization) with sorafenib in patients with hepatocellular carcinoma trial. Int J Cancer. 2013;132(10):2448–58.

41. Zhao Y, Wang WJ, Guan S, Li HL, Xu RC, Wu JB, Liu JS, Li HP, Bai W, Yin ZX, Fan DM, Zhang ZL, Han GH. Sorafenib combined with transarterial chemoembolization for the treatment of advanced hepatocellular carcinoma: a large-scale multicenter study of 222 patients. Ann Oncol. 2013; 24(7):1786–92.

42. Cosgrove DP, Reyes DK, Pawlik TM, Feng AL, Kamel IR, Geschwind J-FH. Open-Label Single-Arm Phase II Trial of Sorafenib Therapy with Drug-eluting Bead Transarterial Chemoembolization in Patients with Unresectable Hepatocellular Carcinoma: Clinical Results. Radiology. 2015;277(2):594–603.

43. Martin RC II, Keck G, Robbins K, Strnad B, Dubel G, et al. (2010) Evaluation of sorafenib in combination with doxorubicin-loaded DC bead as a combination treatment option for HCC. Abstract 216. ASCO Gastrointestinal Cancers Symposium January 22–24.

44. Sansonno D, Lauletta G, Russi S, Conteduca V, Sansonno L, Dammacco F. Transarterial Chemoembolization Plus Sorafenib: A Sequential Therapeutic Scheme for HCV-Related Intermediate-Stage Hepatocellular Carcinoma: A Randomized Clinical Trial. Oncologist. 2012;17(3):359–66.

45. Qu XD, Chen CS, Wang JH, Yan ZP, Chen JM, Gong GQ, Liu QX, Luo JJ, Liu LX, Liu R, et al. The efficacy of TACE combined sorafenib in advanced stages hepatocellullar carcinoma. BMC Cancer. 2012;12:263.

46. Bai W, Wang YJ, Zhao Y, Qi XS, Yin ZX, He CY, Li RJ, Wu KC, Xia JL, Fan DM, Han GH. Sorafenib in combination with transarterial chemoembolization improves the survival of patients with unresectable hepatocellular carcinoma: A propensity score matching study. J Dig Dis. 2013;14(4):181–90.

47. Muhammad A. Comparative effectiveness of traditional chemoembolization with or without sorafenib for hepatocellular carcinoma. World J Hepatol. 2013;5(7):364.

48. Huang YH, Chen W, Li JP, Chen B, Yang JY. Clinical value of continuous administration of sorafenib in combination with modified transarterial chemoembolization in patients with unresectable hepatocellular carcinoma. Chin Med J. 2013;126(2):385–6.

49. Zhang YF, Wei W, Wang JH, Xu L, Jian PE, Xiao CZ, Zhong XP, Shi M, Guo RP. Transarterial chemoembolization combined with sorafenib for the treatment of hepatocellular carcinoma with hepatic vein tumor thrombus. Onco Targets Ther. 2016;9:4239–46.

50. Wan X, Zhai X, Yan Z, Yang P, Li J, Wu D, Wang K, Xia Y, Shen F. Retrospective analysis of transarterial chemoembolization and sorafenib in Chinese patients with unresectable and recurrent hepatocellular carcinoma. Oncotarget. 2016;7(50)

16

Risk factors for hepatic veno-occlusive disease caused by *Gynura segetum*

Yan Wang[1], Dan Qiao[2], Ya Li[1] and Feng Xu[1*]

Abstract

Background: Hepatic veno-occlusive disease (HVOD) caused by *Gynura segetum* has been increasingly reported in China in recent years. The aim of this retrospective study was to identify independent prognostic markers for survival in patients with *Gynura segetum*-induced HVOD and to evaluate the effect of anticoagulants and transjugular intrahepatic portosystemic shunt (TIPS) on survival rate.

Methods: Clinical data including symptoms, signs, imaging characteristics, laboratory test results, results of liver tissue biopsies, type of treatment during follow-up and clinical outcomes were collected. Univariate, multivariate and time-dependent Cox regression analyses were performed.

Results: Survival rates were 91% (95% confidence interval [CI], 82–95%), 64% (95% CI, 53–69%) and 57% (95% CI, 51–65%) at 1, 3 and 60 months, respectively. Total bilirubin, albumin and hepatic encephalopathy were independent prognostic markers of survival. Anticoagulants were administered to 76% of the patients. Among 75 patients treated with anticoagulants, 49 patients (65.3%) were cured, whereas 26 patients (34.7%) died; the cure rate in anticoagulant-treated patients was higher than that of those not treated with anticoagulants ($\chi^2 = 9.129$, $P = 0.004$). Cure rate of the anticoagulation + TIPS treatment group was 64.3%, which was also higher than that of the non-anticoagulation group; however, this was not significantly different ($\chi^2 = 3.938$, $P = 0.096$).

Conclusions: The presence of hepatic encephalopathy, serum bilirubin and albumin levels were major prognostic factors for *Gynura segetum*-induced HVOD. Anticoagulation therapy significantly increased the cure rate; however, TIPS treatment did not have a beneficial effect on the cure rate.

Keywords: Hepatic veno-occlusive disease, *Gynura segetum*, Anticoagulant, Transjugular intrahepatic portosystemic shunt, Prognostic factor

Background

Hepatic veno-occlusive disease (HVOD), also termed hepatic sinusoidal obstruction syndrome, is a rare clinical syndrome caused by several factors including high-dose chemotherapy before haematopoietic stem cell transplantation (HSCT) [1, 2], high-dose chemotherapy and ingestion of herbal compounds containing pyrrolizidine alkaloids (PAs) [3]. In China, HVOD has rarely been reported in patients who received HSCT despite the large number of HSCT cases. HVOD caused by *Gynura segetum* (i.e. Tusanqi)-containing PAs, a Chinese medicinal herb used for self-medication as well as pain relief, hypertension and dissipation of blood stasis [4], has been increasingly reported in China in recent years [5–7].

HVOD is defined as intrahepatic post-sinusoidal portal hypertension caused by stenosis or occlusion of veins, including the central veins of hepatic lobules and the sublobular veins [8]. HVOD is associated with significant mortality due to the severity of the disease and the absence of uniformly effective therapies. Until recently, treatment approaches have largely involved supportive and symptomatic care, such as restriction of water and sodium intake, diuretics, paracentesis and albumin infusion. Other treatment options include anticoagulant

* Correspondence: doctorxuyfy@163.com
[1]Department of Gastroenterology, The First Affiliated Hospital of Zhengzhou University, 1 Jianshe Donglu, Zhengzhou 450052, Henan, China
Full list of author information is available at the end of the article

therapy, transjugular intrahepatic portosystemic shunt (TIPS) [9] and liver transplantation [10].

HSCT-related HVOD differs from that associated with *Gynura segetum* in many aspects, such as aetiology, ethnicity, underlying diseases, clinical findings and treatment. Not much is known about factors that might be relevant in predicting survival in patients with *Gynura segetum*-related HVOD. Most studies are case reports or include limited numbers of patients because of the rarity of this clinical presentation. The aim of this retrospective study was to identify independent prognostic markers for survival in patients with *Gynura segetum*-induced HVOD and to evaluate the effect of anticoagulants and TIPS on survival.

Methods

Patients and database

Between July 2012 and July 2017, 132 patients admitted to the First Affiliated Hospital of Zhengzhou University with a clinical diagnosis of HVOD and stated to have ingested *Gynura segetum* were included in this retrospective study. Previously described diagnostic criteria for Tusanqi-induced HVOD was used [11–13]. Patients with the following conditions were excluded from the study: chronic liver disease due to other causes, hepatocellular carcinoma, Budd–Chiari syndrome, congestive heart disease and incomplete data.

This study was approved by the Ethics Committee of the First Affiliated Hospital of Zhengzhou University in Zhengzhou, China. Written informed consent to participate was obtained from all patients. In all cases, the first available data were used as baseline data. Clinical data including symptoms, signs, imaging characteristics, laboratory test results, results of liver tissue biopsies, types of treatment during follow-up and clinical outcomes were collected. All patients were followed up from the date of diagnosis until death, lost to follow-up or study closure on 31 July 2017.

Treatment

Patients who received treatments other than anticoagulants, such as diuretics, paracentesis, albumin and/or liver unction protection, were categorised in the non-anticoagulation group. After exclusion of contraindications, anticoagulation therapy was administered as follows: oral warfarin at 1.5 mg daily, with dose adjustment to maintain an international normalised ratio between 2 and 3, combined with low-molecular-weight heparin at 4000 IU by subcutaneous injection every 12 h. In patients whose symptoms improved, anticoagulation therapy was maintained until complete remission. In patients whose symptoms did not improve or worsened after 2 weeks of anticoagulation therapy, TIPS was performed following assessment of the patient.

Statistical analysis

All statistical analyses were performed using SPSS statistical software version 17.0 (SPSS, Chicago, Illinois, USA). All continuous variables were expressed as medians (25th–75th percentiles) and compared with Student's t test or non-parametric test according to the distribution characteristics. Categorical variables were expressed as numbers with percentages and compared by the χ^2 test or Fisher's exact

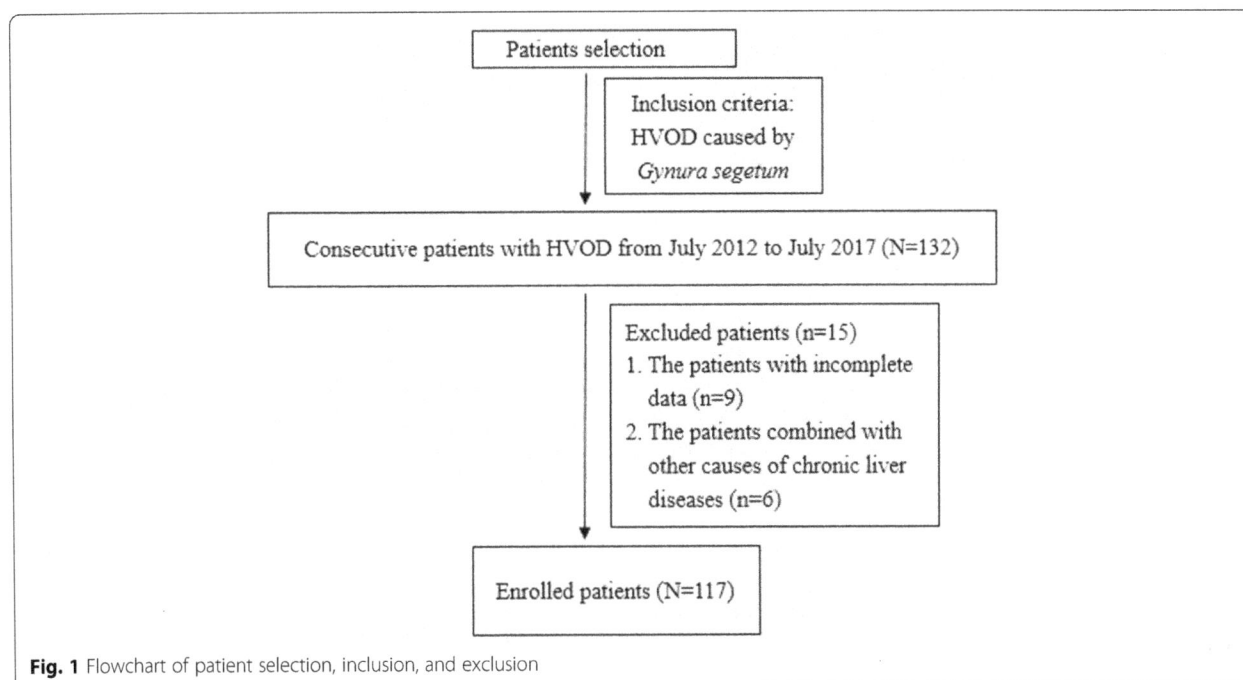

Fig. 1 Flowchart of patient selection, inclusion, and exclusion

test. Survival rates were calculated using the Kaplan–Meier method. Univariate survival analysis to assess the effect of patient characteristics was based on comparison of survival curves by the log-rank test. Statistically significant variables were introduced into a multivariate Cox's proportional hazards analysis. A P value less than 0.05 was considered to indicate a significant difference.

Results

Patient characteristics

After the exclusion of 15 patients who did not fulfil the inclusion criteria, a total of 117 patients who were eligible were included in the analysis (Fig. 1). Patient characteristics at the time of diagnosis are presented in Table 1. Median age was 63 years (range, 18–84 years), and 67% of the patients were male. The most common clinical presentation was ascites (99.1%), followed by abdominal distention (98.3%), hepatomegaly (70%), poor appetite (41%), lower limb oedema (39.3%), splenomegaly (34.2%) and malaise (33.3%).

Survival

In this study, follow-up period ranged from 3 days to 60 months. During the follow-up, 50 patients (43%) died, and causes of death were liver failure ($n = 19$), postoperative multiorgan failure ($n = 2$), cardiovascular disease ($n = 3$), variceal bleeding ($n = 3$), sepsis ($n = 3$), newly developed malignancy ($n = 5$) and combinations of causes ($n = 9$). Information on cause of death could not be retrieved for six patients. Survival rates were 91% (95% confidence interval [CI], 82–95%), 64% (95% CI, 53–69%) and 57% (95% CI, 51–65%) at 1, 3 and 60 months, respectively (Fig. 2).

Prognostic factors

Univariate analysis revealed that hepatic encephalopathy ($P = 0.005$), total bilirubin ($P < 0.001$), direct bilirubin ($P = 0.001$), albumin ($P = 0.044$), blood urea nitrogen ($P = 0.022$) and treatment ($P = 0.009$) were significantly associated with survival (Table 2).

These variables as well as age, sex and platelet count were introduced into a multivariate Cox regression model. Variables were selected using a forward and backward elimination procedure with a significance level of 0.10. The final Cox model showed that total bilirubin ($P = 0.004$), albumin ($P = 0.024$) and hepatic encephalopathy ($P = 0.018$) were independent prognostic markers for survival in this cohort of 117 patients who had complete data for these variables (Table 3).

Interventions

In this study, 28 of the 117 patients (24%) were managed medically with supportive and diuretic therapeutic approaches such as diuretics, paracentesis, albumin and/or liver function protection only for control of ascites.

Table 1 Characteristics of 117 patients with hepatic veno-occlusive disease at the time of diagnosis

Characteristic	Obtained data
Age (years)	63.0 (52.5–69.0)
Male/female (%)	67/33
Clinical manifestations, n (%)	
Ascites	116 (99.1)
Abdominal distention	115 (98.3)
Poor appetite	48 (41.0)
Nausea, vomiting	19 (16.2)
Malaise	39 (33.3)
Lower limb oedema	46 (39.3)
Hepatomegaly	82 (70.0)
Splenomegaly	40 (34.2)
Right upper quadrant pain	23 (19.7)
Weight gain	21 (18.0)
Encephalopathy	19 (16.2)
Variceal bleeding	3 (2.6)
Laboratory tests	
WBC (10^9/L)	6.1 (5.0–8.7)
RBC (10^{12}/L)	4.4 (3.9–4.9)
PLT (10^9/L)	113 (78–153)
ALT (U/L)	49.0 (25.0–152.5)
AST (U/L)	75.0 (39.0–158.5)
GGT (U/L)	100.7 (61.8–164.8)
ALP (U/L)	122.0 (86.8–191.3)
TB (μmol/L)	33.3 (19.7–47.0)
DB (μmol/L)	21.5 (12.7–30.5)
ALB (g/L)	30.6 (27.7–33.6)
PT (s)	14.8 (12.7–17.0)
BUN (mmol/L)	5.5 (3.8–7.9)
CR (μmol/L)	74.0 (60.0–90.0)
CA-125 (U/ml)	259.9 (182.1–458.4)
CA199	13.04 (7.9–34.2)
Treatment, n (%)	
Non-anticoagulation	26 (22.2)
Anticoagulation	74 (63.2)
Anticoagulation + TIPS	17 (14.5)

WBC white blood cell count, *RBC* red blood cell count, *PLT* platelet count, *AST* aspartate aminotransferase, *ALT* alanine aminotransferase, *GGT* λ-glutamyl transferase, *ALP* alkaline phosphatase, *TB* total bilirubin, *DB* direct bilirubin, *TP* total protein, *ALB* albumin, *BUN* blood urea nitrogen, *CR* creatinine, *PT* prothrombin time, *TIPS* transjugular intrahepatic portosystemic shunt

Conversely, 89 patients of 117 (76%) were treated with anticoagulants in addition to the above mentioned non-anticoagulation therapeutic approaches. None of the patients who were treated with anticoagulant therapy developed complications due to the combination of

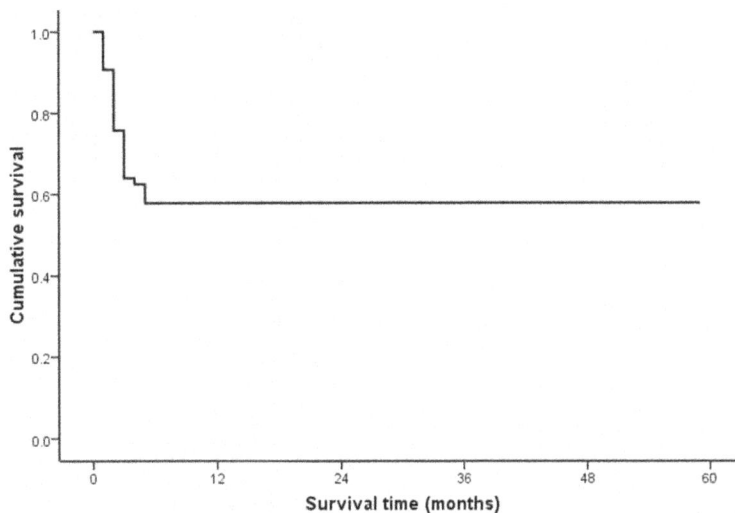

Fig. 2 Overall survival in 117 patients with hepatic veno-occlusive disease caused by *Gynura segetum*

warfarin and low-molecular-weight heparin, such as severe bleeding. TIPS was performed in 14 patients (12%) during follow-up; five of the patients died because of complications or multiple organ failure. None of the patients received liver transplantation (Table 2).

Benefit of anticoagulation and TIPS

The use of anticoagulants to prevent thrombosis was found to yield a significant beneficial effect on survival in the current study cohort. Among 28 patients who received non-anticoagulation treatment, 9 (32.1%) were cured, whereas 19 patients (67.9%) died during treatment period. Among a total of 75 patients treated with anticoagulants, 49 patients (65.3%) were cured and 26 patients (34.7%) died (Table 4). The cure rate was higher in the anticoagulation group than in the non-anticoagulation group (χ^2 = 9.129, P = 0.004). The cure rate in the anticoagulation + TIPS treatment group was 64.3%, which was also higher than that in the non-anticoagulation group, albeit without a statistical significance (χ^2 = 3.938, P = 0.096). Furthermore, there was no statistical difference in the cure rates between the anticoagulation group and anticoagulation + TIPS group (χ^2 = 0.006, P = 1.00).

Discussion

HVOD, first described by Willmot and Robertson in 1920, is a clinical syndrome characterised by hepatomegaly, weight gain, ascites and jaundice [14, 15]. In Western countries, HVOD is most commonly associated with HSCT and high-dose chemotherapy [3, 16], whereas there is growing concern in developing countries over the use of *Gynura segetum*, which can also cause HVOD. Although hepatic impairment due to conventional pharmaceutical drug use is widely acknowledged, the potential hepatotoxicity of herbal preparations is underestimated because of the public misconception that they are harmless. Importantly, these herbal compounds are commonly used for self-medication without supervision.

Clinically, HVOD diagnosis is usually achieved on the basis of the criteria put forth by the Baltimore and Seattle groups [2, 17], which are based on clinical findings that include painful hepatomegaly, weight gain, hyperbilirubinemia and ascites [14]. The specificity of these two criteria is about 92%; however, their sensitivity is relatively low [10].The current study showed that the most prominent clinical manifestations of *Gynura segetum*-induced HVOD were abdominal distention (98.3%), ascites (99.1%) and hepatomegaly (70%), whereas only about half of the patients exhibited jaundice, and only 19.7% of the patients had right upper quadrant pain. These results are consistent with the previous studies [18]. Thus, the diagnosis in patients of the current study was based on the history of *Gynura segetum* intake, clinical manifestations, imaging results and pathological features. Histological assessment of liver biopsy specimen remains the gold standard for the diagnosis of HVOD; the pathology often includes expansion and congestion of the hepatic sinus, endothelial swelling, wall thickening and incomplete luminal occlusion of the hepatic vein [19]. However, liver biopsy is usually delayed because of extensive ascites, clotting abnormalities and thrombocytopaenia [10]. Recent studies showed that contrast-enhanced computed tomography and magnetic resonance imaging were effective non-invasive methods for the early diagnosis of Tusanqi-induced HVOD and could replace histological examination of the liver in patients with typical clinical data and imaging findings. Patchy enhancement, heterogeneous hypoattenuation in portal phase of the computed tomography or non-homogeneous signal by magnetic resonance imaging are main imaging signs of HVOD [6–8].

Table 2 Univariate analysis of risk factors associated with survival in 117 patients with hepatic veno-occlusive disease

Variable	Rehabilitation Group (n = 67)	Death Group (n = 50)	Statistic	P value
Age (years)	63.0 (52.3–69.0)	61.5 (48.3–67.8)	$t = 0.871$	0.385
Male/female (%)	67/33	64/36	$x^2 = 0.008$	0.565
Clinical manifestations, n (%)				
Ascites	67 (100)	49 (98.0)	$x^2 = 1.352$	0.427
Abdominal distention	66 (98.5)	49 (98.0)	$x^2 = 0.044$	0.834
Poor appetite	22 (32.8)	26 (52.0)	$x^2 = 4.346$	0.057
Nausea, vomiting	7 (10.4)	11 (22.0)	$x^2 = 2.935$	0.120
Malaise	22 (32.8)	17 (34.0)	$x^2 = 0.895$	0.525
Lower limb oedema	23 (34.3)	23 (46.0)	$x^2 = 1.653$	0.252
Hepatomegaly	45 (67.2)	37 (74.0)	$x^2 = 0.638$	0.541
Splenomegaly	22 (32.8)	18 (36.0)	$x^2 = 0.127$	0.844
Right upper quadrant pain	14 (20.9)	9 (18.0)	$x^2 = 0.152$	0.815
Weight gain	11 (16.4)	10 (20.0)	$x^2 = 0.249$	0.634
Encephalopathy	5 (7.5)	14 (28.0)	$x^2 = 8.878$	0.005
Variceal bleeding	0	3 (6.0)	$x^2 = 4.126$	0.075
Laboratory tests				
WBC (10^9/L)	6.1 (5.4–9.3)	6.4 (4.5–8.6)	$t = 0.171$	0.864
RBC (10^{12}/L)	4.4 (4.0–4.8)	4.4 (3.3–5.1)	$Z = 0.933$	0.349
PLT (10^9/L)	115.0 (77.0–148.0)	105 (76–144)	$Z = 0.676$	0.750
ALT (U/L)	69.0 (25.0–201.0)	38.0 (23.0–86.0)	$Z = 1.040$	0.230
AST (U/L)	100.0 (44.0–189.0)	72.0 (38.0–158.0)	$Z = 0.902$	0.389
GGT (U/L)	97.0 (61.5–161.0)	113.1 (49.8–176.6)	$Z = 0.746$	0.635
ALP (U/L)	111.0 (82.5–148.0)	137.0 (84.8–202.0)	$Z = 1.002$	0.267
TB (μmol/L)	26.7 (19.7–36.4)	43.75 (37.0–83.0)	$Z = 2.163$	<0.001
DB (μmol/L)	15.1 (12.8–26.1)	27.9 (21.6–59.4)	$Z = 1.914$	0.001
ALB (g/L)	30.6 (28.9–34.4)	29.8 (27.1–32.5)	$t = 2.052$	0.044
PT (s)	14.8 (12.4–16.5)	15.2 (13.1–18.5)	$t = -0.774$	0.442
BUN (mmol/L)	5.0 (3.8–6.3)	7.0 (3.6–9.51)	$Z = 1.503$	0.022
CR (μmol/L)	71.0 (58.0–84.0)	71.0 (53.5–94.0)	$t = -0.088$	0.930
CA-125 (u/ml)	224.5 (136.6–430.7)	270.1 (181.9–429.5)	$t = -0.083$	0.935
CA199	11.9 (7.8–25.0)	17.6 (8.3–38.8)	$Z = 0.672$	0.757
Treatment, n (%)				
Non-anticoagulation	9 (13.4)	19 (38.0)	$x^2 = 9.498$	0.009
Anticoagulation	49 (73.1)	26 (52.0)		
Anticoagulation + TIPS	9 (13.4)	5 (10.0)		

Table 3 Results of the multivariate Cox regression analysis of 117 patients with hepatic veno-occlusive disease

Variable	P value	Risk Ratio	95% CI
TB (μmol/L)	0.004	1.006	1.002–1.010
ALB (g/L)	0.024	0.932	0.816–1.063
Encephalopathy	0.018		
Present		3.440	1.240–9.543
Absent			

Table 4 The effects of different treatment approaches on prognosis of patients with *Gynura segetum*-induced hepatic veno-occlusive disease

Group	n	Clinical Cure		Death	
		n	rate (%)	n	rate (%)
Non-anticoagulation	28	9	32.1	19	67.9
Anticoagulation	75	49	65.3	26	34.7
Anticoagulation + TIPS	14	9	64.3	5	35.7

In the present study, 5 year survival was 57%, which is higher than those reported from Western countries [20–22]. This difference can be explained by the severe underlying haematological disorders associated with stem cell transplantation in HVOD patients in those studies; development of HVOD following pre-treatment for transplantation is more serious and can easily lead to liver and multiorgan failure and death. In contrast, the patients with *Gynura segetum*-induced HVOD do not necessarily have serious underlying diseases. Moreover, 70% of the current study cohort were treated with anticoagulants, which were reported to contribute to improved HVOD prognosis [23].

The aim of the present study was to assess prognostic determinants of survival in HVOD patients. We identified three important factors that were independently associated with survival: serum bilirubin, serum albumin and encephalopathy. Child–Pugh is a well-known and widely used classification of liver disease. These three prognostic factors identified in the current study are included in the Child–Pugh staging system. Conversely, ascites and prothrombin time did not exhibit a significant impact on survival.

Unlike other common causes of HVOD including high-dose chemotherapy before HSCT, *Gynura segetum*-induced HVOD is unpredictable. It is critical to avoid further contact with the suspicious toxin as soon as possible once symptoms appear or when a definitive diagnosis is reached. Currently, there are no effective therapies for HVOD, and supportive care remains the cornerstone of management, including restriction of water and sodium intake, albumin infusion, abdominal paracentesis and diuretics. Defibrotide is a promising agent with anti-ischaemic, anti-inflammatory and antithrombotic activity [24]; however, the results of defibrotide therapy are conflicting and are not shown to be cost-effective [25]. Our results suggested that anticoagulation therapy significantly increased the cure rate of HVOD, compared with the symptomatic treatment. TIPS is used to relieve portal hypertension and refractory ascites; however, many studies reported that its efficacy in HVOD was poor [26, 27]. Our study also revealed that the cure rate of anticoagulation therapy was comparable with that of anticoagulation therapy in combination with TIPS, with no statistical difference between the two groups, which might be due to the small number of patients receiving the combination treatment. Therefore, future studies with larger cohort sizes are necessary to assess the efficacy and outcomes of combination treatment with anticoagulation therapy and TIPS.

Conclusions

Major prognostic factors for *Gynura segetum*-induced HVOD were the presence of hepatic encephalopathy and serum bilirubin and albumin levels. Compared with symptomatic treatment, anticoagulation therapy was associated with a significant increased cure rate, but TIPS treatment had no additional effect on improving the cure rate. No uniformly effective treatments are available for HVOD, and the mortality remains high; therefore, prevention of the potent toxicity of *Gynura segetum* is critical. Future studies are necessary to investigate the mechanisms of HVOD to improve the survival rate.

Abbreviations
CI: Confidence interval; HSCT: Haematopoietic stem cell transplantation; HSOS: Hepatic sinusoidal obstruction syndrome; HVOD: Hepatic veno-occlusive disease; PAs: Pyrrolizidine alkaloids; TIPS: Transjugular intrahepatic portosystemic shunt

Author' contributions
YW participated in the collection and analysis of data and wrote the manuscript. DQ and YL participated in the data collection and analysis. FX participated in conception and oversight of the study, supervision, data analysis and manuscript editing. All authors read and approved the final version of the manuscript.

Funding
Not applicable

Consent for publication
Not applicable

Competing interests
The authors declare that they have no competing interest.

Author details
¹Department of Gastroenterology, The First Affiliated Hospital of Zhengzhou University, 1 Jianshe Donglu, Zhengzhou 450052, Henan, China. ²Department of Zhengzhou Center for Disease Control and Prevention, Zhengzhou, China.

References

1. Cacchione A, LeMaitre A, Couanet DV, Benhamou E, Amoroso L, Simonnard N, Hartmann O. Risk factors for hepatic veno-occlusive disease: a retrospective unicentric study in 116 children autografted after a high-dose BU-thiotepa regimen. Bone Marrow Transplant. 2008;42(7):449–54.
2. Mohty M, Malard F, Abecassis M, Aerts E, Alaskar AS, Aljurf M, Arat M, Bader P, Baron F, Bazarbachi A, et al. Sinusoidal obstruction syndrome/veno-occlusive disease: current situation and perspectives-a position statement from the European Society for Blood and Marrow Transplantation (EBMT). Bone Marrow Transplant. 2015;50(6):781–9.
3. Gozdzik J, Krasowska-Kwiecien A, Wedrychowicz A. sinusoidal obstruction disease (SOS), previous hepatic venoocclusive disease (VOD)--still serious complication after hematopoietic stem cell transplantation. Przegl Lek. 2008; 65(4):203–8.
4. Cheng Y, Liang D, Zhan Y. Morphological and histological studies of herba sedum aizoon. Zhong Yao Cai. 2001;24(5):330–2.
5. Lin G, Wang JY, Li N, Li M, Gao H, Ji Y, Zhang F, Wang H, Zhou Y, Ye Y, et al. Hepatic sinusoidal obstruction syndrome associated with consumption of Gynura segetum. J Hepatol. 2011;54(4):666–73.
6. Kan X, Ye J, Rong X, Lu Z, Li X, Wang Y, Yang L, Xu K, Song Y, Hou X. Diagnostic performance of contrast-enhanced CT in pyrrolizidine alkaloids-induced hepatic sinusoidal obstructive syndrome. Sci Rep. 2016;6:37998.
7. Li X, Yang X, Xu D, Li Q, Kong X, Lu Z, Bai T, Xu K, Ye J, Song Y. Magnetic resonance imaging findings in patients with pyrrolizidine alkaloid-induced

hepatic sinusoidal obstruction syndrome. Clin Gastroenterol Hepatol. 2017; 15(6):955–7.

8.   Shao H, Chen HZ, Zhu JS, Ruan B, Zhang ZQ, Lin X, Gan MF. Computed tomography findings of hepatic veno-occlusive disease caused by Sedum aizoon with histopathological correlation. Braz J Med Biol Res. 2015;48(12):1145–50.

9.   Boyer TD, Haskal ZJ, American Association for the Study of liver D. The role of transjugular intrahepatic portosystemic shunt in the management of portal hypertension. Hepatology. 2005;41(2):386–400.

10.   Chen Z, Huo JR. Hepatic veno-occlusive disease associated with toxicity of pyrrolizidine alkaloids in herbal preparations. Neth J Med. 2010;68(6):252–60.

11.   Zhou H, Wang YX, Lou HY, Xu XJ, Zhang MM. Hepatic sinusoidal obstruction syndrome caused by herbal medicine: CT and MRI features. Korean J Radiol. 2014;15(2):218–25.

12.   Gao H, Li N, Wang JY, Zhang SC, Lin G. Definitive diagnosis of hepatic sinusoidal obstruction syndrome induced by pyrrolizidine alkaloids. J Dig Dis. 2012;13(1):33–9.

13.   Gao H, Ruan JQ, Chen J, Li N, Ke CQ, Ye Y, Lin G, Wang JY. Blood pyrrole-protein adducts as a diagnostic and prognostic index in pyrrolizidine alkaloid-hepatic sinusoidal obstruction syndrome. Drug Design Dev Ther. 2015;9:4861–8.

14.   McDonald GB, Sharma P, Matthews DE, Shulman HM, Thomas ED. Venocclusive disease of the liver after bone marrow transplantation: diagnosis, incidence, and predisposing factors. Hepatology. 1984;4(1):116–22.

15.   Bayraktar UD, Seren S, Bayraktar Y. Hepatic venous outflow obstruction: three similar syndromes. World J Gastroenterol. 2007;13(13):1912–27.

16.   Kumar S, DeLeve LD, Kamath PS, Tefferi A. Hepatic veno-occlusive disease (sinusoidal obstruction syndrome) after hematopoietic stem cell transplantation. Mayo Clin Proc. 2003;78(5):589–98.

17.   Fan CQ, Crawford JM. Sinusoidal obstruction syndrome (hepatic veno-occlusive disease). J Clin Exp Hepatol. 2014;4(4):332–46.

18.   Wang X, Qi X, Guo X. Tusanqi-related sinusoidal obstruction syndrome in China: a systematic review of the literatures. Medicine. 2015;94(23):e942.

19.   Wang JY, Gao H. Tusanqi and hepatic sinusoidal obstruction syndrome. J Dig Dis. 2014;15(3):105–7.

20.   Coppell JA, Richardson PG, Soiffer R, Martin PL, Kernan NA, Chen A, Guinan E, Vogelsang G, Krishnan A, Giralt S, et al. Hepatic veno-occlusive disease following stem cell transplantation: incidence, clinical course, and outcome. Biol Blood Marrow Transpl. 2010;16(2):157–68.

21.   Richardson PG, Riches ML, Kernan NA, Brochstein JA, Mineishi S, Termuhlen AM, Arai S, Grupp SA, Guinan EC, Martin PL, et al. Phase 3 trial of defibrotide for the treatment of severe veno-occlusive disease and multi-organ failure. Blood. 2016;127(13):1656–65.

22.   Richardson PG, Smith AR, Triplett BM, Kernan NA, Grupp SA, Antin JH, Lehmann L, Shore T, Iacobelli M, Miloslavsky M, et al. Defibrotide for patients with hepatic Veno-occlusive disease/sinusoidal obstruction syndrome: interim results from a treatment IND study. Biol Blood Marrow Transpl. 2017;23(6):997–1004.

23.   Yang D, Yang J, Shi D, Deng R, Yan B. Scoparone potentiates transactivation of the bile salt export pump gene and this effect is enhanced by cytochrome P450 metabolism but abolished by a PKC inhibitor. Br J Pharmacol. 2011;164(5):1547–57.

24.   Palomo M, Mir E, Rovira M, Escolar G, Carreras E, Diaz-Ricart M. What is going on between defibrotide and endothelial cells? Snapshots reveal the hot spots of their romance. Blood. 2016;127(13):1719–27.

25.   Aziz MT, Kakadiya PP, Kush SM, Weigel K, Lowe DK. Defibrotide: an oligonucleotide for sinusoidal obstruction syndrome. Ann Pharmacother. 2017. https://doi.org/10.1177/1060028017732586.

26.   Azoulay D, Castaing D, Lemoine A, Hargreaves GM, Bismuth H. Transjugular intrahepatic portosystemic shunt (TIPS) for severe veno-occlusive disease of the liver following bone marrow transplantation. Bone Marrow Transplant. 2000;25(9):987–92.

27.   Rajvanshi P, McDonald GB. Expanding the use of transjugular intrahepatic portosystemic shunts for veno-occlusive disease. Liver Transpl. 2001;7(2): 154–7.

17

Clinical characteristics of hepatic Arterioportal shunts associated with hepatocellular carcinoma

Huiyong Wu[1], Wei Zhao[2], Jianbo Zhang[3], Jianjun Han[1] and Shuguang Liu[4*] 🔵

Abstract

Background: Hepatic arterioportal shunt (A-P shunt) is defined as the direct blood flow established between hepatic artery and portal venous system; it is frequently observed in patients with hepatocellular carcinoma (HCC). Clinically, it is important to diagnose HCC associated A-P shunts, as it may impact the treatment strategy of the patients. In the present study, we described the imaging findings of the HCC associated A-P shunts and discussed the treatments strategy of such patients. From the findings, we also discussed the potential cause of A-P shunts.

Methods: Clinical data of HCC patients ($n = 560$), admitted to the hospital between April 2012 to April 2014, were reviewed. Hepatic angiography was used to examine the presence of A-P shunts. Of the 137 patients with A-P shunts, grading of the A-P shunts was performed, and statistical analysis of the different grades of A-P shunts and clinical characteristics was performed.

Results: The hepatic angiography confirmed that 99 patients had typical A-P shunts (Grade 1–3), and 38 patients had atypical A-P shunts. Embolization was the main strategy used to treat A-P shunts, in which liquid embolic agents appeared to provide a better treatment outcome. The correlation analysis showed that the grading of portal vein tumor thrombus was significantly associated with the grading of A-P shunt ($p = < 0.001$, Spearman correlation coefficient was 0.816 ± 0.043).

Conclusions: We characterized A-P shunts and proposed treatment strategy for treating HCC patients with various levels of A-P shunts. The findings supported the hypothesis that the formation of HCC associated A-P shunts was caused by tumor thrombus.

Keywords: Hepatocellular carcinoma, Hepatic arterioportal shunts, Portal vein tumor embolus, Transarterial chemoembolization

Background

Transcatheter arterial chemoembolization (TACE) is one of the important treatment strategies for patients with hepatocellular carcinoma (HCC). It is not only used as a standard treatment for middle-stage tumor but also as a necessary treatment for early stage patients after surgery [1, 2]. Hepatic arterioportal shunts (A-P shunts) are frequently observed in patients with HCC. The presence of A-P shunt often complicates the HCC cases and severely affects the efficacy and safety of TACE. For example, the A-P shunts may cause the chemotherapy drug and embolic agent to run-off through the shunt path. The hepatic A-P shunts may also lead to the tumor thrombus detached from hepatic artery, resulting in a blockage of portal vein. The tumor thrombus detached may also block the hepatic small arteries, leading to hepatic tissue necrosis [3–6]. As such, the best treatment strategy for HCC complicated with the hepatic A-P shunts remains to be determined.

There are various causes of A-P shunts, such as liver cirrhosis, hepatic neoplasms, hepatic trauma, obstruction of the portal or hepatic vein, and inflammatory diseases [7]. For HCC patients, it was suggested that A-P shunts were caused by the invasion of HCC into the

* Correspondence: jinanwhy@163.com
[4]Department of Thoracic Oncology Surgery, Shandong Tumor Hospital Affiliated to Shandong University, No. 440, Jiyan Road, Jinan 250117, China
Full list of author information is available at the end of the article

portal vein system. When the hepatic vein is obstructed (e.g. due to rumor thrombus), the pressure gradient between the sinusoids and portal veins is reversed, resulting in a functional A-P shunt [8, 9]. The hemodynamics in such cases seem to be very complex and remain to be fully investigated. Histological findings have shown that when tumor tissues invaded along the portal vein cavity, the portal vein structure was generally complete, and structural changes of the portal vein have rarely been observed. On the basis of the hepatic artery angiography findings, direct circulation between hepatic artery and portal vein was not found in cases of tumor invasion. We hypothesized that hepatic A-P shunts of HCC patients were caused by the portal vein tumor thrombus. In this study, we analyzed characteristics of hepatic artery angiography images of A-P shunts in 137 HCC patients, and described the treatment strategy for such patients. We also performed statistical analysis to investigate the correlation of portal vein tumor thrombus and A-P shunts.

Patients and methods

Patients

Clinical data of 560 HCC patients, admitted to Shandong Tumor Hospital Affiliated to Shandong University between April 2012 and April 2014, were reviewed. All of these patients received TACE or transcatheter arterial embolization (TAE) treatment. Among these patients, 137 of them (124 male and 13 female) had A-P shunts. The age of patients with A-P shunts ranged from 32 to 83 years old, with median at 55 years old. The eligibility criteria include: 1) confirmed diagnosis of HCC by biopsy or imaging according to accepted guideline [10]; 2) observation of hepatic A-P shunt in hepatic arteriography; 3) if A-P shunt was not found on hepatic arteriography, observation of iodized oil flowing from hepatic artery to the portal vein must be observed during TAE under X-ray examination; 4) patients with no history of hepatic resection. In this cohort, 127 patients had history of hepatitis B virus infection, 2 patients had hepatitis C virus infection, and the rest had no liver disease of clinical significance. Table 1 summarized the baseline clinical characteristics of the patients. The A-P shunts were divided into four grades: the atypical A-P shunts were classified as Grade 0, while the typical A-P shunts were further classified into three grades (Grade 1–3) according to severity (Table 2).

Treatment with TACE/TAE

Digital subtraction angiography was performed on hepatic artery or superior mesenteric artery in all patients.

Table 1 Characteristics of patients with typical and atypical A-P shunts

Characteristics	Number of patients or Mean/Median	Atypical A-P Shunt	Typical A-P Shunt	p
Sex, n (%)				0.945
Male	124 (90.51)	35 (92.11)	89 (89.90)	
Female	13 (9.49)	3 (7.89)	10 (10.10)	
Age, mean ± sd	54.91 ± 9.47	56.45 ± 8.0	54.32 ± 9.94	0.241
Etiology, n (%)				0.837
HBV	127 (92.70)	35 (92.11)	92 (92.93)	
HCV	2 (1.46)	1 (2.63)	1 (1.01)	
Others	8 (5.84)	2 (5.26)	6 (6.06)	
Number of tumors, n (%)				0.055
Multiple	86 (62.77)	19 (50.00)	67 (67.68)	
Single	51 (37.23)	19 (50.00)	32 (32.32)	
Child-Pugh score, n (%)				0.898
A	102 (74.45)	28 (73.68)	74 (74.75)	
B	35 (25.55)	10 (26.32)	25 (25.25)	
AFP(ng/ml), median (quartile)	309.0(13.85, 1210.0)	57.0 (7.2,1210.0)	579 (15.7,1210.0)	**0.035**
Albumin(g/L), mean ± sd	40.11 ± 5.34	39.59 ± 5.71	40.32 ± 5.21	0.827
Bilirubin (mmol/L), median (quartile)	22.0 (15.5,29.6)	20.95 (14.3,28.5)	22.2 (15.5,30)	0.644
Creatinine (umol/L),median (quartile)	62.0 (54.2, 71.0)	60.65 (53.7,68)	63.1 (54.2,73.1)	0.701
AST(U/L),median(quartile)	41.0 (28.0, 65.0)	32.05 (26.4,58.5)	43.3 (30.0,67.0)	**0.025**
ALT(U/L),median(quartile)	49.0 (36.0, 74.9)	39.5 (29.3, 74.0)	53 (37.8, 77.0)	0.106
Platelets (10^9/L) median(quartile)	125 (88, 282)	109 (91, 161)	128 (87, 182)	0.341
Tumor size (cm), median (quartile)	6.5 (3.8, 9.5)	5 (3.3, 7.0)	7.1 (4.5, 10.5)	**0.007**

Table 2 Grading of A-P shunt

Grade	Definition	Number of patients
0	A-P shunt was not observed in hepatic arterial angiography. The iodized oil was dispersed from hepatic artery into the portal vein, leading to the deposition of iodized oil in intrahepatic portal vein unrelated to tumor.	38
1	Segmental branches of the portal vein portal was observed due to A-P shunt	21
2	Portal vein trunk was observed due to A-P shunt located in the same hepatic lobe	47
3	Portal vein trunk was observed due to A-P shunt located in a different hepatic lobe	31

Iodized oil (5–20 mL) and doxorubicin (40–60 mg) were used in arterial embolization. According to the timing of visualization of the venous structures on imagining, embolic agents including microsphere, absolute ethanol, and coils were used for shunt embolization. After embolization, hepatic artery angiography and liver-enhanced CT/MR were performed to examine the portal vein, specifically to observe the presence of tumor thrombus in the main trunk or branches of the portal vein.

Statistical analysis

Categorical variables were presented in frequency (%), and continuous variables were presented in mean ± standard deviation, or median. Categorical data between two groups were compared using the chi-square test or Fisher exact test. Continuous data between two groups were compared using t-test if the data were normally distributed; otherwise, Wilcoxon two-sample test was used. The association of the grading of A-P shunt and the grading of portal vein tumor thrombus was analyzed using Spearman rank correlation analysis. All statistical analyses were performed using SAS9.3. Two-tailed testing was used, and $p < 0.05$ was defined as statistically significant.

Results

Imaging and clinical characteristics of typical and atypical A-P shunt

A-P shunts were classified into two types (typical and atypical) according to the hepatic arteriogram images. In typical A-P shunt, early enhancement of portal vein was observed (Fig. 1). The detail of the blood flow of the A-P shunts was displayed clearly, with the images showing 'thread and streaks' signs, corresponding to the blood flow and vessels. According to the conditions of the blood supply of tumor and the severity of A-P shunts, embolic agents including microsphere, absolute ethanol, and spring coils were used for shunt embolization.

In atypical A-P shunt, portal vein was not enhanced during the hepatic arteriogram examination. In these patients, when iodized oil was injected, the flow of oil from portal artery through the A-P shunt and through the

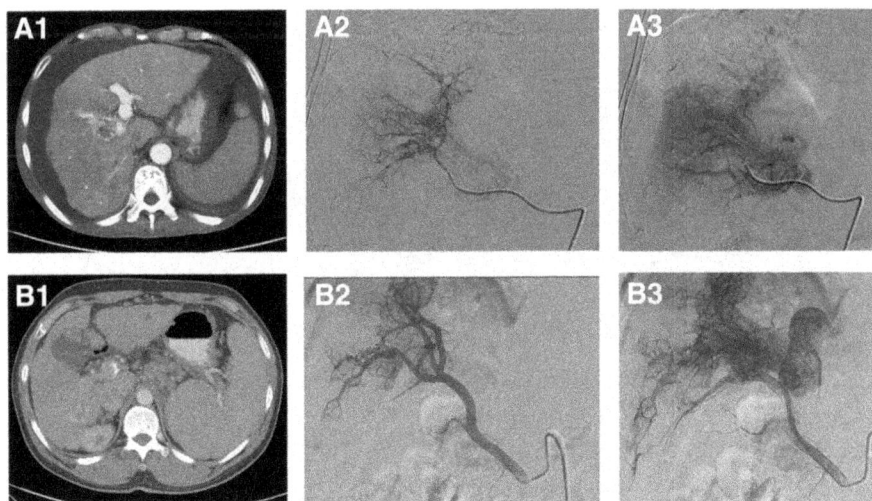

Fig. 1 A. A patient with tumor thrombus and A-P shunt. (A1) Liver CT image showed the presence of right portal vein tumor thrombus. Arteries around the tumor thrombus were filled with contrast agent, suggesting the presence of A-P shunt. The intra-luminal filling of embolus indicated the internal blood flow. (A2) Early phase hepatic angiography showed 'thread and streaks' signs, corresponding to the blood spaces and vessels, which run longitudinally in and around the tumor thrombus. (A3) Late phase hepatic angiography showed that the blood flow of the tumor thrombus reached the portal vein, leading to the enhancement of portal vein. **B**. CT images of another patient with tumor thrombus and A-P shunt. (B1) CT image showed tumor thrombus in the right portal vein branch. Staining of the arteries around thrombus suggested the presence of A-P shunt. (B2) Early phase hepatic angiography showed the hepatic arteries run longitudinally in the hepatic portal vein. (B3) Late phase hepatic angiography: blood vessels in the embolus showed 'tread and streaks' signs. Enhancement of the left branch of the portal vein and segment of portal vein proximal to the embolus

portal vein was observed. Also, the short-term retention of iodized oil in the portal vein and diffused distribution of iodized oil in the liver were observed. This observation was different from the over-embolization of iodized oil, in which the iodized oil was first accumulated in the tumor and then in the peripheral portal vein. Of the 137 patients, 99 of them had typical A-P shunts and 38 had atypical A-P shunts. The comparison the clinical characteristics of the two groups of patients showed that patients with typical A-P shunts had significantly higher levels of serum AFP ($p = 0.035$) and AST ($p = 0.025$). Also, they had significantly larger tumor ($p = 0.007$), suggesting the advanced HCC stage of these typical A-P shunt patients (Table 1).

Grading of A-P shunts and portal vein tumor thrombus

We further classified the A-P shunts into four grades (Table 2). For the 99 cases of typical A-P shunts, 21 of them were Grade 1, 47 patients were Grade 2, and 31 patients were Grade 3 (Fig. 2). We also examined the presence of portal vein tumor thrombus in all patients, and found 85.4% (117/137) of them had tumor thrombus. The tumor thrombus was classified into three grades (Grade 1–3) according to the severity (Table 3). There were 34 patients with Grade 1 tumor thrombus, 50 patients with Grade 2, and 33 patients with Grade 3.

Association of A-P shunt and portal vein tumor thrombus

To investigate if the grading of A-P shunts was associated with the grading of tumor thrombus, a correlation analysis was performed. The grading of portal vein tumor thrombus

was significantly associated with the grading of A-P shunt ($p = < 0.001$, Spearman correlation coefficient was 0.816 ± 0.043) (Table 4). For patients without thrombus, 19/20 of them had Grade 0 A-P shunt. There was only one patient with Grade 2 A-P shunts showed the absence of HCC invasion and absence of portal vein tumor thrombus. This patient had dilated bile duct as shown by the hepatic angiography.

There were 20 patients with no tumor thrombus observed (Grade 0) during the initial imaging examination. However, in the subsequent visits, 18 of these patients had tumor thrombus developed and typical A-P shunts observed. For the 34 patients, who had Grade 1 tumor thrombus, 17 of them had typical A-P shunts observed during the first imaging examination. Along the disease course of HCC and tumor thrombus development, eventually 28/34 patients showed typical A-P shunts by the end of the study.

Discussion

A-P shunts are frequently observed in patients with advanced HCC. In a previous study, hepatic angiogram examination revealed that among the 114 patients with HCC, 63.2% of them had various levels of A-P shunts [11]. A recent study also showed that among 596 patients with HCC, 27% of them had severe A-P shunts [12]. HCC associated A-P shunts may occur in different routes. Okuda et al. reported that shunts could occur 1) through a tumor thrombus in the portal branch, 2) in a retrograde direction via a peripheral tumor nodule, 3) through a small tumor invading or amputating an artery, or 4)

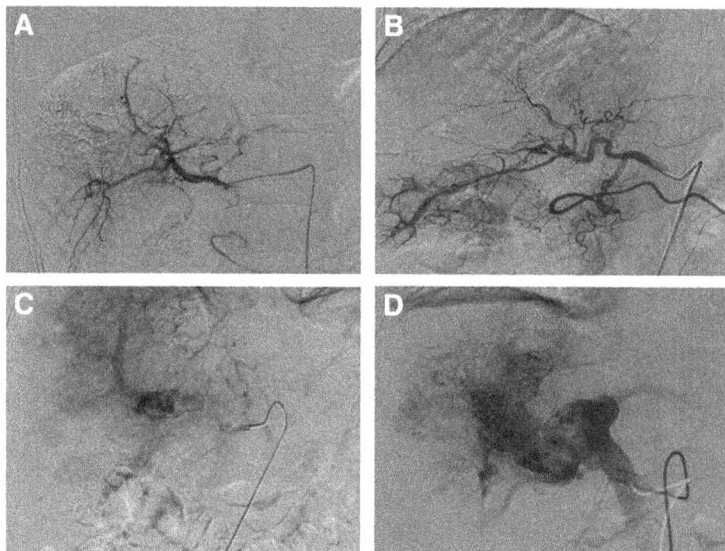

Fig. 2 Representative images of hepatic arteriogram showing different grades of A-P shunts. **a** Grade 0: A-P shunt was not observed. **b** Grade 1: enhancement of the VI segment of the portal vein in the right lobe of the liver. **c** Grade 2: enhancement of the right portal vein and portal vein tumor thrombus. **d** Grade 3: enhancement of right portal vein main branches and trunk, with ill-defined intra-luminal filling defect. A large number of disorganized arteries providing blood supply for the portal vein thrombus was observed

Table 3 Grading of portal vein tumor thrombus

Grade	Definition	Number of patients
0	No tumor thrombus. Only the portal venous invasion was observed.	20
1	Tumor thrombus was observed in branches of portal vein.	34
2	Tumor thrombus was observed in the right or left branches of portal vein.	50
3	Tumor thrombus was observed in the portal vein trunk.	33

through a tumor located near a major portal vein branch and supplied by a large artery [11]. In the present study, almost all the HCC associated A-P shunts were associated with the tumor thrombus.

Digital subtraction angiography has been the gold standard for diagnosis of HCC-associated A-P shunts, but the detail of the blood flow could sometime be difficult to observe using this technique. To date, with the advances in imaging technology, the presence of A-P shunts could easily be detected through hepatic arteriogram. In this study, the detail of the blood flow of the A-P shunts was clearly displayed by imaging examination in majority of the patients with typical A-P shunts (99/137). The imaging showed 'thread and streaks' signs, corresponding to the blood flow and vessels; thrombus located in a large branch and/or trunk of the portal vein was also observed [13]. An increased number and thickening of artery branches in proximity to the bile duct were often observed, indicating an increase of blood supply to the tumor thrombus. Portal vein thrombus is often caused by the HCC tumors that invade through the stroma. The blood supply to the tumor thrombus increased with the growth of the thrombus, leading to the formation of typical A-P shunts.

In this study, most of the patients with atypical A-P had early-stage tumor thrombus. The early-stage thrombus had a relatively small amount of blood supply, thus low-flow of A-P shunts. In some patients with atypical shunt, portal vein thrombus was not found during the initial diagnosis. These patients had the HCC located near the portal vein, with invasion at the portal vein stroma.

This condition is similar to the early-stage tumor thrombus. Indeed, these patients eventually developed tumor thrombus in the course of the disease. Based on the observations, we suggested that majority of HCC associated A-P shunts are related to the development of portal vein tumor thrombus.

It has been suggested that conventional TACE was not effective for HCC patients with significant A-P shunts. Efforts have been made to treat these patients with embolization materials such as gelatin sponges or coils; however, these approaches could only provide short-term benefits [14–16].The embolization materials (e.g. gelatin sponges, coils) are large in size, and are difficult to pass through the shunt and reach the portal vein. It has been reported that the use of iodized oil for embolization was effective in some patients with A-P shunts [14, 15]. We believe it is due to the effective embolization of the blood vessels of tumor thrombus. In our experiences, the use of iodized oil was effective in patients with low or absence of A-P shunts. Retentions of iodized oil in tumor thrombus were often observed in these patients after conventional TACE. Moreover, these patients with low level of A-P shunt may have better liver function. For patients with significant A-P shunts, materials such as sponge particle may first be used to induce shunt occlusion, followed by injection of other embolization agents [17]. Alternatively, the catheter could be inserted into the arteries of the thrombus for injection of embolization agents.

It has been reported that multiple TACE treatments may lead to A-P shunts, thus it is recommended that chemoembolization should be abandoned if A-P shunts appear or the dose of embolic agents should be reduced [18]. In the present study, some of the HCC cases continued to progress after TACE; invasion of the tumor at the portal vein and development of tumor thrombus were found. These conditions lead to an increase of A-P shunt flow. In other cases, TACE treatment did not stop the growth of the existing tumor thrombus, resulting in an increase of A-P shunts. Therefore, embolization of the tumor thrombus should be performed if patients have satisfactory liver function. The embolization of the blood supply of tumor thrombus could reduce the flow of the A-P shunts.

Table 4 Correlations between severity of hepatic A-P shunt and portal vein tumor embolus

Portal Vein Tumor thrombus Grade	Hepatic A-P shunt grade				Total	p	Spearman correlation coefficient
	0	1	2	3			
0	19 (50.00)	0 (0.00)	1 (2.13)	0 (0.00)	20	< 0.001	0.816 ± 0.043
1	17 (44.74)	11 (52.38)	6 (12.77)	0 (0.00)	34		
2	0 (0.00)	10 (47.62)	35 (74.47)	5 (16.13)	50		
3	2 (5.26)	0 (0.00)	5 (10.64)	26(83.87)	33		
Total	38	21	47	31	137		

Conclusions

In conclusion, the findings of the present study supported the hypothesis that the formation of HCC associated A-P shunts was caused by tumor thrombus. The grading of A-P shunts was significantly associated with the grading of tumor thrombus. It is recommended to perform embolization of the tumor thrombus, so that the flow of the A-P shunts may be decreased.

Abbreviations

A-P shunts: Arterioportal shunts; HCC: Hepatocellular carcinoma; TAE: Transcatheter arterial embolization

Acknowledgements

Not applicable.

Funding

None.

Authors' contributions

SG Liu and HY Wu mainly participated in literature search, study design, writing and critical revision. W Zhao, JB Zhang and JJ Han mainly participated in data collection, data analysis and data interpretation. All authors read and approved the final manuscript.

Consent for publication

Not applicable.

Competing interests

All the authors have no conflict of interest for this study.

Author details

[1]Department of Intervention, Shandong Tumor Hospital Affiliated to Shandong University, Jinan 250117, China. [2]Department of Radiotherapy, Shandong Tumor Hospital Affiliated to Shandong University, Jinan 250117, China. [3]Department of pathology, Shandong Tumor Hospital Affiliated to Shandong University, Jinan 250117, China. [4]Department of Thoracic Oncology Surgery, Shandong Tumor Hospital Affiliated to Shandong University, No. 440, Jiyan Road, Jinan 250117, China.

References

1. Montalto G, Cervello M, Giannitrapani L, Dantona F, Terranova A, Castagnetta LA. Epidemiology, risk factors, and natural history of hepatocellular carcinoma. Ann N Y Acad Sci. 2002;963:13–20.
2. Chen X, Liu L, Pan X. Portal vein tumor thrombus in advanced hepatocellular carcinoma: a case report. Oncol Lett. 2015;9(6):2495–8.
3. Llovet JM, Bruix J. Systematic review of randomized trials for unresectable hepatocellular carcinoma: chemoembolization improves survival. Hepatology. 2003;37(2):429–42.
4. Bruix J, Sherman M. American Association for the Study of liver D, *Management of hepatocellular carcinoma: an update.* Hepatology. 2011;53(3):1020–2.
5. Lazaridis KN, Kamath PS. Images in hepatology. Arterio-portal fistula causing recurrent variceal bleeding. J Hepatol. 1998;29(1):142.
6. Okuyama M, Fujiwara Y, Hayakawa T, Shiba M, Watanabe T, Tominaga K, Tamori A, Oshitani N, Higuchi K, Matsumoto T, Nakamura K, Wakasa K, Hirohashi K, Ashida S, Shuin T, Arakawa T. Esophagogastric varices due to arterioportal shunt in a serous cystadenoma of the pancreas in von Hippel-Lindau disease. Dig Dis Sci. 2003;48(10):1948–54.
7. Choi BI, Chung JW, Itai Y, Matsui O, Han JK, Han MC. Hepatic abnormalities related to blood flow: evaluation with dual-phase helical CT. Abdom Imaging. 1999;24(4):340–56.
8. Kanazawa S, Wright KC, Kasi LP, Charnsangavej C, Wallace S. Preliminary experimental evaluation of temporary segmental hepatic venous occlusion: angiographic, pathologic, and scintigraphic findings. J Vasc Interv Radiol. 1993;4(6):759–66.
9. Murata S, Itai Y, Asato M, Kobayashi H, Nakajima K, Eguchi N, Saida Y, Kuramoto K, Tohno E. Effect of temporary occlusion of the hepatic vein on dual blood in the liver: evaluation with spiral CT. Radiology. 1995;197(2):351–6.
10. Bruix J, Sherman M, Llovet JM, Beaugrand M, Lencioni R, Burroughs AK, Christensen E, Pagliaro L, Colombo M, Rodes J, EPoEo HCC. Clinical management of hepatocellular carcinoma. Conclusions of the Barcelona-2000 EASL conference. European Association for the Study of the Liver. J Hepatol. 2001;35(3):421–30.
11. Okuda K, Musha H, Yamasaki T, Jinnouchi S, Nagasaki Y, Kubo Y, Shimokawa Y, Nakayama T, Kojiro M, Sakamoto K, Nakashima T. Angiographic demonstration of intrahepatic arterio-portal anastomoses in hepatocellular carcinoma. Radiology. 1977;122(1):53–8.
12. Huang MS, Lin Q, Jiang ZB, Zhu KS, Guan SH, Li ZR, Shan H. Comparison of long-term effects between intra-arterially delivered ethanol and Gelfoam for the treatment of severe arterioportal shunt in patients with hepatocellular carcinoma. World J Gastroenterol. 2004;10(6):825–9.
13. Okuda K, Musha H, Yoshida T, Kanda Y, Yamazaki T. Demonstration of growing casts of hepatocellular carcinoma in the portal vein by celiac angiography: the thread and streaks sign. Radiology. 1975;117(2):303–9.
14. Luo J, Guo RP, Lai EC, Zhang YJ, Lau WY, Chen MS, Shi M. Transarterial chemoembolization for unresectable hepatocellular carcinoma with portal vein tumor thrombosis: a prospective comparative study. Ann Surg Oncol. 2011;18(2):413–20.
15. Peng BG, He Q, Li JP, Zhou F. Adjuvant transcatheter arterial chemoembolization improves efficacy of hepatectomy for patients with hepatocellular carcinoma and portal vein tumor thrombus. Am J Surg. 2009;198(3):313–8.
16. Tarazov PG. Intrahepatic arterioportal fistulae: role of transcatheter embolization. Cardiovasc Intervent Radiol. 1993;16(6):368–73.
17. Murata S, Tajima H, Nakazawa K, Onozawa S, Kumita S, Nomura K. Initial experience of transcatheter arterial chemoembolization during portal vein occlusion for unresectable hepatocellular carcinoma with marked arterioportal shunts. Eur Radiol. 2009;19(8):2016–23.
18. Ngan H, Peh WC. Arteriovenous shunting in hepatocellular carcinoma: its prevalence and clinical significance. Clin Radiol. 1997;52(1):36–40.

18

Macrocytic anemia is associated with the severity of liver impairment in patients with hepatitis B virus-related decompensated cirrhosis

Jian Yang[1†] 🆔, Bin Yan[1†], Lihong Yang[1], Huimin Li[2], Yajuan Fan[2], Feng Zhu[3], Jie Zheng[1] and Xiancang Ma[2*]

Abstract

Background: Macrocytic anemia is common in liver disease. However, its role in hepatitis B virus (HBV)-related decompensated cirrhosis remains unknown. The aim of the present study was to determine the association between macrocytic anemia and the severity of liver impairment in patients with HBV-related decompensated cirrhosis according to the Model for End Stage Liver Disease (MELD) score.

Methods: A total of 463 participants who fulfilled our criteria were enrolled in this cross-sectional study. Patients were classified into three groups according to anemia types, diagnosed based on their mean corpuscular volume level. Multivariate linear regression analyses were used to determine the association between macrocytic anemia and the MELD score for patients with HBV-related decompensated cirrhosis.

Results: Patients with macrocytic anemia had evidently higher MELD scores (10.8 ± 6.6) than those with normocytic anemia (8.0 ± 5.5) or microcytic anemia (6.3 ± 5.1). The association remained robust after adjusting for age, gender, smoking, drinking, and total cholesterol ($\beta = 1.94$, CI: 0.81–3.07, $P < 0.001$).

Conclusions: Macrocytic anemia was found to be associated with the severity of liver impairment and might be a predictor for short-term mortality in patients with HBV-related decompensated cirrhosis.

Keywords: Macrocytic anemia, HBV-related decompensated cirrhosis, MELD score, Severity of liver impairment

Background

Cirrhosis is an end-stage disease that invariably leads to death. It is the 14th most common cause of death in adults worldwide and results in 1.03 million deaths per year [1]. Chronic infection with hepatitis B virus (HBV) is one of the major causes of cirrhosis and 30% of deaths are attributable to HBV [2, 3]. China is a highly endemic area of HBV, where 78% of patients with cirrhosis are HBsAg positive [4]. In patients with cirrhosis, the 5-year probability of decompensation is 15–20%, while the

* Correspondence: maxiancang@163.com
†Jian Yang and Bin Yan contributed equally to this work.
²Department of Psychiatry, the First Affiliated Hospital, Xi'an Jiaotong University, No.277 Yanta West Road, Yanta District, Xi'an 710061, People's Republic of China
Full list of author information is available at the end of the article

5-year survival rate decreases from 84 to 14–35% once clinical decompensating events occur [5–7].

Anemia is a common comorbidity in cirrhosis that is associated with poor prognosis [8]. Erythrocyte abnormalities were clinically important and frequent findings in patients with chronic disease. Mean corpuscular volume (MCV), a measurement of the average volume of red blood cells (RBCs), has been documented to be associated with an increase in many clinical conditions [9–12]. Typically, anemia can be classified into macrocytic anemia (> 100 fL), normocytic anemia (80–100 fL), and microcytic anemia (< 80 fL) based on the patient's MCV level. A recent study has reported that the elevated MCV level was associated with increased liver cancer mortality, especially in men who are hepatitis B surface antigen (HBsAg) positive [13]. Therefore, in this study, we hypothesized that a common association might exist between macrocytic anemia and the severity of liver impairment in patients with HBV-related decompensated cirrhosis.

We used the Model for End Stage Liver Disease (MELD) score for evaluating the severity of liver impairment of HBV-related decompensated cirrhosis. The MELD score was developed to predict the short-term mortality of end-stage liver disease because of the shortage of donated livers. It had been validated subsequently as an accurate predictor of survival among different populations of patients with advanced liver disease and was adopted for organ allocation for liver transplantation instead of the older Child-Pugh score in the USA since 2002 [14–16]. Liver transplantation is generally recommended for patients with MELD score of > 15, if possible [17].

The goal of the present study is to investigate whether the MELD score is higher in the macrocytic anemia group in patients with HBV-related decompensated cirrhosis.

Methods
Study population
From May 2013 to July 2016, data of 1445 patients diagnosed as having HBV-related decompensated cirrhosis were extracted from the HIS Database at the First Affiliated Hospital of Xi'an Jiaotong University. For patients to be diagnosed as having HBV-related decompensated cirrhosis, the following conditions must be present: HBsAg carrier for ≥6 months; pathological or clinical evidence of cirrhosis; and occurrence of complications, such as ascites, upper gastrointestinal bleeding, spontaneous bacterial peritonitis, or hepatic encephalopathy [6, 18–20]. Anemia was defined according to WHO's haemoglobin thresholds, which is haemoglobin level of < 130 g/L in male and < 120 g/L in female [8]. After strictly screening according to the inclusion criteria and exclusion criteria, 463 patients were enrolled in this hospital-based cross-sectional study (Fig. 1). The study was approved by the Ethics Committee of the First Affiliated Hospital, Xi'an Jiaotong University. Since this is a retrospective study, a written consent is waived by the Ethics Committee and is deemed unnecessary. All methods were carried out in accordance with appropriate clinical practice guidelines and national legal requirements.

Data collection
Demographic characteristics were obtained from an interview during the patients' admission to our hospital. Venous blood samples were collected from the participants after an overnight fasting for laboratory assessments. Smoking was defined as having ≥1 cigarette per day and drinking was defined as alcohol intaking > 20 g per day for at least a year [21, 22]. Estimated glomerular filtration rate (eGFR) was calculated using a formula adapted from the Modification of Diet in Renal Disease (MDRD) equation [23, 24]. Unfortunately, body mass index (BMI) and HBV DNA data were not included in the analysis due to excessive missing values.

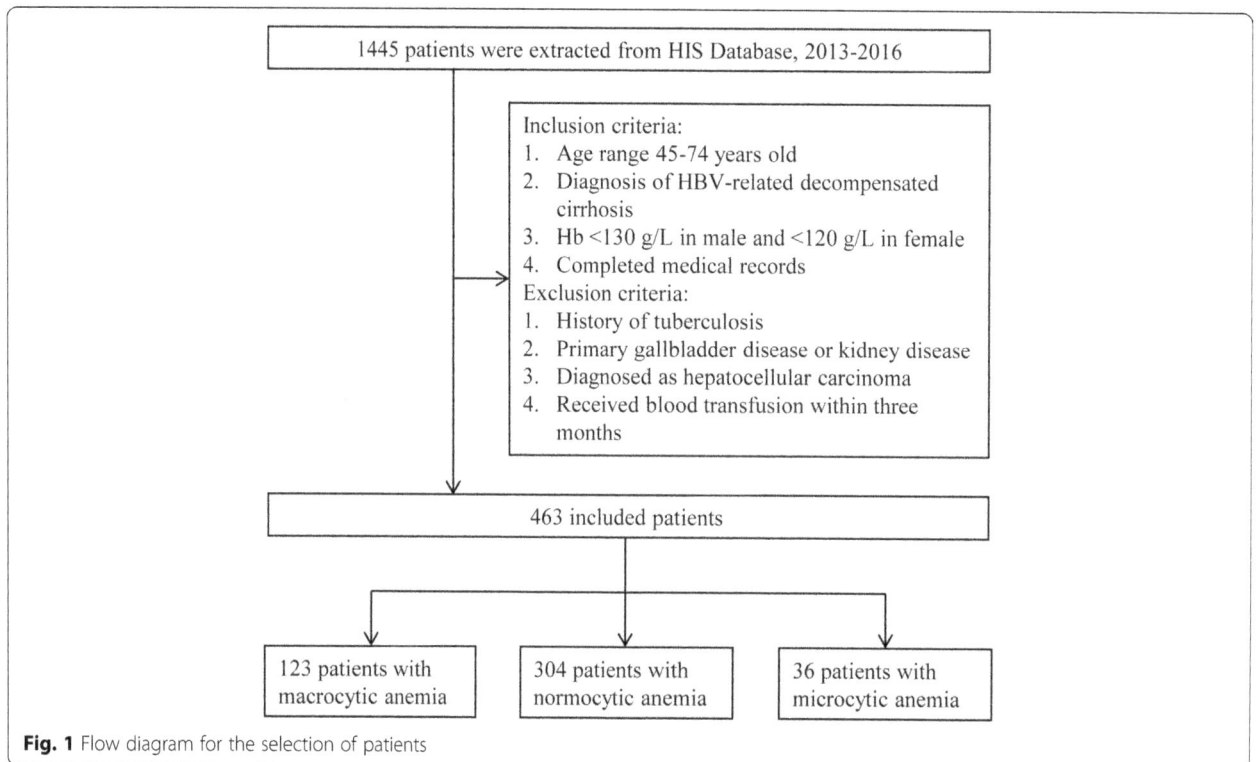

Fig. 1 Flow diagram for the selection of patients

MELD score

The MELD score was calculated using the following formula: $9.57 \times \log_e$ (creatinine mg/dl) $+ 3.78 \times \log_e$ (bilirubin mg/dl) $+ 11.2 \times \log_e$ (INR) $+ 6.43$, where INR is the international normalised ratio and 6.43 is the constant for liver disease aetiology [16].

Statistical analysis

Statistical analyses were conducted using R software (version 3.1.3). Continuous data were presented as mean $\pm$ SD, and categorical variables were presented as count and percentage. All participants were divided into three groups according to their anemia classification. We used one-way ANOVA to determine the differences among the three groups in terms of the continuous variables, because the variables were all normally distributed and homogeneous in variance. Simultaneously, the chi-square test was used for categorical variables. Univariate and multivariate linear regression analyses were used to examine the associations of the MELD score with macrocytic anemia. Variables with P value < 0.05 in univariate models were then included in the multivariate analyses. A two-tailed test was used to calculate the P value, and the results were considered statistically significant when the P value < 0.05.

Results

Characteristics of participants

Table 1 presents the baseline characteristics of the participants, which were divided into three groups according to anemia types. Among the 463 eligible participants, 304 had normocytic anemia, 123 had macrocytic anemia and 36 had microcytic anemia. The average age of participants was 54.3 (SD = 7.3) years and 63.5% of them were male. Our data showed that patients with macrocytic anemia were older and had higher levels of bilirubin, international normalized ratio (INR) and alkaline phosphatase (ALP) compared to patients with normocytic or microcytic anemia. MELD score was also observed to be higher in the macrocytic group. Oppositely, the total cholesterol and albumin were relatively low. There were no significant differences observed in terms of gender, smoking, drinking, hypertension, systolic blood pressure, diastolic blood pressure, creatinine, eGFR, aspartate aminotransferase (AST) and alanine aminotransferase (ALT). The haemoglobin level and prevalence of diabetes in the microcytic group were slightly different from that in the other two groups, but this difference was negligible.

Assessment of the association between MELD score and possible risk factors

We next assessed the correlation between the MELD score and possible risk factors using the univariate linear regression analyses (Table 2). Our results revealed a positive association between the MELD score and male, smoking and drinking. In addition, a negative association between the MELD score and the total cholesterol level was observed.

Association between macrocytic anemia and MELD score

Patients in the macrocytic group had evidently higher MELD scores than patients in the other two groups (Fig. 2). In univariate regression analysis, we found that there was a significant association between macrocytic anemia and the MELD score (estimated coefficient [β] = 2.80, 95% confidence interval [CI]: 1.59–4.01, P value [P] < 0.001), using the normocytic group as the reference. Furthermore, the association remained robust (β = 1.94, CI: 0.81–3.07, P < 0.001) after adjusting for age, gender, smoking, drinking and total cholesterol in multivariate analysis (Table 2).

Discussion

In this retrospective study, we demonstrated that macrocytic anemia, defined as anemia in which the RBCs are larger than their normal volume (100 fL), is associated with the severity of liver impairment in patients with HBV-related decompensated cirrhosis. This finding remains substantial even after adjusting for demographics and laboratory parameters, such as age, gender, smoking, drinking and total cholesterol.

An MCV level greater than 100 fL, which is also known as macrocytosis, may not always be associated with anemia. Moreover, it presents independently from anemia in most cases [10]. Nevertheless, we chose anemia as one of our inclusion criteria because 84.2% of the 1445 pre-screened patients have anemia. This result was consistent with the finding of another study, which reported that about 75% of patients with chronic liver disease have a diverse aetiology of anemia [25]. Furthermore, patients with cirrhosis may have anemia due to a lack of haematopoietic factors, shortened erythrocyte survival, reduced bone marrow function, or gastrointestinal bleeding. All these conditions indicate impaired liver function and a high risk of mortality. Therefore, patients without anemia were excluded from the data analysis to avoid potential bias in our present study.

The importance of macrocytic anemia or macrocytosis seems to be underestimated in the past. Only a few studies focused on its risk of adverse events or death [9–13]. Among these studies, Yoon et al. documented that the elevated MCV level was associated with increased liver cancer mortality in men [13]; this finding was consistent with the result of our study. A small-sample study also found a markedly higher MCV in patients with chronic liver failure than in healthy subjects [26]. These observations, though not directly, provided evidence for our conclusion that patients with HBV-related decompensated cirrhosis

Table 1 Demographic and biochemical characteristics of the study participants ($N = 463$)

Variable	Macrocytic anemia	Normocytic anemia	Microcytic anemia	P value
Number of subjects	123	304	36	
Mean corpuscular volume, fL	102.7 ± 2.6	91.2 ± 5.1[†]	74.2 ± 4.6[†¥]	< 0.001
Age, years	56.1 ± 7.6	53.9 ± 7.1[†]	51.8 ± 6.2[†]	0.002
Male, n(%)	78(63.4)	191(62.8)	25(69.4)	0.738
Drinking, n(%)	24(19.5)	74(24.3)	13(36.1)	0.118
Smoking, n(%)	48(39.0)	107(35.2)	15(41.7)	0.618
Diabetes, n(%)	10(8.1)	39(12.8)	9(25.0) [†]	0.026
Hypertension, n(%)	14(11.3)	36(11.8)	4(11.1)	0.985
Hemoglobin, g/L				
> 90	97(78.9)	230(75.7)	10(27.8)[†¥]	< 0.001
60–90	21(17.1)	63(20.7)	20(55.6)[†¥]	< 0.001
< 60	5(4.1)	11(3.6)	6(16.7)[†¥]	0.002
Total cholesterol, mmol/L	2.4 ± 0.7	2.7 ± 0.9[†]	2.7 ± 0.8	0.012
Systolic blood pressure, mmHg	117.9 ± 17.6	117.8 ± 15.2	113.8 ± 13.8	0.350
Diastolic blood pressure, mmHg	72.6 ± 11.7	73.4 ± 10.0	70.9 ± 8.6	0.354
Bilirubin, mg/dL	3.4 ± 3.4	2.6 ± 3.2[†]	1.8 ± 3.4[†]	0.011
Creatinine, mg/dL	0.8 ± 0.8	0.7 ± 0.4	0.7 ± 0.4	0.147
INR	1.5 ± 0.3	1.4 ± 0.4[†]	1.3 ± 0.1[†]	0.006
eGFR, mL/min/1.73m^2	123.6 ± 54.5	126.9 ± 43.4	130.3 ± 39.1	0.686
Albumin	27.0 ± 4.7	29.1 ± 4.7[†]	31.7 ± 4.8[†¥]	< 0.001
AST	78.3 ± 147.3	84.2 ± 196.6	41.7 ± 39.5	0.394
ALT	45.3 ± 42.4	59.4 ± 114.3	29.3 ± 31.8	0.113
ALP	122.9 ± 55.5	106.4 ± 61.1[†]	85.2 ± 32.7[†]	0.001
MELD score	10.8 ± 6.6	8.0 ± 5.5[†]	6.3 ± 5.1[†]	< 0.001
Complications, n(%)				
UGB	6(4.9)	34(11.2)	5(13.9)	0.093
SBP	36(29.3)	75(24.7)[†]	3(8.3)[†]	0.037
HE	14(11.4)	22(7.2)	3(8.3)	0.377

Values are presented as mean ± standard deviation or numbers (percentage)

INR international normalized ratio, *eGFR* estimated glomerular filtration rate, *AST* aspartate aminotransferase, *ALT* alanine aminotransferase, *ALP* alkaline phosphatase, *MELD* model for end stage liver disease, *UGB* upper gastrointestinal bleeding, *SBP* spontaneous bacterial peritonitis, *HE* hepatic encephalopathy
P indicates the difference among the three groups. [†]Indicates significance ($P < 0.05$) compared to macrocytic anemia; [¥]Indicates significance ($P < 0.05$) compared to normocytic anemia

who have macrocytic anemia were more likely to present worse liver condition.

There are several potential pathological mechanisms that explain why macrocytic anemia is associated with the severity of liver impairment. First, patients with advanced liver damage are more likely to have vitamin B_{12} or folate deficiencies [27], which directly result in macrocytic anemia. Vitamin B_{12} and folate coenzymes are required for thymidylate and purine synthesis, thus, their deficiencies result in retarded DNA synthesis and eventually will develop into macrocytic anemia [28–30]. Second, macrocytic anemia in liver disease may be due to an increased deposition of cholesterol on the membranes of circulating RBCs [31, 32]. This deposition effectively increases the surface area of the

erythrocyte. Third, hemolytic anemias are common in advanced liver failure. In this case, excessive destruction of RBCs and increased reticulocyte count can be observed. The immature erythrocytes are approximately 20% larger compared to the mature erythrocytes, which result in macrocytic anemia [25]. Moreover, erythrocyte morphology is affected by various factors in liver disease, such as causes, degree of liver damage, and drugs used. Complicated mechanisms, which allow the synchronized performance of their independent or collaborative functions, determine the shape of RBCs. Nevertheless, we firmly believe that there is a positive correlation between macrocytic anemia and the severity of liver impairment in patients with HBV-related decompensated cirrhosis.

Table 2 Univariate and multivariate linear regression analysis for MELD score

Variable	Univariate		Multivariate	
	β (CI 95%)	P value	β (CI 95%)	P value
Age	0.05(−0.02,0.13)	0.160	0.07(0.01,0.15)	0.028
Male	2.25(1.15,3.36)	< 0.001	1.49(0.29,2.70)	0.015
Smoking	1.93(0.82,3.03)	< 0.001	0.21(−1.03,1.44)	0.742
Drinking	1.59(0.34,2.85)	0.013	0.73(−0.56,2.01)	0.269
Diabetes	0.53(− 1.11,2.16)	0.527		
Hypertension	0.15(−1.53,1.84)	0.857		
Hemoglobin, g/L				
> 90	Ref	−		
60–90	1.09(−0.21,2.39)	0.100		
< 60	−1.35(−3.90,1.20)	0.298		
Total cholesterol	−2.77(−3.37,-2.16)	< 0.001	−2.53(− 3.14,-1.93)	< 0.001
Systolic blood pressure	−0.01(− 0.04,0.03)	0.863		
Diastolic blood pressure	−0.01(− 0.06,0.05)	0.900		
Anemia classification				
Normocytic anemia	Ref	−	Ref	−
Macrocytic anemia	2.80(1.59,4.01)	< 0.001	1.94(0.81,3.07)	< 0.001
Microcytic anemia	−1.73(−3.72,0.27)	0.089	− 1.77(− 3.59,0.05)	0.057

MELD model for end stage liver disease, *β* estimated coefficient, *95% CI* 95% confidence interval

In addition, we used the MELD score, which is a formula comprising creatinine, bilirubin, and INR values, to evaluate the severity of liver impairment and risk of death. In our study, patients with macrocytic anemia had higher levels of bilirubin and INR, but no significant difference was observed in creatinine levels and eGFR. Thus, macrocytic anemia might be unrelated to kidney damage in patients with HBV-related decompensated cirrhosis.

There were a few limitations in this study. First, we used the MELD score for evaluating the severity of liver impairment in patients with HBV-related decompensated cirrhosis. Although the MELD score could provide an accurate prediction of short-term mortality of patients with cirrhosis, a follow-up data might be better and more credible. Second, the analysis did not include data on serum vitamin B_{12}, folate, reticulocyte count, drugs, and measures of haemolysis, which could

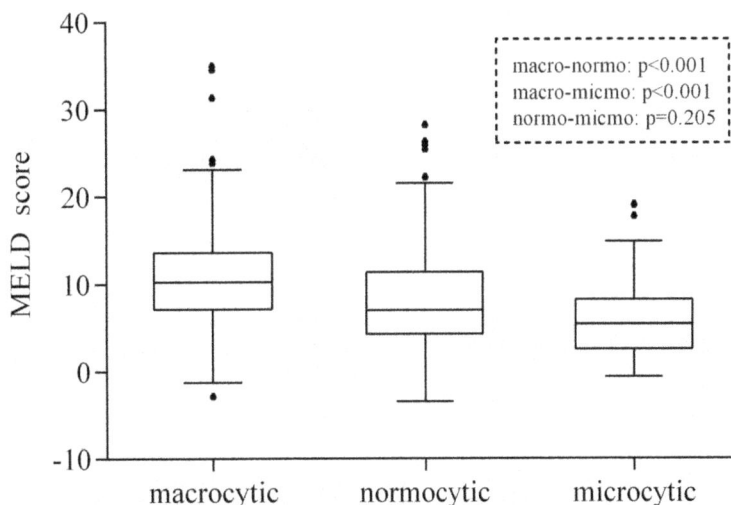

Fig. 2 Anemia types and MELD scores. Patients with macrocytic anemia had evidently higher MELD scores than those with normocytic anemia ($P < 0.001$) or microcytic anemia ($P < 0.001$)

contribute to better understand the mechanisms of macrocytic anemia in patients with cirrhosis.

Conclusions

Macrocytic anemia was found to be associated with the severity of liver impairment and might be a predictor for short-term mortality in patients with HBV-related decompensated cirrhosis. However, a large-scale cohort study is recommended to confirm the present results and to elucidate the mechanisms underlying the observed correlations between macrocytic anemia and the severity of liver impairment in patients with HBV-related decompensated cirrhosis.

Abbreviations
ALP: Alkaline phosphatase; ALT: Alanine aminotransferase; AST: Aspartate aminotransferase; BMI: Body mass index; eGFR: Estimated glomerular filtration rate; HBsAg: Hepatitis B surface antigen; HBV: Hepatitis B virus; HE: Hepatic encephalopathy; INR: International normalised ratio; MCV: Mean corpuscular volume; MDRD: Modification of diet in renal disease; MELD: Model for end stage liver disease; RBCs: Red blood cells; SBP: Spontaneous bacterial peritonitis; UGB: Upper gastrointestinal bleeding

Acknowledgements
We would like to acknowledge the participants in the study. We appreciated the Department of Epidemiology and Biostatistics, Xi'an Jiaotong University Health Science Center for statistical assistance.

Funding
There was no funding for this study.

Authors' contributions
XM, JY and BY designed the study. LY, HL and YF compiled the data and helped with the data interpretation. JY and BY analysed the data and drafted the manuscript. XM, JZ and FZ revised the manuscripts for important intellectual content helped with the data interpretation. All authors reviewed the manuscript.

Consent for publication
Not applicable

Competing interests
The authors declare no competing financial interests.

Author details
[1]Clinical Research Center, the First Affiliated Hospital, Xi'an Jiaotong University, Xi'an 710061, People's Republic of China. [2]Department of Psychiatry, the First Affiliated Hospital, Xi'an Jiaotong University, No.277 Yanta West Road, Yanta District, Xi'an 710061, People's Republic of China. [3]Center for Translational Medicine, the First Affiliated Hospital, Xi an Jiaotong University, Xi'an 710061, People's Republic of China.

References
1. Tsochatzis EA, Bosch J, Burroughs AK. Liver cirrhosis. Lancet. 2014;383(9930): 1749–61.
2. Perz JF, Armstrong GL, Farrington LA, Hutin YJ, Bell BP. The contributions of hepatitis B virus and hepatitis C virus infections to cirrhosis and primary liver cancer worldwide. J Hepatol. 2006;45(4):529–38.
3. Lozano R, Naghavi M, Foreman K, Lim S, Shibuya K, Aboyans V, Abraham J, Adair T, Aggarwal R, Ahn SY, et al. Global and regional mortality from 235 causes of death for 20 age groups in 1990 and 2010: a systematic analysis for the global burden of disease study 2010. Lancet. 2012;380(9859):2095–128.
4. Merican I, Guan R, Amarapuka D, Alexander MJ, Chutaputti A, Chien RN, Hasnian SS, Leung N, Lesmana L, Phiet PH, et al. Chronic hepatitis B virus infection in Asian countries. J Gastroenterol Hepatol. 2000;15(12):1356–61.
5. Srivastava M, Rungta S, Dixit VK, Shukla SK, Singh TB, Jain AK. Predictors of survival in hepatitis B virus related decompensated cirrhosis on tenofovir therapy: an Indian perspective. Antivir Res. 2013;100(2):300–5.
6. Peng CY, Chien RN, Liaw YF. Hepatitis B virus-related decompensated liver cirrhosis: benefits of antiviral therapy. J Hepatol. 2012;57(2):442–50.
7. McMahon BJ. Epidemiology and natural history of hepatitis B. Semin Liver Dis. 2005;25(Suppl 1):3–8.
8. Benoist BD, Mclean E, Egll I, Cogswell M, Benoist BD, Mclean E, Egll I, Cogswell M. Worldwide prevalence of anaemia 1993–2005: WHO global database on anaemia. Geneva, World Health Organization. 2008 2(3):97-100.
9. Ueda T, Kawakami R, Horii M, Sugawara Y, Matsumoto T, Okada S, Nishida T, Soeda T, Okayama S, Somekawa S, et al. High mean corpuscular volume is a new Indicator of prognosis in acute decompensated heart failure. Circ J. 2013;77(11):2766–71.
10. Myojo M, Iwata H, Kohro T, Sato H, Kiyosue A, Ando J, Sawaki D, Takahashi M, Fujita H, Hirata Y, et al. Prognostic implication of macrocytosis on adverse outcomes after coronary intervention. Atherosclerosis. 2012;221(1): 148–53.
11. Tennankore KK, Soroka SD, West KA, Kiberd BA. Macrocytosis may be associated with mortality in chronic hemodialysis patients: a prospective study. BMC Nephrol. 2011;12:19.
12. Kloth JS, Hamberg P, Mendelaar PA, Dulfer RR, van der Holt B, Eechoute K, Wiemer EA, Kruit WH, Sleijfer S, Mathijssen RH. Macrocytosis as a potential parameter associated with survival after tyrosine kinase inhibitor treatment. Eur J Cancer (Oxford, England : 1990). 2016;56:101–6.
13. Yoon HJ, Kim K, Nam YS, Yun JM, Park M. Mean corpuscular volume levels and all-cause and liver cancer mortality. Clin Chem Lab Med. 2016;54(7): 1247–57.
14. Wiesner R, Edwards E, Freeman R, Harper A, Kim R, Kamath P, Kremers W, Lake J, Howard T, Merion RM, et al. Model for end-stage liver disease (MELD) and allocation of donor livers. Gastroenterology. 2003;124(1):91–6.
15. Bambha K, Kim WR, Kremers WK, Therneau TM, Kamath PS, Wiesner R, Rosen CB, Thostenson J, Benson JT, Dickson ER. Predicting survival among patients listed for liver transplantation: an assessment of serial MELD measurements. Am J Transplant Off J Am Soc Transplant Am Soc Transplant Surg. 2004;4(11):1798–804.
16. Kamath PS, Kim WR. Advanced liver disease study G: the model for end-stage liver disease (MELD). Hepatology (Baltimore, MD). 2007;45(3):797–805.
17. Murray KF, Carithers RL Jr. AASLD: AASLD practice guidelines: evaluation of the patient for liver transplantation. Hepatology (Baltimore, MD). 2005;41(6): 1407–32.
18. Shim JH, Lee HC, Kim KM, Lim YS, Chung YH, Lee YS, Suh DJ. Efficacy of entecavir in treatment-naive patients with hepatitis B virus-related decompensated cirrhosis. J Hepatol. 2010;52(2):176–82.
19. Jang JW, Choi JY, Kim YS, Woo HY, Choi SK, Lee CH, Kim TY, Sohn JH, Tak WY, Han KH. Long-term effect of antiviral therapy on disease course after decompensation in patients with hepatitis B virus-related cirrhosis. Hepatology (Baltimore, MD). 2015;61(6):1809–20.
20. Wang FY, Li B, Li Y, Liu H, Qu WD, Xu HW, Qi JN, Qin CY. Entecavir for patients with hepatitis B decompensated cirrhosis in China: a meta-analysis. Sci Rep. 2016;6:32722.
21. Carter BD, Abnet CC, Feskanich D, Freedman ND, Hartge P, Lewis CE, Ockene JK, Prentice RL, Speizer FE, Thun MJ, et al. Smoking and mortality-- beyond established causes. N Engl J Med. 2015;372(7):631–40.
22. Kim HM, Kim BS, Cho YK, Kim BI, Sohn CI, Jeon WK, Kim HJ, Park DI, Park JH, Joo KJ, et al. Elevated red cell distribution width is associated with advanced fibrosis in NAFLD. Clin Mol Hepatol. 2013;19(3):258–65.
23. National Kidney Foundation. K/DOQI clinical practice guidelines for chronic kidney disease: evaluation, classification, and stratification. Am J Kidney Dis. 2002;39(2 Suppl 1):S1–266.
24. Ma YC, Zuo L, Chen JH, Luo Q, Yu XQ, Li Y, Xu JS, Huang SM, Wang LN, Huang W, et al. Modified glomerular filtration rate estimating equation for Chinese patients with chronic kidney disease. J Am Soc Nephrol. 2006; 17(10):2937–44.

25. Gonzalez-Casas R. Spectrum of anemia associated with chronic liver disease. World J Gastroenterol. 2009;15(37):4653.

26. Remkova A, Remko M. Homocysteine and endothelial markers are increased in patients with chronic liver diseases. Eur J Intern Med. 2009;20(5):482–6.

27. Rocco A, Compare D, Coccoli P, Esposito C, Di Spirito A, Barbato A, Strazzullo P, Nardone G. Vitamin B12 supplementation improves rates of sustained viral response in patients chronically infected with hepatitis C virus. Gut. 2013;62(5):766–73.

28. Morris MS, Jacques PF, Rosenberg IH, Selhub J. Folate and vitamin B-12 status in relation to anemia, macrocytosis, and cognitive impairment in older Americans in the age of folic acid fortification. Am J Clin Nutr. 2007; 85(1):193–200.

29. Green R, Dwyre DM. Evaluation of macrocytic anemias. Semin Hematol. 2015;52(4):279–86.

30. Robinson AR, Mladenovic J. Lack of clinical utility of folate levels in the evaluation of macrocytosis or anemia. Am J Med. 2001;110(2):88–90.

31. Owen JS, Bruckdorfer KR, Day RC, McIntyre N. Decreased erythrocyte membrane fluidity and altered lipid composition in human liver disease. J Lipid Res. 1982;23(1):124–32.

32. Grattagliano I, Calamita G, Cocco T, Wang DQ, Portincasa P. Pathogenic role of oxidative and nitrosative stress in primary biliary cirrhosis. World J Gastroenterol. 2014;20(19):5746–59.

19

Ultrasonic assessment of liver stiffness and carotid artery elasticity in patients with chronic viral hepatitis

Jing-Hua Li[†], Ning Zhu[†], Ying-Bin Min, Xiang-Zhou Shi, Yun-You Duan and Yi-Lin Yang[*]

Abstract

Background: This study investigated the relationship between liver stiffness and carotid artery elasticity in patients with chronic viral hepatitis. We used an acoustic radiation force impulse (ARFI) technique to measure stiffness, and a radio frequency (RF) vascular quantitative ultrasound technique to measure changes in common carotid artery elasticity and vascular function.

Methods: Two-hundred seventeen patients with chronic viral hepatitis caused by either hepatitis B virus (HBV) or hepatitis C virus (HCV) were enrolled. We divided the patients into two groups, one comprising 147 patients with chronic hepatitis B (CHB) (98 men and 49 women, average age 46.5 ± 12.2 years) and another comprising 70 patients with chronic hepatitis C (CHC) (47 men and 23 women, average age 47.6 ± 12.1 years). Additionally, 64 healthy age- and sex-matched participants (43 men and 21 women, average age 47.8 ± 5.1 years) were selected as the control group. The ARFI technique was used to measure liver stiffness and the RF ultrasound technique was used to measure carotid artery elasticity parameters including intima-media thickness (IMT), pulse wave velocity (PWV), arterial wall dilation coefficient (DC), compliance coefficient (CC), sclerosis indices α and β, and augmentation index (Aix). Clinical indicators, liver stiffness, and carotid artery elasticity parameters were observed and compared between the different age groups to investigate the correlation between carotid artery elasticity parameters and liver stiffness.

Results: The ARFI values for the CHB and CHC groups were significantly higher than those for the control group (1.84 ± 0.52 vs. 1.04 ± 0.11 m/s; 1.86 ± 0.37 vs. 1.04 ± 0.11 m/s, respectively; $P < 0.001$). When compared to the control group, both CHB and CHC groups showed an IMT of the same order, but had significantly higher elasticity parameters, such as α and β, as well as lower DC and CC values ($P < 0.001$). The PWV of the CHC group was significantly higher than that of the control group (7.98 ± 1.42 vs. 6.09 ± 0.90 m/s, $P < 0.001$). In the CHB group, all parameters including ARFI, IMT, PWV, DC, CC, α and β, were significantly different between the two age groups ($P < 0.05$). Within the CHC group, all parameters including IMT, PWV, DC, α and β, were significantly different between the two age groups ($P < 0.05$), except for ARFI, wherein the difference was not statistically significant. The correlation analysis and stepwise multiple linear regression analysis indicated that for patients with CHB, age was an independent predictor of common carotid artery IMT ($R^2 = 0.468$, F = 54.635, and $P < 0.001$). For patients with CHC, age and blood sugar were independent predictors of common carotid artery IMT ($R^2 = 0.465$, F = 29.118, and $P < 0.001$).

Conclusion: Although based on ARFI and RF ultrasound, the carotid artery IMT in patients with CHB and CHC was not significantly higher than that in the control group, their functional elasticity parameters had already changed. This finding serves as a useful reference for the clinical diagnosis of vascular diseases in patients with viral hepatitis.

Keywords: Ultrasound, HBV, HCV, Carotid artery elasticity

* Correspondence: yangyl66@126.com
[†]Jing-Hua Li and Ning Zhu contributed equally to this work.
Department of Ultrasound Diagnosis, Tangdu Hospital, Fourth Military Medical University, Xi'an 710038, Shaanxi Province, China

Background

Vascular wall elasticity is an important indicator of abnormal lipid metabolism in vascular disease, which is caused by pathogen-mediated chronic liver damage [1, 2]. Signals in the radio frequency (RF) vascular quantitative ultrasound technique quantify the intima-media thickness (IMT) and arterial stiffness within blood vessels and can serve as a sensitive indicator of early changes in vascular wall stiffness. The progression of liver fibrosis changes liver morphology and hepatic haemodynamics and decreases liver function. Liver biopsy has been the gold standard to measure and classify liver fibrosis, but because of its invasiveness, its clinical use is limited. Recently, elastography, a novel non-invasive technique for evaluating the degree of liver fibrosis, has gradually been applied in clinical practice and has been included in several liver disease diagnosis and treatment guidelines [3]. Preliminary experiments found that carotid artery elasticity parameters in patients with coronary artery disease and diabetes differed from those of healthy subjects [4]. However, whether these parameters were correlated with the degree of liver fibrosis in patients with chronic viral hepatitis have not been not studied using the new vascular measurement technologies. As a result, we conducted relevant clinical investigations and experiments to understand the extent of the changes in carotid artery morphology and function in patients with chronic viral hepatitis. These findings would help to determine whether the liver fibrosis is related to macrovascular diseases.

Methods

Research targets and grouping

A total of 217 consecutive patients with chronic viral hepatitis that were treated at our hospital between December 2015 and March 2017 were enrolled. The study population comprised 147 patients with Chronic hepatitis B (CHB) and 70 patients with Chronic hepatitis C (CHC). Patients were admitted into the CHB group according to the standard chronic hepatitis B diagnostic criteria [5], defined as hepatitis B surface antigen-positive without detectable ascites. Decompensated patients with symptoms such as ascites and lower oesophageal varices were excluded from this group. In the CHB group, there were 98 men and 49 women, with an average age of 46.5 ± 12.2 years. Among them, 34 patients had biopsy-proven liver fibrosis. Patients enrolled in the CHC group were hepatitis C virus antibody- (HCVAb) positive and had decompensated liver function. The exclusion criteria for the CHC group were the same as those for the CHB group. The CHC group consisted of 47 men and 23 women, with an average age of 47.6 ± 12.1 years. Among them, a biopsy confirmed liver fibroses in 21 patients. Contemporaneously, 64 healthy subjects comparable in age and sex, which was defined by no history of liver disease, hepatitis

B virus surface antigen (HBsAg) and HCVAb negativity, normal haemogram, liver, and kidney laboratory examinations, and no detection of liver diseases via 2-D ultrasound examination. Patients with disorders, such as high blood pressure, hypercholesterolemia, and dyslipidemia were excluded. The control group included 43 men and 21 women, with an average age of 45.8 ± 10.6 years.

Instruments and methods

Liver Elastography ultrasound

The acoustic radiation force impulse (ARFI) technique uses the 4C1 convex probe from the Color Doppler Diagnostic Ultrasound Scanner (Siemens, Siemens Acuson S2000) with a frequency of 3.0 to 4.5 MHz. During ARFI imaging, measurements were performed with the probe placed between the rib bones with the patient lying in either a dorsal decubitus or left recumbent position, taking normal breaths under a resting state or holding their breath, with displays of real-time 2-D images of the right liver lobe. When the image became clear, the operator used the cursor to locate a 5 mm × 10 mm-sized region of interest that targeted the liver parenchyma area and was free of vessels and bile duct. The measurement depth was fixed at 3 cm. When echoing was uniform within the sampling region, the operator pressed the probe button to freeze the image and display the depth and shear wave velocity (in m/s) in the region of interest. This measurement procedure was repeated 10 times for each patient. The median value of the measurements was recorded as the final result [6] (Fig. 1a).

Quantitative measurement of the common carotid artery

Measurements of the common carotid artery were obtained using the LA523 vascular probe from the Esaote Mylab Color Doppler Diagnostic Ultrasound Scanner with a frequency of 4 to 13 MHz. The ultrasound scanner was equipped with the RF-data technique and the Mylab Desk analysis working station. To take quantitative measurements of the common carotid artery, the patient was placed in the dorsal decubitus position, and instructed to breath normally in a resting state. After the patient's systolic and diastolic blood pressures in the right upper limb were measured, the patient's neck was sufficiently exposed. The ultrasonic probe was moved down longitudinally from the beginning of the common carotid artery, skipping the bifurcation area by 1 cm and the plaque sites. The operator then moved the sampling frame to the region for measurement, and the scanner automatically recorded the IMT and the elasticity parameters during 6 cardiac cycles. When the standard deviation of the IMT was less than 30, the indicator would turn green, suggesting that the measurements were stable. At that time, the values of parameters such as IMT, pulse wave velocity (PWV), arterial wall dilation

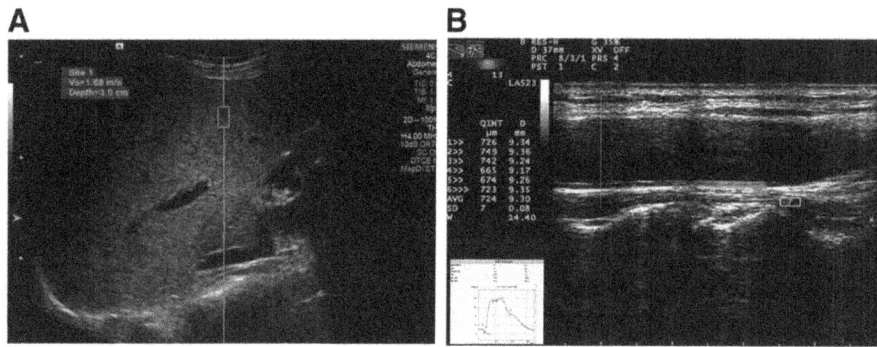

Fig. 1 ARFI liver stiffness images and common carotid artery RF ultrasound images in patients with CHB: **a** Use of the ARFI technique to measure liver stiffness in patients with CHB using a conventional ultrasound interface. **b** Use of QIMT and QAS techniques to quantify the carotid artery intima-media thickness (IMT) and vascular elasticity in patients with CHB

coefficient (DC), arterial wall compliance coefficient (CC), sclerosis indices α and β, and augmentation index (Aix) were exported as the final results [7] (Fig. 1b).

Clinical information

For all subjects, the following information was collected: (1) laboratory indicators including blood sugar, glycated haemoglobin, total cholesterol, triglycerides, low-density lipoprotein, high-density lipoprotein, alanine aminotransferase, aspartate aminotransferase, albumin, globulin, and platelets. (2) blood pressures including systolic and diastolic blood pressures.

Statistical analysis

Statistical analysis was performed using SPSS statistical software (version 19.0, IBM Corp., Armonk, NY, USA). Metrological data were expressed as average ± standard deviation ($\overline{X} \pm S$), while classification data were expressed as percentages (%). Inter-group measurement data were compared using one-way analysis of variance (ANOVA) and Levene's homogeneity of variance test. The average values of the two groups of measurement data were compared using the independent sample t test. A determination of correlation was conducted using Pearson's linear correlation method. Casual relationships of various intra-group parameters were investigated using either linear regression analysis or stepwise multiple linear regression analysis.

Results

General clinical data of the subjects

General clinical data for all study participants are listed in Table 1. We observed that there was no significant difference in age or sex among the three groups. Compared to the control group, the CHB group demonstrated a higher blood sugar level (5.3 ± 1.1 vs. 4.9 ± 0.5 mmol/L; $P = 0.010$) as well as higher levels of other

parameters such as platelets, albumin, AST and ALT, whereas the systolic and diastolic blood pressures were similar. The CHC group demonstrated a higher blood sugar level (5.3 ± 1.1 vs. 4.9 ± 0.5 mmol/L, $P < 0.001$), higher glycated haemoglobin level (6.8 ± 1.6 vs. $5.3 \pm 0.5\%$, $P < 0.001$), and higher levels of other parameters such as AST, ALT, and platelets compared to the control group. However, there was no significant difference in the cholesterol, triglycerides, HDL, and LDL levels.

Comparison of liver stiffness and elasticity parameters among groups

Results measured by the ARFI technique showed that both the CHB group (1.84 ± 0.52 m/s) and the CHC group (1.86 ± 0.37 m/s) had significantly higher liver elasticity parameters than the control group, and the inter-group differences were statistically significant (F = 90.806, $P < 0.001$) (Fig. 2a).

Comparison of carotid artery IMT values measured by RF ultrasound showed statistically significant differences ($P = 0.015$) between the control group (534.08 ± 134.25 μm), the CHB group (529.56 ± 131.04 μm), and the CHC group (587.34 ± 162.70 μm). An intergroup comparison showed significant difference between the CHB and the CHC group ($P = 0.032$) (Fig. 2b).

The PWV measurements of the CHC group (7.98 ± 1.42) were evidently higher than those of the CHB and the control groups, which were 6.70 ± 1.32 and 6.09 ± 0.90 m/s respectively. Differences in the intergroup comparisons were statistically significant (F = 40.310, $P < 0.001$) (Fig. 3a). The α values of the CHC and the CHB group were significantly higher than those of the control group, which were 3.03 ± 0.79, 4.13 ± 1.68, and 5.77 ± 2.29, respectively, with statistically significant differences under intergroup comparisons (F = 44.036, $P < 0.001$) (Fig. 3b). Similarly, the β values of the CHC and the CHB group were significantly higher than those of the control group, which were 6.17 ± 1.58, 8.42 ± 3.37, and

Table 1 General clinical data of all study participants

	Control Group n = 64	Patients with chronic viral hepatitis		F	P
		Patients with CHB n = 147	Patients with CHC n = 70		
Age, Years	45.8 ± 10.6	46.5 ± 12.2	47.6 ± 12.1	0.400	0.670
Men Percentage, Count (%)	43(67)	98(67)	47(67)	–	–
Systolic pressure, mmHg	115.7 ± 11.6	116.2 ± 13.1	119.7 ± 12.8	2.166	0.177
Diastolic, pressure mmHg	71.2 ± 8.7	73.2 ± 8.6	71.2 ± 8.6	1.872	0.156
Blood Glu, mmol/L	4.9 ± 0.5	5.3 ± 1.1	6.0 ± 1.7	15.933	< 0.001
Glycated haemoglobin, %	5.3 ± 0.5	5.5 ± 1.4	6.8 ± 1.6	30.804	< 0.001
BMI, Kg/m^2	23.2 ± 2.6	23.5 ± 3.0	24.4 ± 3.4	2.936	0.055
Cholesterol, mmol/L	3.8 ± 1.1	3.8 ± 1.3	3.7 ± 1.1	0.373	0.689
Triglycerides, mmol/L	1.2 ± 0.7	1.2 ± 0.5	1.2 ± 0.6	0.185	0.831
LDL, mmol/L	1.9 ± 0.8	1.8 ± 0.8	1.7 ± 0.8	0.695	0.500
HDL, mmol/L	1.0 ± 0.3	1.2 ± 0.4	1.1 ± 0.5	3.115	0.046*
Platelets, 10^9 /L	187.6 ± 70.2	137.4 ± 77.8	138.3 ± 64.3	11.598	< 0.001
AST, U/L	23.8 ± 8.7	45.8 ± 34.2	37.7 ± 24.6	13.927	< 0.001
ALT, U/L	28.5 ± 13.8	46.1 ± 38.5	43.1 ± 40.4	5.765	0.004
Albumin, g/L	43.8 ± 7.4	40.9 ± 8.9	40.8 ± 8.2	3.104	0.046*
Globulin, g/L	24.2 ± 6.3	25.3 ± 7.2	24.9 ± 7.1	0.566	0.569

Note: *CHB* chronic hepatitis B, *CHC* chronic hepatitis C, *BMI* Body mass index, *LDL* Low-density lipoprotein, *HDL* High-density lipoprotein, *AST* Aspartate aminotransferase, *ALT* Alanine aminotransferase. * $P < 0.05$ when compared to the control group

11.67 ± 4.53, respectively, with statistically significant differences under intergroup comparisons (F = 44.493, $P < 0.001$) (Fig. 3c). On the contrary, the DC and CC values of the CHC and CHB group were significantly lower than those of the control group. The DC values of the three groups were 0.32 ± 0.008, 0.030 ± 0.008, and 0.017 ± 0.008 1/kPa, respectively (Fig. 3e), with statistically significant intergroup differences (F = 3.897, $P = 0.021$). The CC values were 1.290 ± 0.248, 1.054 ± 0.385, and 0.815 ± 0.378 mm^2/kPa, respectively (Fig. 3d), with statistically significant intergroup differences (F = 29.717, P < 0.001). The DC and CC values of the CHC group were also significantly lower than those of the CHB group ($P < 0.001$). Aix measurements showed no statistically significant differences among the 3 groups (F = 2.237, $P = 0.0109$) (Fig. 3f).

Comparison of liver stiffness and left common carotid elasticity parameters among different age groups

All subjects were divided into two groups according to their age (Tables 2 and 3). with age 50 years being the dividing line. A comparison of the two groups showed no significant difference in ARFI values. However, in terms of carotid elasticity parameters, except for Aix, all other parameters including IMT, PWV, DC, CC, α, and β were significantly different between the two groups (all P values < 0.001). In the CHB group, ARFI values, as well as parameters including IMT, PWV, DC, CC, α, β, and Aix were all significantly different between the two

age groups (all P values < 0.05). In the CHC group, IMT, PWV, DC, α, β, and Aix were significantly different between the two age groups (all P values < 0.05).

Relationship between liver stiffness with carotid artery elasticity in patients with chronic viral hepatitis

Stepwise multiple linear regression analysis indicated that for patients with CHB, age was an independent predictor of common carotid artery IMT ($R^2 = 0.468$, F = 54.635, and $P < 0.001$) (Fig. 4a). For patients with CHC, both age (β = 8.291, $t = 6.847$, $P < 0.001$) and blood glucose (β = 22.436, $t = 2/573$, $P = 0.012$) were independent predictors of common carotid artery IMT ($R^2 = 0.465$, F = 29.118, and $P < 0.001$) (Fig. 4b, c).

Discussions

Chronic liver disease can cause abnormal lipid metabolism, which, in severe cases, can directly change the peripheral blood vessel walls. Timely and convenient measurements of changes in the peripheral blood vessel walls have a positive effect on preventing detrimental cardiovascular and cerebrovascular events [1, 8]. Previous studies reported that HCV infection can alter in vivo glucose homeostasis and lipid metabolism leading to liver and peripheral insulin resistance [9, 10]. Our study found that patients with CHC not only had thickened IMT compared to the control and the CHB groups, but also had higher PWV, α, and β parameters and lower DC and CC values than the control group. This

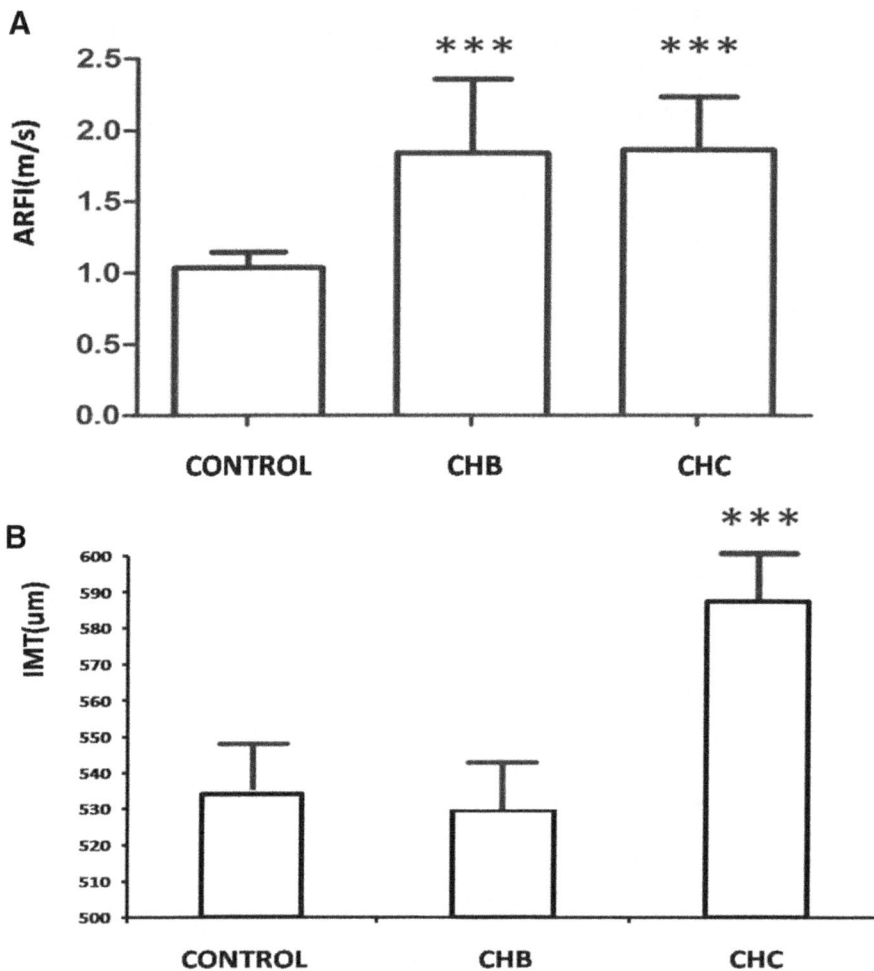

Fig. 2 Comparison of liver stiffness and carotid artery IMT values among the 3 groups: **a** Use of the ARFI technique to measure liver stiffness in patients with CHB, CHC and control group using a conventional ultrasound interface. **b** Use of QIMT and QAS techniques to quantify the carotid artery intima-media thickness (IMT) and vascular elasticity in patients among the 3 groups. Note: ARFI: acoustic radiation force impulse; IMT: intima-media thickness; CHB: chronic hepatitis B; CHC: chronic hepatitis C; ***: when compared to the control group, $P < 0.001$

indicated that both the carotid artery structure and function parameters of the CHC group had changed compared to the control group. This finding was in line with the argument that HCV infection is a risk factor for atherosclerosis [10, 11] . For patients with CHB, although their carotid artery IMT were not thickened, their other parameters such as α and β were higher, and their CC value was lower than those in the control group. These results indicated that, despite normal carotid artery wall structures, their carotid arteries and the elasticity parameters of their carotid artery walls had already changed. A possible explanation is that carotid atherosclerosis could cause both structural and functional changes. One major indicator for structural changes was an increase in the carotid IMT, while functional changes were mainly indicated by changes in carotid artery elasticity [12, 13]. Although structural changes in the carotid artery can cause changes in its elasticity, such elasticity changes

may also indicate that IMT thickening is not the only cause of arterial wall composition changes. It is speculated that carotid artery functional changes in patients with CHB may occur before the structural changes. Therefore, this study showed that patients with viral hepatitis maybe suffer a higher risk of cardiovascular events than healthy people, and this finding can provide some reference value for clinical diagnosis and treatment of these patients.

Age is also a critical factor affecting the potential for development of arteriosclerosis [14, 15]. In this study, participants were divided into two groups according to their age, with those aged 50 or above in one group and those aged under 50 in the other. It was found that within the CHB group, the ARFI value ($P = 0.001$) and the carotid artery elasticity parameters (all P values < 0.05) differed significantly between the two age groups, indicating that these parameters might be related to the

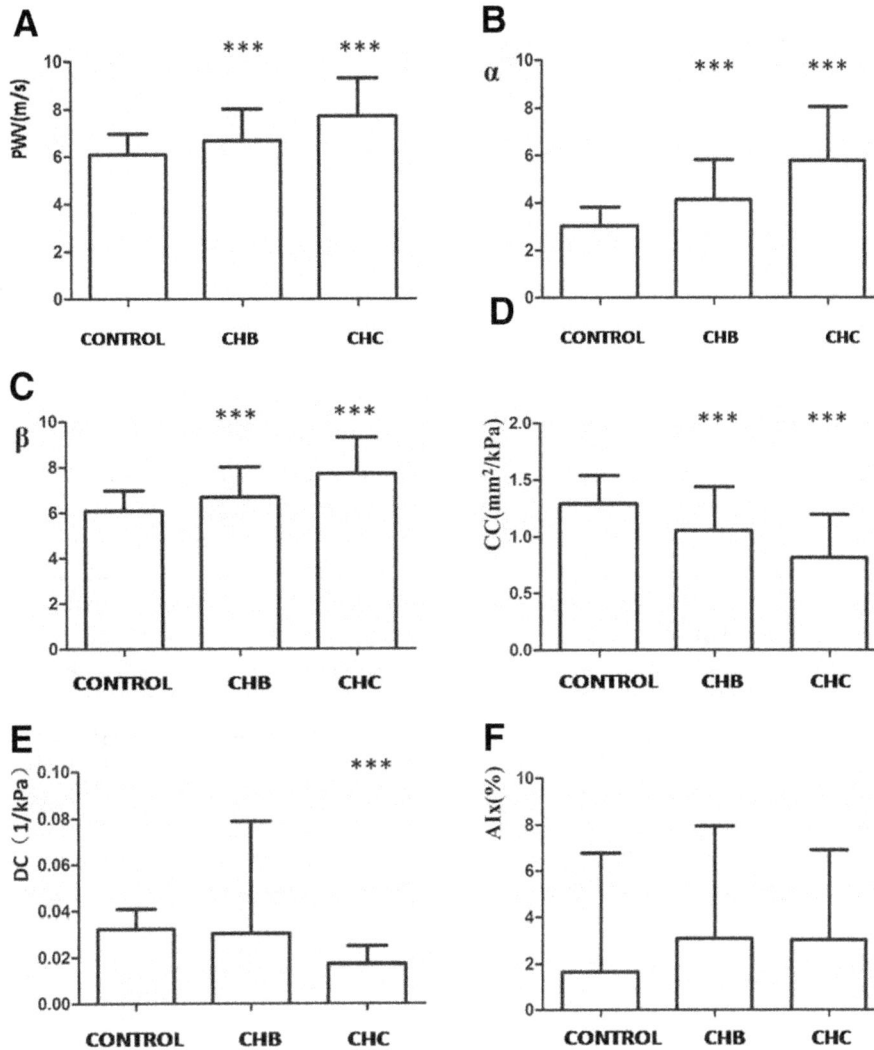

Fig. 3 Carotid elasticity parameters and comparisons among the 3 groups: **a** PWV values and comparisons among the 3 groups; **b** α values and comparisons among the 3 groups; **c** β values and comparisons among the 3 groups; **d** CC values and comparisons among the 3 groups; **e** DC values and comparisons among the 3 groups; **f** Aix values of the 3 groups. CHB: chronic hepatitis B; CHC: chronic hepatitis C; PWV: pulse wave velocity; CC: arterial wall compliance coefficient; DC: arterial wall dilation coefficient; Aix: augmentation index. Note: ***: when compared to the control group, $P < 0.001$

Table 2 Liver stiffness and left common carotid elasticity parameters in the different age groups

	Age, Year	No.	ARFI, m/s	IMT, μm	PWV, m/s	DC, 1/kPa
Control Group	< 50	41	1.02 ± 0.09	478.44 ± 107.86	5.72 ± 0.73	0.035 ± 0.007
	≥50	23	1.06 ± 0.13	633.26 ± 120.02	6.75 ± 0.80	0.026 ± 0.007
	P	–	0.127	< 0.001*	< 0.001*	< 0.001*
CHB Group	< 50	86	1.72 ± 0.50	456.70 ± 87.56	6.26 ± 1.35	0.038 ± 0.062
	≥50	61	2.02 ± 0.50	630.30 ± 112.17	7.32 ± 1.00	0.020 ± 0.007
	P	–	< 0.001*	< 0.001*	< 0.001*	0.009*
CHC Group	< 50	41	1.84 ± 0.38	526.63 ± 130.03	7.70 ± 1.57	0.018 ± 0.009
	≥50	29	1.89 ± 0.36	673.17 ± 167.48	8.36 ± 1.09	0.015 ± 0.006
	P	–	0.569	< 0.001*	0.041*	0.079

ARFI radio frequency, *IMT* intima-media thickness, *PWV* pulse wave velocity, *DC* arterial wall dilation coefficient
* $P < 0.05$ when compared to the control group

Table 3 Liver stiffness and left common carotid elasticity parameters in the different age groups

	Age, Year	No.	CC, mm²/kPa	α	β	Aix,%
Control Group	< 50	41	1.376 ± 0.259	2.70 ± 0.54	5.54 ± 1.10	0.82 ± 5.18
	≥50	23	1.137 ± 0.129	3.63 ± 0.81	7.30 ± 1.70	3.14 ± 4.76
	P	–	< 0.001*	< 0.001*	< 0.001*	0.082
CHB Group	< 50	86	1.139 ± 0.420	3.71 ± 1.69	7.58 ± 3.41	1.55 ± 4.41
	≥50	61	0.935 ± 0.291	4.72 ± 1.51	9.61 ± 2.96	5.25 ± 4.68
	P	–	0.001*	< 0.001*	< 0.001*	< 0.001*
CHC Group	< 50	41	0.854 ± 0.423	5.31 ± 1.97	10.65 ± 3.79	1.75 ± 3.45
	≥50	29	0.761 ± 0.303	6.42 ± 2.57	13.11 ± 5.13	4.84 ± 3.75
	P	–	0.317	0.044*	0.024*	0.001*

CC arterial wall compliance coefficient, *Aix* augmentation index
* $P < 0.05$ when compared to the control group

time span of HBV infection. Older patients with chronic hepatitis B are likely to carry the virus for a longer period of time and, consequently, experience a higher degree of liver stiffness. This difference was not observed in the control group, which indicated that aging is not related to the natural aging and fibrosis of the liver. In a study of 459 chronic HBV carriers, liver biopsies showed that the liver tissue inflammatory activity level and degree of liver fibrosis gradually increased with age [16], which was in line with our findings.

However, within the CHC group, the ARFI did not differ significantly between the two age groups ($P > 0.05$). A possible explanation was that patients with CHC have a higher risk of increased blood glucose levels. Studies on using the ARFI technique to grade liver stiffness and fibrosis showed that fat in the liver is an important factor that affects the accurate measurement of the ARFI value [17, 18]. Since 40% of the patients with CHC in this study had elevated blood glucose, the abnormal lipid metabolism caused by abnormal blood sugar levels led to fat deposition in their liver, thus affecting the ARFI values. Although the accuracy of ARFI measurements were affected by abnormal blood glucose contents, measurements of carotid artery elasticity parameters were also found to be significantly abnormal. This indicated that HCV not only significantly affected liver stiffness but also changed carotid artery elasticity. Stepwise multiple linear regression analysis demonstrated that both

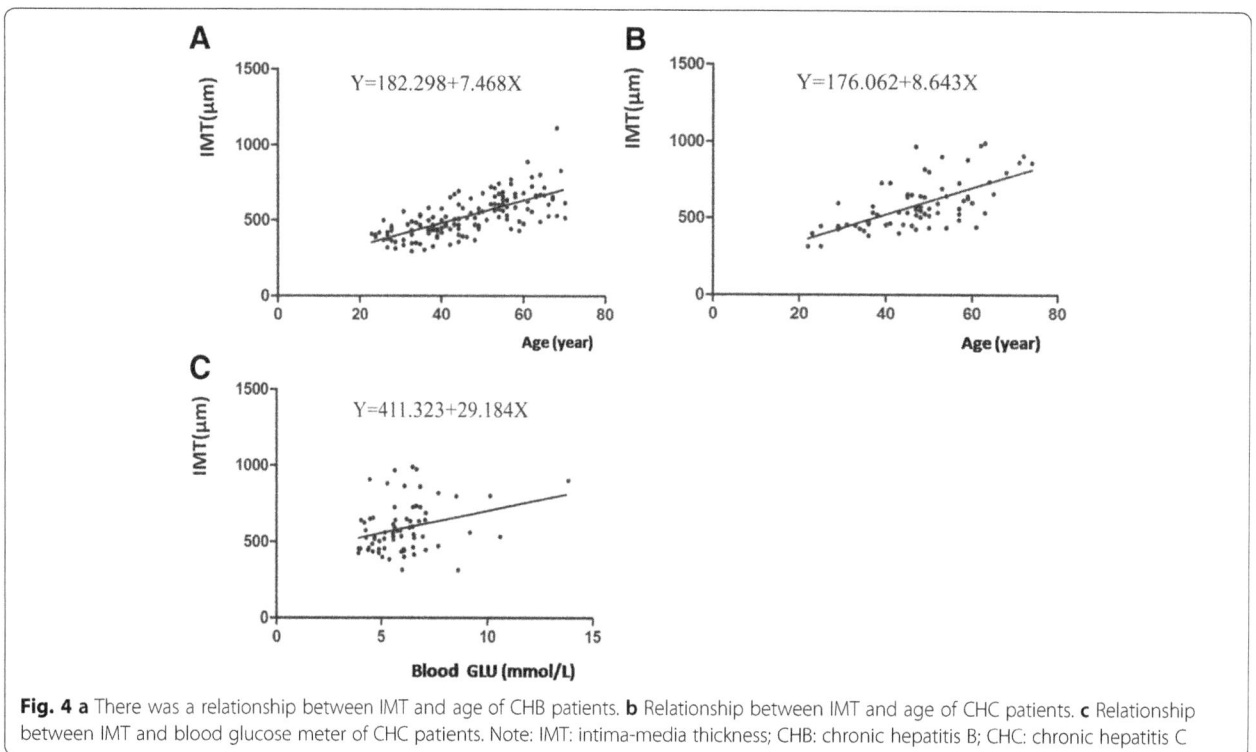

Fig. 4 a There was a relationship between IMT and age of CHB patients. **b** Relationship between IMT and age of CHC patients. **c** Relationship between IMT and blood glucose meter of CHC patients. Note: IMT: intima-media thickness; CHB: chronic hepatitis B; CHC: chronic hepatitis C

age and blood sugar are independent predictors of IMT in patients with CHC. Therefore, we speculated that, in addition to lipid metabolism, patients with chronic viral hepatitis also have metabolic syndromes caused by viral infections. The macrovascular damages caused by blood viscosity and hyperglycaemia also affect the structural changes of the carotid artery.

This study was limited by the fact that patients' diagnoses were made based on clinical diagnosis primarily. Biopsy was used to obtain pathological results in only a limited number of cases. The next step is to obtain results to classify liver fibrosis into different pathological levels, to further exclude any confounding factors.

Conclusions

In summary, using RF ultrasound and ARFI techniques to measure liver stiffness and carotid artery elasticity in patients with chronic viral hepatitis is beneficial for assessing the liver fibrosis and the structural and functional changes of the carotid artery. This serves as a reference for clinicians to monitor any vascular diseases in these patients.

Abbreviations

Aix: Augmentation index; ANOVA: Analysis of variance; ARFI: Acoustic radiation force impulse; CC: Compliance coefficient; CHB: Chronic hepatitis B; CHC: Chronic hepatitis C; DC: Arterial wall dilation coefficient; HBV: Hepatitis B virus; HCV: Hepatitis C virus; HCVAb: Hepatitis C virus antibody; IMT: Intima-media thickness; PWV: Pulse wave velocity; RF: Radio frequency

Acknowledgments

We are grateful to the doctors and nurses working in Tangdu Hospital of Infectious diseases for the help in conducting of this study.

Funding

Project 81371566 supported by National Natural Science Foundation of China. The funders had no role in study design, data collection and analysis, decision to publish, or preparation of the manuscript.

Authors' contributions

YLY conceived the idea. YLY, NZ and JHL was responsible for conception and participation in design, experimental work and collection of data, analysis and interpretation of results, drifting and substantial editing the manuscript. BYM, XZS, YYD were responsible for experimental work and collection of data, analysis and interpretation of results. YLY was responsible for interpretation of results and critically revising the manuscript. All authors read and approved the final manuscript.

Consent for publication

Not applicable.

Competing interests

The authors declare that they have no competing interests.

References

1. Adinolfi LE, Zampino R, Restivo L, Lonardo A, Guerrera B, Marrone A, Nascimbeni F, Florio A, Loria P. Chronic hepatitis C virus infection and atherosclerosis: clinical impact and mechanisms [J]. World J Gastroenterol. 2014;20(13):3410–7.
2. Lorenz MW, Markus HS, Bots ML, Rosvall M, Sitzer M. Prediction of clinical cardiovascular events with carotid intima-media thickness: a systematic review and meta-analysis [J]. Circulation. 2007;115(4):459–67.
3. Castera L, Hepatitis B. Are non-invasive markers of liver fibrosis reliable?[J]. Liver Int. 2014;34:91–6.
4. Wang Y, Duan YY, Zhang L, Yuan LJ, Xu L. The predictive value of carotid intima-media thickness and elasticity for coronary heart disease[J]. Chin J med ultrasound. 2013;10(9):39–45.
5. Wei L, Hou JL. Guideline of chronic hepatitis B prevention (2015 version) [J]. Infect Dis Info. 2015;28(6):321–40.
6. Ferraioli G, Filice C, Castera L, Choi BI, Sporea I, Wilson SR, Cosgrove D, Dietrich CF, Amy D, Bamber JC, Barr R, Chou YH, Ding H, Farrokh A, Friedrich-Rust M, Hall TJ, Nakashima K, Nightingale KR, Palmeri ML, Schafer F, Shiina T, Suzuki S, Guidelines KMWFUMB. Recommendations for clinical use of ultrasound Elastography: part 3: liver [J]. ultrasound in. Medicine and Biology. 2015;41(5):1161–79.
7. Zhang L, Yin JK, Duan YY, Liu X, Xu L. Evaluation of carotid artery elasticity changes in patients with type 2 diabetes [J]. Cardiovasc Diabetol. 2014;13:39–45.
8. Li WC, Lee YY, Chen IC, Sun C, Chiu FH, Chuang CH. Association between the hepatitis B and C viruses and metabolic diseases in patients stratified by age [J]. Liver Int. 2013;33(8):1194–202.
9. Adinolfi LE, Restivo L, Zampino R, Guerrera B, Lonardo A, Ruggiero L, Riello F, Loria P, Florio A. Chronic HCV infection is a risk of atherosclerosis. Role of HCV and HCV-related steatosis [J]. Atherosclerosis. 2012;221(2):496–502.
10. Ishizaka N, Ishizaka Y, Takahashi E, Toda Ei E, Hashimoto H, Ohno M, Nagai R, Yamakado M. Increased prevalence of carotid atherosclerosis in hepatitis B virus carriers [J]. Circulation. 2002;105(9):1028–30.
11. Ishizaka N, Ishizaka Y, Takahashi E, Ei T, Hashimoto H, Nagai R, Yamakado M. association between hepatitis C virus seropositivity, carotid-artery plaque, and intima-media thickening [J]. Lancet. 2002;359(9301):133–5.
12. Patel AK, Suri HS, Singh J, Kumar D, Shafique S, Nicolaides A, Jain SK, Saba L, Gupta A, Laird JR, Giannopoulos A, Suri JSA. Review on atherosclerotic biology, wall stiffness, physics of elasticity, and its ultrasound-based measurement[J]. Curr Atheroscler Rep. 2016;18(12):83–92.
13. Boesen MF, Singh D, Menon BK, Frayne R. a systematic literature review of the effect of carotid atherosclerosis on local vessel stiffness and elasticity[J]. Atherosclerosis. 2015;243(1):211–22.
14. Pelisek J, Wendorff H, Wendorff C, Kuehnl A, Eckstein HH. Age-associated changes in human carotid atherosclerotic plaques[J]. Ann Med. 2016;48(7):541–51.
15. Maloberti A, Meani P, Varrenti M, Giupponi L, Stucchi M, Vallerio P, Structural GC. Functional abnormalities of carotid artery and their relation with EVA phenomenon[J]. High Blood Press Cardiovasc Prev. 2015;22(4):373–9.
16. Xing YF, Tong GD, Zhou DQ, He JS, Shao MM, Wei CS, Chen YJ. Liver histological features analysis of 459 cases chronic hepatitis B virus carriers[J]. Chinese Journal of Integrated Traditional and Western Medicine on Liver Diseases. 2015;6:324–7.
17. Karlas T, Petroff D, Sasso M, Fan JG, Mi YQ, de Lédinghen V, Kumar M, Lupsor-Platon M, Han KH, Cardoso AC, Ferraioli G, Chan WK, Wong VW, Myers RP, Chayama K, Friedrich-Rust M, Beaugrand M, Shen F, Hiriart JB, Sarin SK, Badea R, Lee HW, Marcellin P, Filice C, Mahadeva S, Wong GL, Crotty P, Masaki K, Bojunga J, Bedossa P, Keim V, Wiegand J. Impact of controlled attenuation parameter on detecting fibrosis using liver stiffness measurement[J]. Aliment Pharmacol Ther. 2018;15:1–12.
18. Kelly ML, Riordan SM, Bopage R, Lloyd AR, Post JJ. Capacity of non-invasive hepatic fibrosis algorithms to replace transient elastography to exclude cirrhosis in people with hepatitis C virus infection: a multi-Centre observational study[J]. PLoS One. 2018;13(2):e0192763.

20

Characterization of intrahepatic cholangiocarcinoma after curative resection: outcome, prognostic factor, and recurrence

Kun-Ming Chan[*][iD], Chun-Yi Tsai, Chun-Nan Yeh, Ta-Sen Yeh, Wei-Chen Lee, Yi-Yin Jan[*] and Miin-Fu Chen

Abstract

Background: Intrahepatic cholangiocarcinoma (ICC) is a relatively rare subtype of cholangiocarcinoma. The study herein gathered experience of surgical treatment for ICC, and aimed to analyze the prognosis of patients who had received curative-intent liver resection.

Methods: A total of 216 patients who had undergone curative-intent liver resection for ICC between January 1977 and December 2014 was retrospectively reviewed.

Results: Overall, the rates of 5-years recurrence-free survival (RFS) and overall survival (OS) were 26.1 and 33.9% respectively. Based on multivariate analysis, four independent adverse prognostic factors including morphology patterns, maximum tumor size > 5 cm, pathological lymph node involvement, and vascular invasion were identified as affecting RFS after curative-intent liver resection for ICC. Among patients with cholangiocarcinoma recurrence, only 27 (16.9%) were able to receive surgical resection for recurrent cholangiocarcinoma that had a significantly better outcome than the remaining patients.

Conclusion: Despite curative resection, the general outcome of patients with ICC is still unsatisfactory because of a high incidence of cholangiocarcinoma recurrence after operation. Tumor factors associated with cholangiocarcinoma remain crucial for the prognosis of patients with ICC after curative liver resection. Moreover, aggressive attitude toward repeat resection for the postoperative recurrent cholangiocarcinoma could provide a favorable outcome for patients.

Keywords: Intrahepatic cholangiocarcinoma, Curative resection, Recurrence, Prognostic factors, Outcome

Background

Intrahepatic cholangiocarcinoma (ICC) is a primary liver malignancy arising from the epithelial cells of the distal branch intrahepatic bile duct. The incidence of ICC exhibits wide geographical variation and generally accounts for between 5 and 30% of primary liver cancers [1–4]. There has been a noticeable increase in the incidence of ICC in Western countries in recent years [5].

* Correspondence: chankunming@adm.cgmh.org.tw;
janyy@adm.cgmh.org.tw
Department of General Surgery, Chang Gung Memorial Hospital at Linkou, Chang Gung University College of Medicine, 5 Fu-Hsing Street, Kwei-Shan District, Taoyuan City 33305, Taiwan

Currently, surgical resection with curative intent remains the most effective treatment for ICC. However, because of vague symptomatic presentation, most patients are at an advanced stage by the time of diagnosis, and only nearly one-third of patients are eligible for surgical resection [6]. As a result, the overall outcome of ICC remains extremely poor, in which patients who are unable to undergo surgical resection have a less than 10% survival rate at 5 years. Moreover, the reported outcome after hepatic resection is also not optimistic, with a 5-year survival rate of 30 to 35% [7]. The principal reason for the dismal outcome of surgical treatment is the high incidence of postoperative ICC recurrence, in which more than 60% of patients may subsequently develop cancer recurrence after hepatic resection.

As a noteworthy malignancy, predictors for ICC recurrence and long-term outcome following hepatic resection remains entirely elusive. In addition, this remains an issue of great concern despite a growing experience and literature. Therefore, here we retrospectively reviewed our experience with surgical resection for ICC patients with the aim of providing additional information about the prognostic factors associated with those patients undergoing curative-intent liver resection, as well as the outcomes of ICC recurrence after surgical treatment.

Materials and methods
Patients
This study included patients with ICC who underwent surgical treatment with curative resection between January 1977 and December 2014 at Chang Gung Memorial Hospital, Linkou Medical Center, Taoyuan, Taiwan. A retrospective review of all medical records was performed under the approval of the Institutional Review Board of Chang Gung Memorial Hospital (Approval No.: 201701127B0). The medical records, including clinical characteristics, surgical management, and outcomes were thoroughly reviewed and analyzed. Patients who had no curative resection with macroscopically and/or microscopically positive of carcinoma at the resection margin were not included in the study. Therefore, a total of 225 patients who had pathological confirmation of cholangiocarcinoma were retrieved. After exclusion of 9 patients (4%) with postoperative hospital mortality, 216 patients [99 men (45.8%) and 117 women (54.2%)] were recruited and analyzed for this study.

Liver resection and follow-up
Transection of hepatic parenchymal was performed using either the surgical clamp-crush technique or a Cavitron Ultrasonic Surgical Aspirator (CUSA; Valleylab, Inc., Integra LifeSciences, Plainsboro, NJ). However, liver resection was mostly performed by CUSA transection after it was introduced into our institute in 2002. After the operation, all patients were followed-up at regular intervals until death or the end of the current study. The clinical assessments included physical examination, blood chemistry tests, measurement of tumor-markers, and abdominal ultrasonography every 3–6 months. A comprehensive assessment was done using computed tomography (CT) and/or magnetic resonance imaging (MRI) on an annual basis or when suspicious of cancer recurrence.

Based on the pathological examination, cancer was staged according to the 7th edition of tumor-node-metastasis (TNM) classification proposed by the Union for International Cancer Control (UICC) and the American Joint Committee on Cancer (AJCC) to classify the extent of

cholangiocarcinoma. Patients who had cancer staged by former version of classification system were restaged by the 7th edition of UICC/AJCC classification. The administration of postoperative adjuvant chemotherapy was optional and mainly based on tumor characteristics, patient's physical condition, and availability or affordability of chemotherapeutic regimens. The chemotherapeutic options were mostly fluorouracil plus leucovorin and/or a combination of regimens such as cisplatin, mitomycin, oxaliplatin, gemcitabine, and so on.

Disease recurrence was determined by a tissue sample from either a biopsy or surgical resection confirming cholangiocarcinoma, and/or by serial imaging examinations. Generally, the treatment algorithm of recurrent cholangiocarcinoma after surgical resection was the same as that for the initial management of cholangiocarcinoma. Repeat surgical resection was the preferred treatment whenever the recurrent tumor was considered to be resectable. Palliative chemotherapy was usually recommended for patients who had unresectable recurrent tumor or not received reoperation unless a patient was unsuitable for chemotherapy or unwilling to receive chemotherapy.

Outcome and statistical analysis
The end-point outcome measures included recurrence-free survival (RFS) and overall survival (OS). RFS was defined as the date of liver resection to the date of detected cholangiocarcinoma recurrence or the date of the last follow-up if there was no cancer recurrence. OS was measured from the date of liver resection to the date of death or the date of the last follow-up by the end of this study. Survival curves were constructed using the Kaplan–Meier method and analyzed by means of the log-rank test. The categorical variables were assessed using the χ^2 or Fisher exact test as appropriate, and the independent samples t-test was used for continuous data. Variables were analyzed using a Cox regression proportional hazards model to identify factors influencing RFS and OS. All significant factors determined by univariate analysis were then entered into a multivariate analysis using the Cox proportional hazards regression model. All statistical analyses were performed using SPSS statistical software version 20.0 (SPSS, Inc., Chicago, IL) for Windows. A P-value of less than 0.05 was considered to be statistically significant.

Results
Clinical features of patients
Table 1 summarizes the clinical features of the 216 patients who underwent curative-intent liver resection for ICC in this study. The median age of patients at the time of initial diagnoses was 60-years-old and ranged from 29 to 90-years-old. The majority of patients (90.3%) were not associated with liver cirrhosis, and 23.2% of patients were noted as having the simultaneous presence of

Table 1 Clinical characteristics of patients undergoing curative resection for intrahepatic cholangiocarcinoma

Characteristics	Patients n = 216(%)
Age (years), median (range)	60.0 (29–90)
Gender	
Male	99 (45.8)
Female	117 (54.2)
Liver cirrhosis	
Yes	21 (9.7)
No	195 (90.3)
Hepatolithiasis	
Yes	51 (23.2)
No	165 (76.8)
Virus hepatitis	
HBV positive	48 (22.2)
HCV positive	19 (8.8)
Extent of hepatic resection	
≥ 3 segments	126 (58.3)
< 3 segments	90 (41.7)
Extrahepatic bile duct resection	11 (5.1)
Years of liver resection	
1977–1994	31 (14.4)
1995–2004	75 (34.7)
2005–2014	110 (50.9)
Morphology type	
Intraductal growth	42 (19.4)
Mass-forming	123 (56.9)
Mix type	21 (9.7)
Periductal-infiltrating	30 (13.9)
TNM stage	
I	103 (47.7)
II	18 (8.3)
III	24 (11.1)
IVA	71 (32.9)

HBV Hepatitis B virus, *HCV* Hepatitis C virus

hepatolithiasis in the biliary tree. Of these, major hepatectomy (≥ 3 hepatic segments according to Couinaud's definition) was performed for 126 patients (58.3%), and the remaining 90 patients (41.7%) underwent minor hepatectomy (< 3 hepatic segments). Meanwhile, 11 patients (5.1%) underwent simultaneous bile duct resection. The majority of patients (50.9%) underwent liver resection during the last decade of the study period.

Patient's outcome
The median follow-up time for all patients was 26.9 months (range, 1.7 to 268). Overall, 160 patients (74.1%) encountered cancer recurrence after liver resection, and 56 (25.9%) patients had no cancer recurrence by the date of last follow-up or the end of this study. Meanwhile, 168 (77.8%) patients had died during the follow-up period, in which 145 (67.1%) patients died of cholangiocarcinoma, and 23 (10.6%) patients died of diseases other than cholangiocarcinoma. Only 42 (19.4%) patients were still alive by the end of the study, including 28 (13.0%) patients who were cancer free and 14 (6.5%) patients alive with recurrent cholangiocarcinoma. The remaining 6 (2.8%) patients were lost during the follow-up period. The RFS and OS curves are shown in Fig. 1. The 1-, 3-, and 5-year RFS rates were 57.5, 33.0, and 26.1% respectively, and the 1-, 3-, and 5-year OS rates were 84.2, 45.7, and 33.9% respectively.

Prognostic factors affecting cancer recurrence
The prognostic factors affecting cholangiocarcinoma recurrence after curative-intent liver resection were analyzed and summarized in Table 2. Univariate analysis identified nine significant factors including morphology patterns, histologic differentiation, maximum tumor size, pathological T stage, pathological N stage, vascular invasion, perineural invasion, and postoperative adjuvant chemotherapy. Subsequently, multivariate regression analysis of these significant factors showed that morphology patterns, maximum tumor size > 5 cm, pathological lymph node involvement, and vascular invasion were independent risk factors for cholangiocarcinoma recurrence after liver resection.

Recurrence after curative-intent liver resection
Of the 160 patients who developed cancer recurrence after curative-intent liver resection, 38 (23.8%) patients occurred only at the intrahepatic area, 57 (35.6%) patients had locoregional recurrence with (n = 22) or without (n = 35) intrahepatic recurrence, and 65 (40.6%) patients had distant metastasis at the detection of cancer recurrence. Table 3 summarizes the location of cholangiocarcinoma recurrence. Only 27 (16.9%) patients were able to receive surgical resection for recurrent lesions. The overall survival based on recurrent patterns showed that patients with intrahepatic recurrence had better survival than those with the other recurrence types. The 5-year survival rates were 14.5, 8.3, and 0% for intrahepatic recurrence, locoregional recurrence, and distant metastasis respectively (Fig. 2). The survival curve of patients who had undergone repeat surgical resection for recurrent cholangiocarcinoma was better than that of patients who were unable to undergo surgical resection, in which the 5-year survival rates after cholangiocarcinoma recurrence were 32.5%. With regard to patients without surgical treatment for recurrent cholangiocarcinoma, the survival curve of patients who had received palliative chemotherapy was better than that of

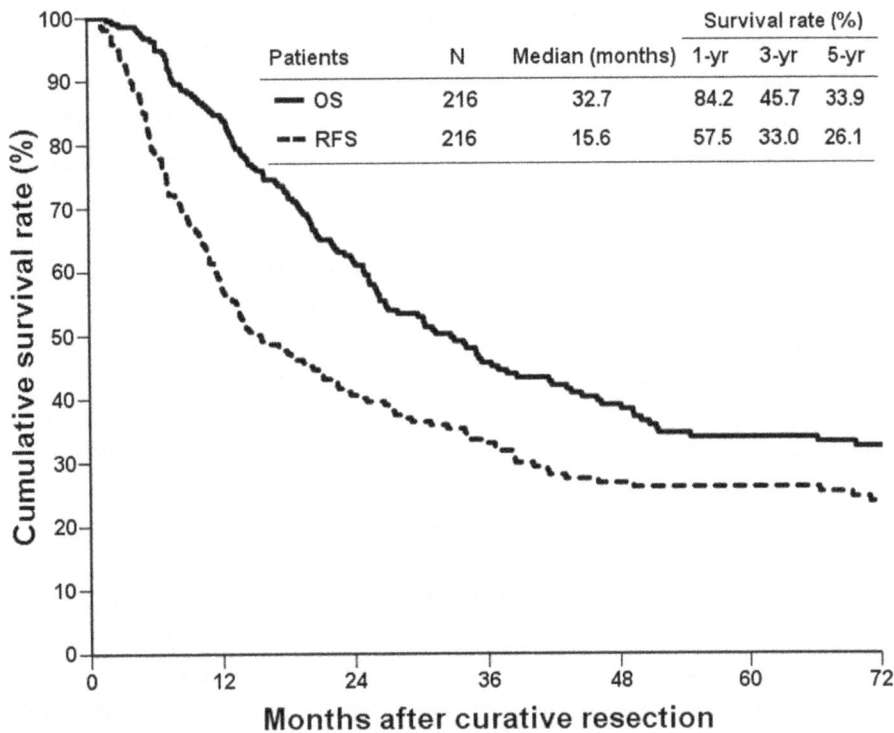

Patients	N	Median (months)	Survival rate (%)		
			1-yr	3-yr	5-yr
— OS	216	32.7	84.2	45.7	33.9
-- RFS	216	15.6	57.5	33.0	26.1

Fig. 1 Kaplan-Meier cumulative survival curves of the patients who underwent curative resection for intrahepatic cholangiocarcinoma by recurrence-free survival (RFS) and overall survival (OS)

patients without palliative chemotherapy. The 5-year survival rate of patients with palliative chemotherapy was 5.4%, and patients without palliative chemotherapy could not survive more than 5 years reflected by 0% of 5-year survival rate (Fig. 3).

Discussion

Cholangiocarcinoma is the second most common primary liver cancer following hepatocellular carcinoma despite being rare in clinical practice, and generally accounting for 10–15% of primary hepatic malignancy. ICC is a relatively rare subtype and represents less than 10% of cholangiocarcinoma cases [2, 8]. Although surgical resection is undoubtedly the most effective treatment for ICC, its low resectability and high incidence of postoperative recurrence affect the overall outcome of patients with ICC. Here we gathered data from decades of treating ICC and show that the rate of long-term cancer recurrence remains high (up to 74%). Meanwhile, prognostic factors affecting cancer recurrence after curative resection and outcome of patients after recurrent disease were also elucidated, providing further understanding in terms of the therapeutic strategies of ICC.

Cholangiocarcinoma usually arises from epithelial cells of the biliary tract and could be distinguished by anatomic location and classified as intrahepatic, perihilar, or extrahepatic types. Additionally, outcomes based on these classifications are also varied in a clinical setting. Among the three types, ICC accounts for less than 10% of all cholangiocarcinoma but seems to have the best outcome of the three types [8]. Currently, no specific risk factors are identified association with cholangiocarcinoma, and most cancer arises de novo. Although numerous studies have recognized that cirrhosis, viral hepatitis B and C, primary sclerosing cholangitis, and hepatolithiasis could be risk factors for cholangiocarcinoma, data reported from eastern and western countries are not identical [9–14]. Therefore, there is a lack of consensus on the guideline of risk stratification for disease surveillance.

Additionally, the high incidence of disease recurrence after surgical resection remains a major concern. Numerous studies have reported several prognostic factors that affect the outcomes of patients who undergo surgical resection for ICC [15–18], and similar factors were also noted in this study. The size of the primary tumor and presence of lymph node involvement seem to be important risk factors for cholangiocarcinoma recurrence after surgical resection. Although the 7th edition of UICC/AJCC TNM staging system does not mention tumor diameter, tumor diameter remains an important prognostic factor of tumor behavior, as shown in the current study. Therefore, the 8th edition of UICC/AJCC staging system for cholangiocarcinoma has re-inserted tumor size into the TNM system again.

Table 2 Univariate and multivariate analyses of clinicopathological factors affecting RFS after curative resections of patients with ICC

Factors	Univariate analysis			Multivariate analysis	
	medium RFS months	95%CI	p value	HR(95%CI)	p value
Age (years)					
≤ 65	13.5	8.6–18.5	0.320	–	
> 65	18.3	11.0–25.7			
Gender					
Male	18.0	10.4–25.5	0.962	–	
Female	13.8	8.8–18.8			
Liver cirrhosis					
Yes	14.0	3.6–24.5	0.963	–	
No	15.6	10.5–20.8			
Hepatolithiasis					
Yes	21.0	5.4–36.7	0.856	–	
No	14.2	9.8–18.7			
Years of liver resection					
1977–1994	38.4	12.7–64.2	0.688	–	
1995–2004	13.0	10.3–15.6			
2005–2014	15.7	1.6–20.7			
Morphology patterns					
Intraductal growth	71.0	6.7–135.3	< 0.0001	1	
Mass-forming	7.0	4.8–9.3		1.87 (1.11–3.13)	< 0.001
Mix type	16.4	10.5–20.3		2.59 (1.13–5.95)	0.018
Periductal-infiltrating	10.3	2.2–18.3		4.43 (2.09–9.38)	0.025
Histologic differentiation					
Well, moderate	19.6	11.9–27.3	0.004	1	
Poor, undifferentiated	10.1	6.7–13.6		1.13 (0.78–1.62)	0.522
Maximum tumor size					
≤ 5 cm	25.1	13.0–37.2	< 0.0001	1	
> 5 cm	10.7	8.2–13.3		1.52 (1.07–2.15)	0.019
Pathological T stage					
T1–2	32.4	19.6–45.1	< 0.0001	1	
T3–4	8.0	5.4–10.6		1.02 (0.63–1.66)	0.931
Pathological N stage					
N0	22.5	15.4–29.6	< 0.0001	1	
N1	6.1	4.3–8.0		2.67 (1.59–4.48)	< 0.001
Vascular invasion					
No	20.3	14.3–26.2	< 0.0001	1	
Yes	6.9	3.7–10.0		2.43 (1.54–3.84)	< 0.001
Perineural invasion					
No	22.3	15.0–29.6	< 0.0001	1	
Yes	10.3	6.0–14.6		1.02 (0.65–1.62)	0.921
Adjuvant chemotherapy					
No	20.3	14.0–26.6	0.023	1	0.517
Yes	12.5	10.7–14.3		0.89 (0.62–1.26)	

ICC Intrahepatic cholangiocarcinoma, *RFS* Recurrence-free survival, *HR* Hazard ratio, *CI* Confidence interval

Table 3 Surgical resection of recurrent lesions based on the recurrent patterns

Recurrent features	Recurrence[a]	Surgical resection[b]
Number of patients	160	27 (16.9%)
Recurrent patterns		
Intrahepatic only	38 (23.8%)	12 (57.9%)
Locoregional		
with intrahepatic lesion	22 (13.8%)	2 (9.1%)
without intrahepatic lesion	35 (21.9%)	9 (25.7%)
Distant metastasis	65 (40.6%)	4 (6.2%)

[a]percentages represent the ratio among total recurrences; [b]percentages represent the ratio among recurrent cases

Cancer spreading through the lymphatic system is a common characteristic of cholangiocarcinoma, which is different from primary hepatocellular carcinoma that is rarely associated with lymph node metastasis. Hence, lymphadenectomy during the resection of ICC is highly recommended by most reports, despite no sufficient data supporting the true benefit of prophylactic lymphadenectomy [19]. This study also confirmed that lymph node involvement was a prognostic factor for cancer recurrence in patients after curative resection of ICC, indicating that lymphadenectomy might potentially provide benefit for these patients. Interestingly, the study also showed that vascular invasion was an independent prognostic factor for RFS of ICC. Vascular invasion is always a crucial prognostic factor for primary hepatocellular carcinoma after hepatic resection [20, 21]. However, vascular invasion is rarely reported as a prognostic factor for ICC after curative resection. To our knowledge, our current study might be the few to identify vascular invasion as a prognostic factor of ICC. Although this study might be limited by a relatively small number of patients in a single institute, we believe this observation to be valid. Additionally, further researches involving basic science and a larger number of patients should be conducted to confirm the significance of our results.

Although the study evaluated patients treated over four decades, the concept in terms of treatment strategies and surgical resection for ICC has not markedly changed during this period. As the study had analyzed patient outcomes based on different timeframes, the results showed that no significance was observed along with the time period at least in the institute. As such, early diagnosis accompanied by surgical resection is the gold standard for providing long term survival. Nonetheless, the majority of patients with ICC was initially asymptomatic or with vague symptoms that lead to late detection of malignancy and few patients eligible for curative surgical resection at early cancer stage. Although numerous risk factors were identified possibly association with the development of cholangiocarcinoma, none of the risk factors is specific to

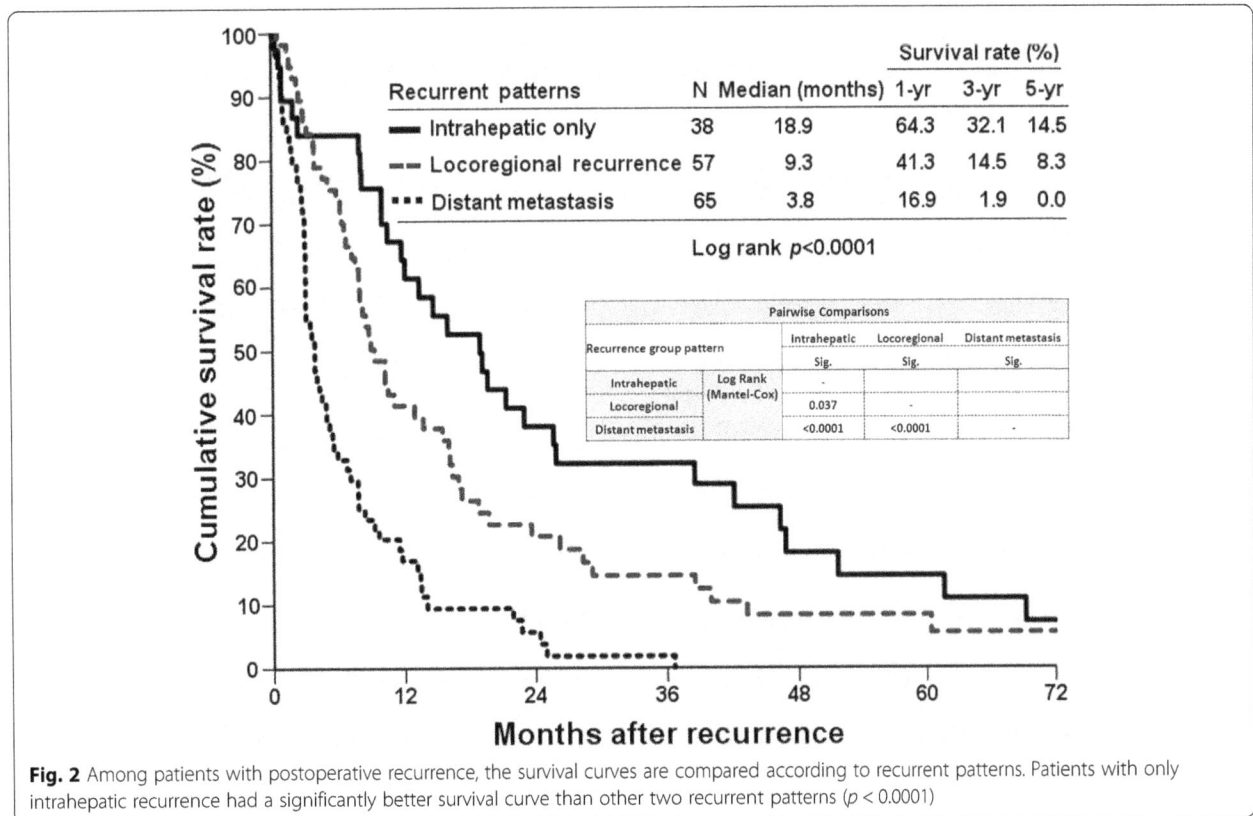

Fig. 2 Among patients with postoperative recurrence, the survival curves are compared according to recurrent patterns. Patients with only intrahepatic recurrence had a significantly better survival curve than other two recurrent patterns (p < 0.0001)

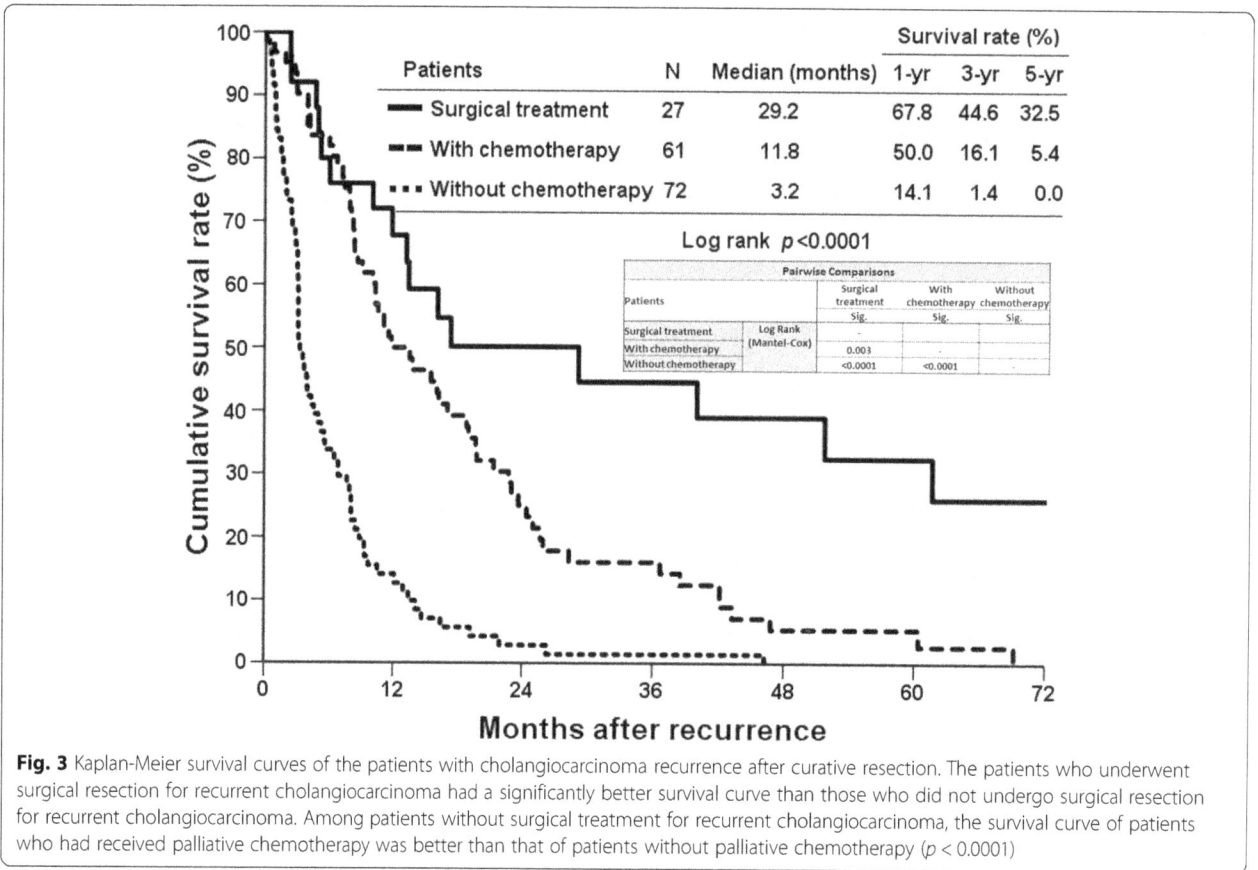

Fig. 3 Kaplan-Meier survival curves of the patients with cholangiocarcinoma recurrence after curative resection. The patients who underwent surgical resection for recurrent cholangiocarcinoma had a significantly better survival curve than those who did not undergo surgical resection for recurrent cholangiocarcinoma. Among patients without surgical treatment for recurrent cholangiocarcinoma, the survival curve of patients who had received palliative chemotherapy was better than that of patients without palliative chemotherapy ($p < 0.0001$)

the disease. Currently, consensus on the implementation of risk stratification for disease surveillance is still unsettled despite current advancement of diagnostic tools. Therefore, the general outcome of patients with ICC remains not optimistic.

However, the high incidence of postoperative recurrence as this study is a major concern influencing the overall outcome of patients with ICC after surgical resection. Although postoperative adjuvant chemotherapy might be beneficial for patients following surgical resection, there is no consensus of adjuvant treatment strategies in terms of chemotherapeutic protocol and regimens to diminish the risk of postoperative recurrence nowadays [22]. Despite not being an independent prognostic factor, patients who received adjuvant chemotherapy after liver resection had a shorter disease free interval than those without adjuvant chemotherapy in the univariate analysis of the study. The theoretical explanation of this phenomenon could possibly be related to patient selection, in which patients who were subjected to chemotherapy had a considerable severe tumor status than other patients in the clinical practice. As a result, patients who had received adjuvant chemotherapy after liver resection had a relative poor outcome in terms of RFS. However, the present study was unable to clarify this issue, and further detailed analysis will need to confirm the validity of this observation.

Given the high incidence of recurrence after surgical resection, the management of postoperative recurrent cholangiocarcinoma has become more important. Although it remains arguable that the prognosis of patients who are suitable to undergo surgical resection for recurrent cancer is naturally better than that of patients who are unable to undergo surgical resection, an aggressive attitude in terms of surgical resection for postoperative recurrent cholangiocarcinoma still seems to be beneficial. As shown in this study, patients who had undergone repeat surgical resection for the recurrent disease would enjoy a better chance of survival. Nonetheless, for patients without surgical resection of postoperative recurrent cholangiocarcinoma, there is no doubt that palliative chemotherapy is better recommended. Palliative chemotherapy could also provide certain survival benefit for patients who are unable to receive surgical treatment for recurrent cholangiocarcinoma after adequate resection.

Conclusion

The vague initial presentation of ICC may result in late detection at an advanced stage and lead to a low proportion of patients eligible for curative surgical resection. Meanwhile, the long-term incidence of postoperative cholangiocarcinoma recurrence is high, accounting for 74% of patients regardless of whether curative resection was performed. In line with previous studies, here the study identified many well-known prognostic factors that influence cancer recurrence after operation. Although patients with only intrahepatic recurrence had a better survival, the predictor of recurrent patterns after surgical resection was not identifiable based on the present study. Apart from that, the results suggest that an aggressive attitude in terms of surgical resection for postoperative recurrence might also be beneficial for the long-term outcome of a patient with ICC. Therefore, it is essential to regularly and frequently follow-up patients in the first few years after the operation to ensure early detection of recurrence at an operable stage. Eventually, in order to achieve better long-term outcomes for patients with ICC, the development of a treatment protocol that involves multidisciplinary modalities might be helpful in the future.

Abbreviations
AJCC: American Joint Committee on Cancer; CT: Computed tomography; CUSA: Cavitron Ultrasonic Surgical Aspirator; ICC: Intrahepatic cholangiocarcinoma; MRI: Magnetic resonance imaging; OS: Overall survival; RFS: Recurrence-free survival; UICC: Union for International Cancer Control

Acknowledgments
The authors would like to thank Ms. Shu-Fang Huang from Department of General Surgery, Chang Gung Memorial Hospital at Linkou for the statistical support.

Funding
This manuscript is made by author's own work without receiving any funding. There was no financial support for this research and publication.

Authors' contributions
KMC conceived the study concept and design and drafted the manuscript. KMC, CYT, CNY, TSY, WCL, YYJ, and MFC performed the acquisition of data and critical revision of the manuscript for important intellectual content. All authors have read and approved the final manuscript.

Consent for publication
Not applicable.

Competing interests
The authors declare that they have no competing interests.

References
1. Chen MF. Peripheral cholangiocarcinoma (cholangiocellular carcinoma): clinical features, diagnosis and treatment. J Gastroenterol Hepatol. 1999; 14:1144–9.
2. Razumilava N, Gores GJ. Cholangiocarcinoma. Lancet. 2014;383:2168–79.
3. Shaib Y, El-Serag HB. The epidemiology of cholangiocarcinoma. Semin Liver Dis. 2004;24:115–25.
4. Jan YY, Yeh CN, Yeh TS, Hwang TL, Chen MF. Clinicopathological factors predicting long-term overall survival after hepatectomy for peripheral cholangiocarcinoma. World J Surg. 2005;29:894–8.
5. Patel T. Increasing incidence and mortality of primary intrahepatic cholangiocarcinoma in the United States. Hepatology. 2001;33:1353–7.
6. Moeini A, Sia D, Bardeesy N, Mazzaferro V, Llovet JM. Molecular pathogenesis and targeted therapies for intrahepatic Cholangiocarcinoma. Clin Cancer Res. 2016;22:291–300.
7. de Jong MC, Nathan H, Sotiropoulos GC, Paul A, Alexandrescu S, Marques H, Pulitano C, et al. Intrahepatic cholangiocarcinoma: an international multi-institutional analysis of prognostic factors and lymph node assessment. J Clin Oncol. 2011;29:3140–5.
8. DeOliveira ML, Cunningham SC, Cameron JL, Kamangar F, Winter JM, Lillemoe KD, Choti MA, et al. Cholangiocarcinoma: thirty-one-year experience with 564 patients at a single institution. Ann Surg. 2007;245:755–62.
9. El-Serag HB, Engels EA, Landgren O, Chiao E, Henderson L, Amaratunge HC, Giordano TP. Risk of hepatobiliary and pancreatic cancers after hepatitis C virus infection: a population-based study of U.S. veterans. Hepatology. 2009; 49:116–23.
10. Lee TY, Lee SS, Jung SW, Jeon SH, Yun SC, Oh HC, Kwon S, et al. Hepatitis B virus infection and intrahepatic cholangiocarcinoma in Korea: a case-control study. Am J Gastroenterol. 2008;103:1716–20.
11. Welzel TM, Mellemkjaer L, Gloria G, Sakoda LC, Hsing AW, El Ghormli L, Olsen JH, et al. Risk factors for intrahepatic cholangiocarcinoma in a low-risk population: a nationwide case-control study. Int J Cancer. 2007;120:638–41.
12. Zhou YM, Yin ZF, Yang JM, Li B, Shao WY, Xu F, Wang YL, et al. Risk factors for intrahepatic cholangiocarcinoma: a case-control study in China. World J Gastroenterol. 2008;14:632–5.
13. Chapman MH, Webster GJ, Bannoo S, Johnson GJ, Wittmann J, Pereira SP. Cholangiocarcinoma and dominant strictures in patients with primary sclerosing cholangitis: a 25-year single-centre experience. Eur J Gastroenterol Hepatol. 2012;24:1051–8.
14. Huang MH, Chen CH, Yen CM, Yang JC, Yang CC, Yeh YH, Chou DA, et al. Relation of hepatolithiasis to helminthic infestation. J Gastroenterol Hepatol. 2005;20:141–6.
15. Jiang W, Zeng ZC, Tang ZY, Fan J, Sun HC, Zhou J, Zeng MS, et al. A prognostic scoring system based on clinical features of intrahepatic cholangiocarcinoma: the Fudan score. Ann Oncol. 2011;22:1644–52.
16. Ribero D, Pinna AD, Guglielmi A, Ponti A, Nuzzo G, Giulini SM, Aldrighetti L, et al. Surgical approach for long-term survival of patients with intrahepatic Cholangiocarcinoma: a multi-institutional analysis of 434 patients. Arch Surg. 2012;147:1107–13.
17. Wang Y, Li J, Xia Y, Gong R, Wang K, Yan Z, Wan X, et al. Prognostic nomogram for intrahepatic cholangiocarcinoma after partial hepatectomy. J Clin Oncol. 2013;31:1188–95.
18. Ni Q, Shen W, Zhang M, Yang C, Cai W, Wu M, Yang J. Prognostic analysis of radical resection for intrahepatic cholangiocarcinoma: a retrospective cohort study. Oncotarget. 2017;8(43):75627-37.
19. Amini N, Ejaz A, Spolverato G, Maithel SK, Kim Y, Pawlik TM. Management of lymph nodes during resection of hepatocellular carcinoma and intrahepatic cholangiocarcinoma: a systematic review. J Gastrointest Surg. 2014;18:2136–48.
20. Chan KM, Chou HS, Wu TJ, Lee CF, Yu MC, Lee WC. Characterization of hepatocellular carcinoma recurrence after liver transplantation: perioperative prognostic factors, patterns, and outcome. Asian J Surg. 2011;34:128–34.
21. Lee WC, Jeng LB, Chen MF. Estimation of prognosis after hepatectomy for hepatocellular carcinoma. Br J Surg. 2002;89:311–6.
22. Bupathi M, Ahn DH, Bekaii-Saab T. Therapeutic options for intrahepatic cholangiocarcinoma. Hepatobiliary Surg Nutr. 2017;6:91–100.

21

Peripheral blood toll-like receptor 4 correlates with rapid virological response to pegylated-interferon and ribavirin therapy in hepatitis C genotype 1 patients

Chuan-Mo Lee[1,2], Tsung-Hui Hu[1,2], Sheng-Nan Lu[1,2], Jing-Houng Wang[1,2], Chao-Hung Hung[1,2], Chien-Hung Chen[1,2] and Yi-Hao Yen[1,2]*

Abstract

Background: Toll-like receptors (TLRs) are effectors of the innate immune system that are able to recognize hepatitis C virus (HCV) and give rise to an immune response. Failure of interferon (IFN)-α-based treatment is related to host immunity. Therefore, we sought to study the clinical importance of TLRs in HCV genotype 1 patients who received pegylated IFN (PEG-IFN) plus ribavirin (RBV) therapy.

Methods: We enrolled 79 treatment-naïve patients with HCV genotype 1. Patients completed a 24- to 48-week course of response-guided therapy. Peripheral blood monocyte (PBMC) expression of mRNA for TLRs 2, 3, 4, 7, and 9 was quantified by real-time PCR before therapy. TLR mRNA expression is shown as a log ratio relative to GAPDH mRNA (log $2^{-(\Delta Ct)}$).

Results: Forty-five patients (57.0 %) showed a rapid virological response (RVR). Univariate analysis revealed that TLR 2, 3, 4, 7, and 9 were significantly lower in the RVR group than in the non-RVR group ($P = 0.001$, 0.014, < 0.001, 0.008, and 0.001, respectively). Multivariate analysis revealed that TLR 4 < −2 log (OR: 7.17, 95 % CI: 1.70–30.34, $P = 0.007$) was an independent predictor for RVR. In addition, levels of TLR 2, 3, 4, 7, and 9 were positively correlated with HCV viral load ($P = 0.009$, 0.013, < 0.001, 0.007, and 0.001, respectively).

Conclusions: A low level of TLR 4 mRNA in PMBCs was correlated with RVR, which indicates that TLR4 may play a critical role in HCV recognition and activation of innate immunity. TLR expression levels were correlated with HCV viral load, indicating that TLR activation upon exposure to HCV may subsequently limit HCV replication.

Keywords: Hepatitis C virus, Toll-like receptor, Rapid virological response

Background

Hepatitis C virus (HCV) is a blood-borne, hepato-trophic virus that establishes a chronic HCV infection in up to 85 % of cases [1]. With an estimated 2 % of the global population infected with HCV [2], which carries the potential for chronic infection leading to cirrhosis, end-stage liver diseases, and hepatocellular carcinoma (HCC), it poses a considerable health risk [3–6].

Non-alcoholic fatty liver disease (NAFLD) is now increasingly being recognized as a cause of end-stage liver disease and is associated with increased rates of HCC, liver transplantation, and death [7–9]. Current population based prevalence of NAFLD is approximately 70 % in people with type 2 diabetes mellitus (DM) [10]. Further, a recent study showed that liver transplant recipients with non-alcoholic steatohepatitis (NASH) have a higher risk of de novo post-transplant DM. This suggests the presence of an underlying metabolic disorder beyond fatty liver that may be causative for both NASH and type 2 diabetes [11].

* Correspondence: cassellyen@yahoo.com.tw
[1]Division of Hepatogastroenterology, Department of Internal Medicine, Kaohsiung Chang Gung Memorial Hospital, 123 Ta Pei Road, Niao Sung Dist. 833, Kaohsiung City, Taiwan
[2]School of Medicine, College of Medicine, Chang Gung University, Taoyuan, Taiwan

Infection with HCV genotype 1, the prevalent genotype in Taiwan, Japan, and Southern and Eastern Europe [12–16], is predictive of a poor response to interferon (IFN)-based therapy. The sustained virological response (SVR) is 50–80 % following combination therapy with pegylated interferon (peg-IFN) plus ribavirin (RBV) for 48 weeks [17–20].

The European Association for the Study of the Liver (EASL) and the American Association for the Study of Liver Diseases (AASLD) guidelines [21, 22] both suggest direct antiviral agents (DAAs) as the first line of therapy for patients infected with genotype 1. However, the SVR rate can reach 76 % after 48 weeks of peg-IFN plus RBV therapy in Taiwanese patients with genotype 1 [20], and peg-IFN plus RBV therapy remains the standard of care in Taiwan. Therefore, it is crucial to determine the mechanism of treatment failure for IFN-based therapy in Taiwan.

Host immunity is an important factor that is related to the failure of IFN-α-based treatment. The innate immune system is particularly relevant in viral infections [23]. Toll-like receptors (TLRs), as effectors of the innate immune system, are activated immediately upon exposure to infectious agents and may subsequently limit replication of infectious agents [24].

TLRs belong to a family of cell receptors that are present on mammalian cells, and that are able to recognize several pathogen-associated molecular patterns (PAMPs) present on microbes [25]. Various viral components (RNA, viral proteins, and intact virions) can be recognized as PAMPs by the immune system; recognition can give rise to an immune response [25], including up-regulation of IFN-α production [23]. This may induce enhanced expression of IFN-α-inducible genes, most of which perform important antiviral and immune regulatory functions. In vitro studies have indicated that, of the 11 human TLRs identified so far, TLR 2, 3, 4, 7, and 9 recognize specific HCV viral components as PAMP ligands [26–33].

Whether TLR expression is associated with a virological response in patients infected with HCV genotype 1 remains unclear. In this study, we investigated whether TLR expression on peripheral blood monocytes (PBMCs) is associated with virological responses to peg-IFN plus RBV therapy in patients infected with HCV genotype 1.

Methods

Patients

We enrolled 79 treatment-naïve patients with HCV genotype 1, who then completed a 24- to 48-week course of response-guided therapy (RGT) with peg-IFN plus RBV. The RGT received was simply part of standard care in Taiwan and was funded by the Bureau of National Health Insurance, Department of Health, Taiwan. RGT was performed as follows: 24-week therapy for patients with rapid

virological response (RVR) (defined as undetectable HCV RNA at week 4); 48-week therapy for patients with early virological response (EVR) (defined as detectable HCV RNA at week 4 and a > 2-log decrease in HCV RNA at week 12); therapy was stopped at week 12 for patients with a null response (defined as a > 2-log decrease in HCV RNA at week 12). PegIFN α-2b (Peg-Intron, Schering-Plough Corporation, Kenilworth, NJ) at 1.5 μg/kg or PegIFN α-2a (Pegacys, Roche, Basel, Switzerland) at 180 μg was given subcutaneously once weekly. RBV was given at 1000 mg/day for patients with a body weight of ≤ 75 kg and 1200 mg/day for those > 75 kg. Forty five patients achieved RVR, 34 patients did not. The characteristics of non-RVR group patients were as follow: there were 19 male and 15 female, the median age was 53.4 years, the median body mass index (BMI) was 26.4 Kg/m^2, the median Alanine Aminotransferase (ALT) was 84.5 IU/L, 28 patients had high viral load ($\geq 4 \times 10^5$ IU/ml), 6 patients had liver crrhosis, 24 patients had rs12979860 CC genotype, and 24 patients with good drug adherence.

Patients who were positive for anti-HCV antibody, assessed by third-generation enzyme-linked immunosorbent assay, were diagnosed with chronic hepatitis C; the diagnosis was confirmed by detection of serum HCV-RNA. Patients were excluded if they tested positive for serum hepatitis B surface antigens, anti-HIV antibodies, or exhibited other causes of hepatocellular injury (e.g., any history of alcoholism, autoimmune hepatitis, primary biliary cirrhosis, or treatment with hepatotoxic drugs).

HCV RNA was qualitatively detected using a PCR-based assay (Cobas Amplicor Hepatitis C Virus Test, version 2.0, Roche Molecular Systems, Branchburg, NJ, USA), which has a lower limit of detection of approximately 50 IU/mL. HCV RNA was quantified by real-time PCR-based assay (COBAS AmpliPrep/COBAS TaqMan HCV Test, Roche), with a dynamic range of 43 to 69,000,000 IU/ml. Genotyping of HCV was performed using a Siemens Diagnostics Versant HCV Genotype Assay. SVR was defined as serum HCV RNA undetectable at week 24 after treatment.

PBMC preparation and RNA extraction

PBMCs were isolated by Ficoll-Hypaque density gradient centrifugation from the peripheral venous blood of the subjects before antiviral therapy. Total cellular RNA was extracted using the TRizol Reagent (Invitrogen, Carlsbad, CA) in accordance with the manufacturer's instructions. RNA yield and purity were determined by measuring the absorbance at 260/280 nm on a NanoDrop spectrophotometer (Thermo Fisher Scientific, Waltham, Massachusetts, USA).

mRNA expression of TLR genes in PBMCs

To quantify mRNA expression of TLR genes (including TLR 2, 3, 4, 7, and 9) in PBMCs, we performed quantitative reverse transcription polymerase chain reactions (QRT-PCR) with a LightCycler 480 system (Roche Diagnostics GmbH, Mannheim, Germany). The reagent mixture was prepared according to the protocol provided by the manufacturer (Roche Diagnostics GmbH, Mannheim, Germany). Total RNA (2 μg) was extracted from PMBCs and cDNA was generated using an oligo(dT)$_{18}$ primer (GeneMark Taiwan). PCR was performed in a 10-μl reaction mixture containing 2× LightCycler 480 SYBR Green I Master mix (5 μl) (Roche Diagnostics GmbH, Mannheim, Germany), forward and reverse primers (0.5 μM each), and cDNA (1 μl). The conditions for amplification were as follows: one cycle of 95 °C for 10 min and 40 cycles of 95 °C for 10 s, 60 °C for 12 s, and 72 °C for 20 s. After amplification was completed, a final melting-curve analysis was performed by denaturation at 95 °C, re-annealing at 65 °C for 1 min, and then slow heating (0.1 °C/s) to 95 °C to determine the product-specific melting temperature. The reaction chamber was then cooled to 40 °C for 30 s prior to opening the chamber to remove the plate, as recommended by the manufacturer. Data were analyzed using the LightCycler Software 1.5 (Roche Diagnostics GmbH, Mannheim, Germany). The threshold cycle value (Ct) was determined using the following equation: $\Delta Ct = Ct$ (target gene) - Ct (GAPDH). The expression of target genes in each sample was tested in triplicate. mRNA expression of target genes is shown as a log ratio relative to GAPDH mRNA (log $2^{-(\Delta Ct)}$).

Genetic variation in interleukin (IL)28B

Patient IL28B genotypes ere determined with ABI TaqMan SNP genotyping assays (Applied Biosystems, Foster City, CA) and with predesigned commercial genotyping assays (ABI assay ID: C__11710096_10). Briefly, PCR primers and two allele-specific probes were designed to detect a specific Single-nucleotide polymorphism (SNP) target. PCR reactions were performed in 96-well microplates with a StepOnePlus™ Real-Time PCR System (Applied Biosystems). Allele discrimination was achieved by fluorescence detection using the StepOne™ Software v2.1.

Statistical analysis

We analyzed differences between virological responders and non-responders using the chi-square test and Student's t-test. Independent factors that may have influenced the response to combination therapy were identified using stepwise multiple logistic regression analysis. We used Pearson's correlation coefficient analysis to evaluate the correlation between mRNA expression of TLRs and baseline clinical variables. A P-value of <0.05 was considered statistically significant.

Results

Comparison of baseline features in patients with RVR and non-RVR

Forty-five patients (57 %) achieved RVR. The proportion of patients with a low viral load (< 4 × 10^5 IU/ml), rs12979860 CC genotype, and rs8099917 TT genotype was higher in the RVR group than in the non-RVR group. In addition, the median body mass index (BMI) was lower and mRNA expression of TLR 2, 3, 4, 7, and 9 was lower in the RVR group, compared with the non-RVR group.

There were no significant differences between the RVR and non-RVR patient groups in terms of gender, ALT levels, rates of adherence to treatment, or the proportion of patients with liver cirrhosis (Table 1).

Multivariate analysis of pretreatment factors associated with RVR

Stepwise multiple logistic regression analysis revealed that mRNA expression of TLR 4 < −2 log (odds ratio (OR), 7.17; 95 % confidence interval (CI), 1.70–30.34; P = 0.007), a viral load <4 × 10^5 IU/ml (OR, 7.08; 95 % CI, 1.17–30.09; P = 0.008), and rs 8099917 TT genotype (OR, 38.8; 95 % CI, 2.65–568.63; P = 0.008) were independent predictors for RVR.

Comparison of baseline features in patients with SVR and non-SVR

Four patients who completed the treatment but not the follow-up were excluded. The remaining 75 patients were analyzed. Of these 75 patients, 45 (60 %) achieved SVR. The proportion of males and the rate of liver cirrhosis were both lower in the SVR group than in the non-SVR group. The proportion of patients with RVR, rs 12979860 CC genotype, and rs 8099917 TT genotype were higher in the SVR group than in the non-SVR group. There were no significant differences between the SVR and non-SVR patient groups in terms of TLR expression (Table 2).

Multivariate analysis of pretreatment factors associated with SVR

Stepwise multiple logistic regression analysis revealed that non-liver cirrhosis (OR, 6.94; 95 % CI, 1.22–40.0; P = 0.029), rs 12979860 CC genotype (OR, 6.53; 95 % CI, 1.18–36.01; P = 0.031), and RVR (OR, 3.06; 95 % CI, 1.01–9.28; P = 0.048) were independent predictors for SVR.

Table 1 Comparisons of baseline features of patients with rapid virological response (RVR) and those with non-RVR

Variables	RVR (N = 45)	Non-RVR (N = 34)	P value
Sex (M:F)	23:22	19:15	0.674
Age (median,IQR)	60.5 (52.9 ~ 67.8)	53.4 (43.9 ~ 63.0)	0.003
BMI, Kg/m^2 (median,IQR)	23.5 (21.8 ~ 24.7)	26.4 (23.0 ~ 29.4)	0.001
ALT, IU/L(median,IQR)	71.0 (48.0 ~ 138.5)	84.5 (56.3 ~ 115.5)	0.801
HCV viral load (≥ vs < 4x10^5 IU/ml)	17:28	28:6	< 0.001
Liver cirrhosis (yes vs. no)	4:41	6:28	0.313
> 80 % adherence (yes vs. no)	32:13	24:10	0.960
rs12979860 (CC vs. CT + TT)	43:2	24:10	0.002
rs 8099917 (TT vs. GG + GT)	44:1	25:9	0.002
TLR2 mRNA (median,IQR)	−1.36 (−2.52 ~ 0.76)	0.82 (0.55 ~ 0.96)	0.001
TLR3 mRNA (median,IQR)	−2.66 (−3.13 ~ −1.28)	−1.47 (−1.90 ~ −1.27)	0.014
TLR4 mRNA (median,IQR)	−1.85 (−2.53 ~ 0.57)	0.66 (0.31 ~ 0.86)	< 0.001
TLR7 mRNA (median,IQR)	−2.41 (−3.19 ~ −0.07)	−0.77 (−1.18 ~ −0.57)	0.008
TLR9 mRNA (median,IQR)	−2.44 (−3.17 ~ −1.01)	−0.98 (−1.26 ~ −0.84)	0.001

BMI body mass index, *ALT* alanine aminotransferase, *TLR* toll like receptor, *TLR* mRNA expressions were shown as log ratios relative to GAPDH mRNA (log 2 $^{-(\Delta Ct)}$).
> 80 % adherence: patients who received more than 80 % of standard dose and duration

Correlation between mRNA expression of TLRs and baseline clinical features

mRNA expression of TLR 2, 3, 4, 7, and 9 was correlated with HCV viral load, but was not correlated with ALT levels or liver cirrhosis (Table 3).

Discussion

In this study, we found that low TLR4 mRNA expression in PBMCs was associated with RVR in patients with HCV genotype 1 who received peg-IFN and RBV therapy. Univariate analysis also revealed that TLR 4

expression is lower in the SVR group than in the non-SVR group (P = 0.067), although it is not statistically significant. The case number in our study is limited, may be more case number is needed to reach statistically significant.

TLR4, a lipopolysaccharide-receptor, plays a critical role in pathogen recognition and activation of innate and adaptive immunity. Ten et al. studied the release of soluble TLR2 and TLR4 in plasma of 394 patients with infections (infectious mononucleosis, measles, respiratory tract infections, bacterial sepsis and candidemia) or

Table 2 Comparisons of baseline features of patients with sustained virological response (SVR) and those with non-SVR

Variables	SVR (N = 45)	Non-SVR (N = 30)	P value
Sex (M:F)	19:26	20:10	0.038
Age (median,IQR)	59.7 (51.1 ~ 67.4)	56.6 (45.9 ~ 64.7)	0.176
BMI, Kg/m^2 (median,IQR)	23.9 (22.4 ~ 27.1)	23.7 (21.4 ~ 27.8)	0.787
ALT, IU/L(median,IQR)	84.0 (52.0 ~ 134.5)	77.0 (44.8 ~ 14.8)	0.423
Viral load (≥ vs < 4 × 10^5 IU/ml)	25:20	19:11	0.503
RVR (yes vs. no)	31:14	10:20	0.002
Liver cirrhosis (yes vs. no)	2:43	8:22	0.012
> 80 % adherence (yes vs. no)	32:13	21:9	0.918
rs12979860 (CC vs CT + TT)	43:2	20:10	0.002
rs 8099917 (TT vs GG + GT)	45:0	20:10	< 0.001
TLR2 mRNA (median,IQR)	−1.07 (−4.05 ~ −0.74)	−0.96 (−3.39 ~ −0.67)	0.304
TLR3 mRNA (median,IQR)	−3.39 (−4.53 ~ −2.86)	−3.28 (−4.10 ~ −2.90)	0.607
TLR4 mRNA (median,IQR)	−1.24 (−4.05 ~ −0.96)	−1.02 (−3.54 ~ −0.78)	0.067
TLR7 mRNA (median,IQR)	−2.76 (−4.53 ~ −2.19)	−2.42 (−4.18 ~ −2.20)	0.545
TLR9 mRNA (median,IQR)	−2.85 (−4.57 ~ −2.59)	−2.62 (−4.12 ~ −2.47)	0.124

RVR rapid virological response, *BMI* body mass index, *ALT* alanine aminotransferase, *TLR* toll like receptor. TLR mRNA expression levels were shown as log ratios relative to GAPDH mRNA (log 2 $^{-(\Delta Ct)}$)

Table 3 Correlation between TLR mRNA expression levels and baseline clinical factors ($N = 79$)

	TLR2		TLR3		TLR4		TLR7		TLR9	
	R value	P value	R value	P value	R value	P value	R value	P value	R value	P value
HCV RNA	0.292	0.009	0.277	0.013	0.386	< 0.0001	0.301	0.007	0.354	0.001
ALT	−0.126	0.269	0.046	0.688	−0.009	0.934	0.097	0.393	−0.05	0.663
Cirrhosis	−0.124	0.278	0.087	0.447	−0.024	0.832	0.014	0.901	−0.901	0.425

Spearman correlation. HCV RNA (log IU), *ALT* alanine aminotransferase (U/dl). Cirrhosis:yes vs. no. TLR mRNA expression levels were shown as log ratios relative to GAPDH mRNA (log 2 $^{-(\Delta Ct)}$)

non-infectious inflammation (Crohn's disease, gout, rheumatoid arthritis, autoinflammatory syndromes and pancreatitis). They found that soluble TLR4 had a similar capacity for differentiating infectious and non-infectious inflammation compared to C reactive protein (CRP), and suggest the possibility to use soluble TLRs as diagnostic tool in inflammatory conditions [34].

Machida et al. reported that HCV non-structural 5A (NS5A) protein, which plays a potential role in resistance to IFN-α treatment, transactivates the TLR4 promoter in vitro, resulting in increased transcription of TLR4 [29].

He et al. enrolled 15 HCV infected patients who had received a 48-week treatment with peg-IFN and RBV. They found that baseline PBMC TLR 2 and 3 mRNA levels were significantly higher in patients with SVR than in non-responders. They suggested that TLR 2/3, which was up-regulated in PBMCs, might act as an adjuvant receptor, increasing not only the sensitivity to HCV PAMPs but also the sensitivity to INF-α treatment, and subsequently increased effective antiviral responses [35]. However, the number of cases examined was small.

Yuki et al. reported that low hepatic TLR3 expression was a predictor of SVR to peg-IFN plus RBV in patients with HCV genotype 1 [36]. TLRs are known to be intra-hepatic interferon stimulated genes (ISGs) and these results were consistent with previous studies which found that pre-activation of intra-hepatic ISGs was associated with non-response in HCV-infected patients [37–40]. Activation of the endogenous IFN system in HCV-infected patients was ineffective in clearing the infection and even impeded the response to therapy, most likely by inducing a refractory state in the IFN signaling pathway [37–40]. However, analyzing gene expression in liver biopsy specimens requires an invasive procedure.

In this study, we found that mRNA expression of TLR 2, 3, 4, 7, and 9 was correlated with HCV viral load. TLR activation upon exposure to HCV may subsequently limit HCV replication [25, 26, 28, 31, 32]. However, HCV can escape host immunity via several methods and sustain a chronic infection [30, 41, 42]. These interactions between HCV and TLRs may be one reason for the correlation between TLR expression and HCV viral load observed in our study.

Conclusion

Low PMBC TLR 4 levels were correlated with RVR, which indicates that TLR4 may play a critical role in HCV recognition and activation of innate and adaptive immunity. mRNA expression of TLRs was correlated with HCV viral load, which indicates that TLR activation upon exposure to HCV may subsequently limit HCV replication.

Abbreviations
AASLD, American Association for the Study of Liver Diseases; ALT, Alanine Aminotransferase; BMI, body mass index; CRP, C reactive protein; Ct, threshold cycle value; DAAs, direct antiviral agents; DM, diabetes mellitus; EASL, European Association for the Study of the Liver; EVR, early virological response; HCC, hepatocellular carcinoma; HCV, hepatitis C virus; IFN, interferon; ISGs, interferon stimulated genes; NAFLD, Non-alcoholic fatty liver disease; NASH, non-alcoholic steatohepatitis; NS5A, non-structural 5A; PAMPs, pathogen-associated molecular patterns; PBMCs, peripheral blood monocytes; PEG-IFN, pegylated interferon; QRT-PCR, quantitative reverse transcription polymerase chain reactions; RBV, ribavirin; RGT, response-guided therapy; RVR, rapid virological response; SVR, sustained virological response; TLRs, Toll-like receptors

Acknowledgments
This study was supported by Grant CMRPG8A0071 from the Chang Gung Memorial Hospital-Kaohsiung Medical Center, Taiwan.

Funding
This study was supported by Grant CMRPG8A0071 from the Chang Gung Memorial Hospital-Kaohsiung Medical Center, Taiwan. The funders had no role in study design, data collection and analysis, decision to publish, or preparation of the manuscript.

Authors' contributions
Conception and design of study: YH-Y. Acquisition of data: TH-H. Analysis and interpretation of data: SN-L. Drafting the manuscript: CM-L. Revising the manuscript critically for important intellectual content: JH-W, CH-H and CH-C. All authors read and approved the final manuscript.

Competing interests
The authors declare that they have no competing interests.

Consent for publication
The use of study data was approved by the ethical committee of Chang Gung Memorial Hospital.

References

1. Alberti A, Vario A, Ferrari A, Pistis R. Review article: chronic hepatitis C–natural history and cofactors. Aliment Pharmacol Ther. 2005;22 Suppl 2:74–8.
2. Shepard CW, Finelli L, Alter M. Global epidemiology of hepatitis C virus infection. Lancet Infect Dis. 2005;5:558–67.
3. El Serag HB. Hepatocellular carcinoma and hepatitis C in the United States. Hepatology. 2002;36:S74–83.
4. Lauer GM, Walker BD. Hepatitis C virus infection. N Engl J Med. 2001;345:41–52.
5. Seeff LB. Natural history of chronic hepatitis C. Hepatology. 2002;36:S35–46.
6. Lee CM, Lu SN, Changchien CS, Yeh CT, Hsu TT, Tang JH, et al. Age, gender, and local geographic variations of viral etiology of hepatocellular carcinoma in a hyperendemic area for hepatitis B virus infection. Cancer. 1999;86:1143–50.
7. Charlton MR, Kondo M, Roberts SK, Steers JL, Krom RA, Wiesner RH. Liver transplantation for cryptogenic cirrhosis. Liver Transpl Surg. 1997;3:359–64.
8. McCullough AJ. Update on nonalcoholic fatty liver disease. J Clin Gastroenterol. 2002;34:255–62.
9. Sass DA, Chang P, Chopra KB. Nonalcoholic fatty liver disease: a clinical review. Dig Dis Sci. 2005;50:171–80.
10. Blachier M, Leleu H, Peck-Radosavljevic M, Valla DC, Roudot-Thoraval F. The burden of liver disease in Europe: a review of available epidemiological data. J Hepatol. 2013;58:593–608.
11. Stepanova M, Henry L, Garg R, Kalwaney S, Saab S, Younossi Z. Risk of de novo post-transplant type 2 diabetes in patients undergoing liver transplant for non-alcoholic steatohepatitis. BMC Gastroenterol. 2015;15:175.
12. Nousbaum JB, Pol S, Nalpas B, Landais P, Berthelot P, Bréchot C, et al. Hepatitis C virus type 1b (II) infection in France and Italy. Collaborative Study Group. Ann Intern Med. 1995;122:161–8.
13. McOmish F, Yap PL, Dow BC, Follett EA, Seed C, Keller AJ, et al. Geographical distribution of hepatitis C virus genotypes in blood donors: an international collaborative survey. J Clin Microbiol. 1994;32:884–92.
14. Kao JH, Chen PJ, Lai MY, Yang PM, Sheu JC, Wang TH, et al. Genotypes of hepatitis C virus in Taiwan and the progression of liver disease. J Clin Gastroenterol. 1995;21:233–7.
15. Lee CM, Lu SN, Hung CH, Tung WC, Wang JH, Tung HD, et al. Hepatitis C virus genotypes in southern Taiwan: prevalence and clinical implications. Trans R Soc Trop Med Hyg. 2006;100:767–74.
16. Lee CM, Hung CH, Lu SN, Wang JH, Tung HD, Huang WS, et al. Viral etiology of hepatocellular carcinoma and HCV genotypes in Taiwan. Intervirology. 2006;49:76–81.
17. Manns MP, McHutchison JG, Gordon SC, Rustgi VK, Shiffman M, Reindollar R, et al. Peginterferon alfa-2b plus ribavirin compared with interferon alfa-2b plus ribavirin for initial treatment of chronic hepatitis C: a randomised trial. Lancet. 2001;358:958–65.
18. Fried MW, Shiffman ML, Reddy KR, Smith C, Marinos G, Gonçales Jr FL, et al. Peginterferon alfa-2a plus ribavirin for chronic hepatitis C virus infection. N Engl J Med. 2002;347:975–82.
19. Hadziyannis SJ, Sette Jr H, Morgan TR, Balan V, Diago M, Marcellin P, et al. PEGASYS International January 2006 American Gastroenterological Association 253 Study Group. Peginterferon-α-2a and ribavirin combination therapy in chronic hepatitis C: a randomized study of treatment duration and ribavirin dose. Ann Intern Med. 2004;140:346–55.
20. Liu CH, Liu CJ, Lin CL, Liang CC, Hsu SJ, Yang SS, et al. Pegylated interferon-alpha-2a plus ribavirin for treatment-naive Asian patients with hepatitis C virus genotype 1 infection: a multicenter, randomized controlled trial. Clin Infect Dis. 2008;47:1260–9.
21. European Association for the Study of the Liver. EASL recommendations on treatment of hepatitis C 2015. J Hepatol. 2015;63:199–236.
22. AASLD/ISDA HCV Guidance Panel. Hepatitis C guidance: AASLD-IDSA recommendations for testing, managing, and treating adults infected with hepatitis C virus. Hepatology. 2015;62:932–54.
23. Fearon DT, Locksley RM. The instructive role of innate immunity in the acquired immune response. Science. 1996;272:50–3.
24. Biron CA. Role of early cytokines, including α and β interferons (IFN-α/β), in innate and adaptive immune responses to viral infections. Semin Immunol. 1998;10:383–90.
25. Meylan E, Tschopp J. Toll-like receptors and RNA helicases: two parallel ways to trigger antiviral responses. Mol Cell. 2006;22:561–9.
26. Kawai T, Akira S. Innate immune recognition of viral infection. Nat Immunol. 2006;7:131–7.
27. Kawai T, Akira S. TLR signaling. Cell Death Differ. 2006;13:816–25.
28. Dolganiuc A, Oak S, Kodys K, Golenbock DT, Finberg RW, Kurt-Jones E, Szabo G, et al. Hepatitis C core and nonstructural 3 proteins trigger toll-like receptor 2-mediated pathways and inflammatory activation. Gastroenterology. 2004;127:1513–24.
29. Machida K, Cheng KT, Sung VM, Levine AM, Foung S, Lai MM, et al. Hepatitis C virus induces toll-like receptor 4 expression, leading to enhanced production of beta interferon and interleukin-6. J Virol. 2006;80:866–74.
30. Li K, Foy E, Ferreon JC, Nakamura M, Ferreon AC, Ikeda M, et al. Immune evasion by hepatitis C virus NS3/4A protease-mediated cleavage of the Toll-like receptor 3 adaptor protein TRIF. Proc Natl Acad Sci. 2005;102:2992–7.
31. Lee J, Wu CC, Lee KJ, Chuang TH, Katakura K, Liu YT, et al. Activation of anti-hepatitis C virus responses via Toll-like receptor 7. Proc Natl Acad Sci. 2006;103:1828–33.
32. Takeshita F, Suzuki K, Sasaki S, Ishii N, Klinman DM, Ishii KJ, et al. Transcriptional regulation of the human TLR9 gene. J Immunol. 2004;173:2552–61.
33. Fukuda K, Tsuchihara K, Hijikata M, Nishiguchi S, Kuroki T, Shimotohno K, et al. Hepatitis C virus core protein enhances the activation of the transcription factor, Elk1, in response to mitogenic stimuli. Hepatology. 2001;33:159–65.
34. Ten Oever J, Kox M, van de Veerdonk FL, Mothapo KM, Slavcovici A, Jansen TL, et al. The discriminative capacity of soluble Toll-like receptor (sTLR)2 and sTLR4 in inflammatory diseases. BMC Immunol. 2014;15:55.
35. He Q, Graham CS, Durante Mangoni E, Koziel MJ, et al. Differential expression of toll-like receptor mRNA in treatmen t non-responders and sustained virologic responders at baseline in patients with chronic hepatitis C. Liver Int. 2006;26:1100–10.
36. Yuki N, Matsumoto S, Kato M, Yamaguchi T. Hepatic Toll-like receptor 3 expression in chronic hepatitis C genotype 1 correlates with treatment response to peginterferon plus ribavirin. J Viral Hepat. 2010;17:130–8.
37. Sarasin-Filipowicz M, Oakeley EJ, Duong FH, Christen V, Terracciano L, Filipowicz W, et al. Interferon signaling and treatment outcome in chronic hepatitis C. Proc Natl Acad Sci. 2008;105:7034–9.
38. Chen L, Borozan I, Feld J, Sun J, Tannis LL, Coltescu C, et al. Hepatic gene expression discriminates responders and nonresponders in treatment of chronic hepatitis C viral infection. Gastroenterology. 2005;128:1437–44.
39. Asselah T, Bieche I, Narguet S, Sabbagh A, Laurendeau I, Ripault MP, et al. Liver gene expression signature to predict response to pegylated interferon plus ribavirin combination therapy in patients with chronic hepatitis C. Gut. 2008;57:516–24.
40. Sarasin-Filipowicz M, Wang X, Yan M, Duong FH, Poli V, Hilton DJ, et al. Alpha interferon induces long-lasting refractoriness of JAK-STAT signaling in the mouse liver through induction of USP18/UBP43. Mol Cell Biol. 2009;29:4841–51.
41. Otsuka M, Kato N, Moriyama M, Taniguchi H, Wang Y, Dharel N, et al. Interaction between the HCV NS3 protein and the host TBK1 protein leads to inhibition of cellular antiviral responses. Hepatology. 2005;41:1004–12.
42. Abe T, Kaname Y, Hamamoto I, Tsuda Y, Wen X, Taguwa S, et al. Hepatitis C virus nonstructural protein 5A modulates the toll-like receptor-MyD88-dependent signaling pathway in macrophage cell lines. J Virol. 2007;81:8953–66.

22

Implementation of baby boomer hepatitis C screening and linking to care in gastroenterology practices

Zobair M. Younossi[1,2,9*], Louis L. LaLuna[3], John J. Santoro[4], Flavia Mendes[5], Victor Araya[6], Natarajan Ravendhran[7], Lisa Pedicone[8], Idania Lio[8], Fatema Nader[2], Sharon Hunt[2], Andrei Racila[2] and Maria Stepanova[2]

Abstract

Background: Estimates suggest that only 20 % of HCV-infected patients have been identified and <10 % treated. However, baby boomers (1945-1965) are identified as having a higher prevalence of HCV which has led the Centers for Disease Control and Prevention to make screening recommendations. The aim of this study was to implement the CDC's screening recommendations in the unique setting of gastroenterology practices in patients previously unscreened for HCV.

Methods: After obtaining patient informed consent, demographics, clinical and health-related quality of life (HRQOL) data were collected. A blood sample was screened for HCV antibody (HCV AB) using the OraQuick HCV Rapid Antibody Test. HCV AB-positive patients were tested for presence of HCV RNA and, if HCV RNA positive, patients underwent treatment discussions.

Results: We screened 2,000 individuals in 5 gastroenterology centers located close to large metropolitan areas on the East Coast (3 Northeast, 1 Mid-Atlantic and 1 Southeast). Of the screened population, 10 individuals (0.5 %) were HCV AB-positive. HCV RNA testing was performed in 90 % (9/10) of HCV AB-positive individuals. Of those, 44.4 % (4/9) were HCV RNA-positive, and all 4 (100 %) were linked to caregiver. Compared to HCV AB negative subjects, HCV AB-positive individuals tended to be black (20.0 vs. 5.2 %, $p = 0.09$) and reported significantly higher rates of depression: 60.0 vs. 21.5 %, $p = 0.009$. These individuals also reported a significantly lower HRQOL citing having more fatigue, poorer concentration, and a decreased level of energy ($p < 0.05$).

Discussion: Although the prevalence of HCV AB-positive was low in previously unscreened subjects screened in the gastroenterology centers, the linkage to care was very high. The sample of patients used in this study may be biased, so further studies are needed to assess the effectiveness of the CDC screening recommendations.

Conclusion: Implementation of the Baby Boomer Screening for HCV requires identifying screening environement with high prevalence of HCV+ individuals as well as an efficient process of linking them to care.

Background

Hepatitis C viral (HCV) infection is the leading cause of cirrhosis and hepatocellular carcinoma in the United States, and the most common indication for liver transplantation [1–4]. There is increasing evidence that HCV is a systemic disease with both hepatic and extrahepatic manifestations [1]. There is also significant evidence that HCV infection is associated with tremendous economic burden including both direct and indirect costs associated with management of HCV-related hepatic and extrahepatic manifestations as well as lost years of life, impaired quality of life and work productivity [1–9] On the other hand, sustained viral response (SVR) of HCV infection has been reported to improve morbidity and mortality as well as health-related quality of life and work productivity in patients with HCV [10–13]. With the current all-oral second generation direct-acting antiviral agents, over 95 % of treated patients can achieve SVR with an excellent safety profile [14–29].

* Correspondence: zobair.younossi@inova.org
[1]Center for Liver Diseases, Inova Fairfax Hospital, Falls Church, VA, USA
[2]Center for Outcomes Research in Liver Diseases, Washington, DC, USA

Despite substantial gains in treating HCV with these new highly effective antiviral regimens, there are a number of barriers which still exist [30–34]. Of these, the two most notable barriers are difficulty in obtaining insurance funding for the new regimens and the identification of all HCV infected patients [30–34]. The current estimates suggest that only between 10–50 % of HCV infected patients in the US are currently diagnosed [31]. This is partly due to health care providers' lack of enthusiasm about the previous anti-HCV treatment regimens and their substantial side effect profile. Additionally, the recommended risk-based screening has not been effective in identifying infected patients [35]. Since 1998, the CDC has suggested HCV antibody screening of individuals with past behaviors or health indicators associated with HCV infection (e.g., history of injection drug use, hemodialysis, etc.). Despite these recommendations, more than 50 % of individuals with chronic hepatitis C (CHC) continue to be unaware of their infections, leading to questions about the effectiveness of such "risk-based" screening [36, 37].

In the United States, HCV infection is most prevalent among individuals born between 1945 and 1965 accounting for approximately 75 % of hepatitis C-associated mortality [38]. Since more than 50 % of infected individuals are unaware of their infection, the number of adults with CHC that will progress to cirrhosis, liver failure, hepatocellular carcinoma, and death is expected to increase dramatically in the coming decades [38, 39]. Without changes to CH-C screening, diagnosing and treatment paradigms, over the next 20 years, the total medical costs for individuals with HCV infection are expected to more than double, from $30 billion to over $85 billion [40]. Therefore, in 2012, CDC adjusted their recommendations to include a one-time hepatitis C screening of all individuals born between 1945 and 1965 [41]. The US Preventive Services Task Force has stepped forward and supported the CDC's recommendation for birth cohort screening as well [42].

With therapies achieving SVR in >90 % of patients, targeted testing and link to care for infected persons in this birth cohort are expected to reduce HCV-related morbidity and mortality [35]. Therefore, the aim of this study was to implement a pilot screening project in 5 real world Gastroenterology Practices to identify baby boomers infected with HCV and to test the feasibility of screening and linking patients to care in a specialized practice setting.

Methods

Study population

This is a multi-center study sponsored by Chronic Liver Disease Foundation that involved 5 gastroenterology practices selected by the American College of Gastroenterology. The sites were large clinical practices within metropolitan

areas that had familiarity with standard preventative screening procedures (e.g., colon cancer screening) and Good Clinical Practices (i.e., informed consent, data privacy, data collection). Enrollment started in 2014 and was completed in June 2015; it was competitive and not capped at any given site. Inclusion criteria were as follows: male and female patients born between 1945 and 1965, inclusive; willingness to give written informed consent; ability to read and understand English. Patients with documented history of HCV antibody (HCV Ab) or HCV RNA screening were excluded. To obtain baseline information, all patients were asked to fill out two questionnaires - one with their demographic and basic clinical history and one with health-related quality of life information (HRQL). Each patient underwent a blood draw to obtain a sample of blood for HCV screening. If the patient tested positive for HCV Ab, a standard of care confirmatory test was performed.

Clinical and HRQL data

After informed consent, demographic, clinical and quality of life data were obtained. In particular, all enrolled individuals reported their age, gender, race/ethnicity and zip code. Medical history questionnaire asked about history of diabetes mellitus, hypertension, hyperlipidemia (that or high cholesterol or high triglycerides), heart disease (not specified), and about experiencing anxiety, depression, and fatigue. Individuals were also asked about recent alcohol consumption (3 or more drinks a week for a year) and about their current smoking status.

To assess fatigue, vitality, and exertion, 20 items from three widely used and extensively validated HRQL assessment instruments were selected and included into one questionnaire [43–47]. Specifically, the items were chosen from the physical functioning domain (PF) of the SF-36, the activity/energy (AE) and emotional (EM) domains of CLDQ-HCV, and the fatigue scale domain (FS) of FACIT-F [43–47]. The questionnaire was in English and self-administered. The responses to individual items were collected and, after transformation to a universal scale, were averaged to a total generic HRQL score (0–100).

Screening for HCV infection

Sites were provided with commercially approved OraQuick HCV Rapid Antibody Test kits (OraSure Technologies). Each subject's blood sample was screened for HCV Ab using Oraquick anti-HCV test. An adverse event was defined as any medical occurrence in response to the administration of the OraQuick Rapid HCV Test.

Individuals who were HCV Ab-negative were no longer followed-up for this study. For HCV Ab-positive individuals, a standard of care confirmatory testing was ordered by the screening site (as per standard medical practice) such as HCV RNA test, and results were collected. Individuals were also counseled and educated on HCV, including the use of alcohol, acetaminophen, and receiving hepatitis A and B vaccinations. The HCV Ab-positive individuals who consented to be followed also completed a four week follow-up HRQL survey. Finally, HCV RNA positive individuals were linked to care within the site practice or the geographical area and the date of the scheduled visit was recorded. The site also followed instructions regarding the local state requirements on whether a positive result had to be reported to a state health department.

The study outcomes and statistical analysis

The primary endpoint of this study was the percentage of individuals with a positive HCV Ab. The secondary endpoints were the percentages of HCV Ab-positive individuals who underwent confirmatory testing and were linked to care, and HRQL scores at baseline and at follow-up.

The demographic and clinical parameters of individuals who were HCV Ab-positive or HCV Ab-negative were compared using Fisher exact test or Mann-Whitney non-parametric test. Individual HRQL items were treated as ordinal parameters; the total HRQL score was considered continuous. A p-value of less than 0.05 was considered significant. Independent predictors of a positive HCV Ab result were evaluated by a logistic regression using all collected clinico-demographic parameters as predictors. All analyses were run in SAS 9.3

(SAS Institute, Cary, NC). The study was approved by Copernicus IRB Board.

Results

Two thousand baby boomer individuals were consented and screened in 5 gastroenterology practices selected by American College of Gastroenterology (regions: 3 Northeast, 1 Mid-Atlantic and 1 Southeast). The demographic and clinical data is summarized in Table 1, and HRQL data is summarized in Table 2.

Screened individuals were, on average, 60 ± 6 years old, 40 % male, 72 % Caucasian, 21 % Hispanic and 5 % African-American. Also, 30 % reported history of anxiety, 22 % reported depression and 38 % reported clinically overt fatigue. Furthermore, 16 % had a history of diabetes, 43 % had a history of hypertension, and 48 % had history of hyperlipidemia. Additionally, 27.5 % reported drinking alcohol ≥ 3 drinks per week, and 10.2 % reported current smoking (Table 1).

Of the screened population, 10 individuals (0.5 %) had positive serology for HCV. Of those, 4 (40 %) reported history of IV drug use and 2 (20 %) a history of intranasal drug use, 4 (40 %) had an unregulated tattoo, 1 (10 %) had a history of incarceration, and 1 (10 %) reported a history of blood transfusion before 1992 (Table 3).

The HCV RNA testing was done in 90 % (9/10) of HCV-antibody positive individuals, and 44.4 % (4/9)

Table 1 Demographics and medical history of the screened birth cohort

	HCV Ab+	HCV Ab-	p	All subjects
N	10	1,990		2,000
Age, years	58.4 ± 3.2	59.8 ± 6.0	0.41	59.8 ± 6.0
Race or ethnicity				
Caucasian	8 (80.0 %)	1429 (71.8 %)	0.73	1437 (71.9 %)
African-American	2 (20.0 %)	103 (5.2 %)	0.0933	105 (5.3 %)
Hispanic	0 (0.0 %)	418 (21.0 %)	0.13	418 (20.9 %)
Asian	0 (0.0 %)	26 (1.3 %)	1.00	26 (1.3 %)
Other	0 (0.0 %)	14 (0.7 %)	1.00	14 (0.7 %)
Male gender	4 (40.0 %)	793 (39.8 %)	1.00	797 (39.9 %)
History of:				
Type 2 diabetes	3 (30.0 %)	308 (15.5 %)	0.20	311 (15.6 %)
Hypertension	5 (50.0 %)	858 (43.4 %)	0.75	863 (43.4 %)
Hyperlipidemia	4 (40.0 %)	951 (47.9 %)	0.76	955 (47.8 %)
Anxiety	4 (40.0 %)	600 (30.3 %)	0.50	604 (30.3 %)
Depression	6 (60.0 %)	424 (21.5 %)	0.0094	430 (21.7 %)
Fatigue	6 (60.0 %)	742 (37.5 %)	0.19	748 (37.6 %)
Heart disease	2 (20.0 %)	219 (11.1 %)	0.31	221 (11.1 %)
Alcohol consumption > 30 g/week	3 (30.0 %)	545 (27.5 %)	1.00	548 (27.5 %)
Current smoking	3 (30.0 %)	199 (10.1 %)	0.0731	202 (10.2 %)

Table 2 Quality of life in the screened birth cohort

Question text	Range [a]	Instrument, item (domain)	HCV Ab + (N = 10)	HCV Ab- (N = 1,889)	p	All subjects
How much have you been tired or fatigued during the last 2 weeks?	1–7	CLDQ-HCV Q1 (AE)	3.60 ± 1.96	4.82 ± 1.70	0.0412	4.82 ± 1.70
How much difficulty have you had with bending, lifting, or stooping in the last 2 weeks?	1–7	CLDQ-HCV Q4 (AE)	5.10 ± 1.85	5.53 ± 1.69	0.37	5.53 ± 1.69
How often during the last 2 weeks have you felt a decreased level of energy?	1–7	CLDQ-HCV Q7 (AE)	3.80 ± 2.10	4.98 ± 1.69	0.0155	4.97 ± 1.69
How often during the last 2 weeks have you felt depressed?	1–7	CLDQ-HCV Q16 (EM)	4.40 ± 2.12	5.88 ± 1.49	0.0144	5.87 ± 1.50
How much of the time during the last 2 weeks have you had problems concentrating?	1–7	CLDQ-HCV Q18 (AE)	4.80 ± 1.75	5.70 ± 1.47	0.0471	5.70 ± 1.47
The following questions are about activities you might do during a typical day. Does your health now limit you in these activities? If so, how much?						
Vigorous activities, such as running, lifting heavy objects, participating in strenuous sports	1–3	SF-36 PF01	2.10 ± 0.99	2.13 ± 0.82	0.41	2.13 ± 0.82
Moderate activities, such as moving a table, pushing a vacuum cleaner, bowling, or playing golf	1–3	SF-36 PF02	2.20 ± 1.03	2.60 ± 0.67	0.0122	2.59 ± 0.67
Lifting or carrying groceries	1–3	SF-36 PF03	2.30 ± 0.95	2.67 ± 0.60	0.0450	2.67 ± 0.60
Climbing several flights of stairs	1–3	SF-36 PF04	2.20 ± 0.92	2.47 ± 0.72	0.29	2.47 ± 0.72
Climbing one flight of stairs	1–3	SF-36 PF05	2.20 ± 1.03	2.69 ± 0.60	0.0064	2.68 ± 0.61
Bending, kneeling, or stooping	1–3	SF-36 PF06	2.40 ± 0.84	2.47 ± 0.70	0.65	2.47 ± 0.70
Walking more than a mile	1–3	SF-36 PF07	2.20 ± 0.79	2.46 ± 0.76	0.22	2.46 ± 0.76
Walking several hundred yards	1–3	SF-36 PF08	2.10 ± 0.88	2.66 ± 0.64	0.0195	2.66 ± 0.64
Walking one hundred yards	1–3	SF-36 PF09	2.10 ± 0.99	2.73 ± 0.58	0.0063	2.72 ± 0.59
Bathing or dressing yourself	1–3	SF-36 PF10	2.60 ± 0.84	2.86 ± 0.44	0.10	2.86 ± 0.44
Please indicate how true each statement has been for you during the past 7 days.						
I feel fatigued	4–0	FACIT-F HI7 (FS)	2.10 ± 1.45	1.11 ± 1.20	0.0107	1.11 ± 1.20
I feel tired	4–0	FACIT-F An2 (FS)	2.00 ± 1.49	1.25 ± 1.16	0.15	1.25 ± 1.16
I have trouble starting things because I am tired	4–0	FACIT-F An3 (FS)	1.70 ± 1.64	0.80 ± 1.12	0.0148	0.80 ± 1.13
I have energy	0–4	FACIT-F An5 (FS)	1.80 ± 0.63	2.41 ± 1.18	0.0352	2.41 ± 1.18
I need help doing my usual activities	4–0	FACIT-F An14 (FS)	0.80 ± 0.79	0.37 ± 0.86	0.0100	0.37 ± 0.86
Average score	0–100	generic	58.9 ± 32.5	76.3 ± 21.3	0.071	76.2 ± 21.4

[a] the range is from the worst to the best health status. Higher scores indicate better HRQOL

were found to be HCV RNA-positive, 100 % of whom were counseled and linked to care by establishing an appointment regarding their HCV. Compared to HCV-antibody negative individuals, those who were HCV-antibody positive tended to be African-Americans (20.0 vs. 5.2 %, $p = 0.09$) and report more frequently a history of depression: 60.0 vs. 21.5 % ($p = 0.009$) (Table 1). Multivariate analysis with logistic regression showed that depression was the only clinical parameter independently associated with being HCV-antibody positive [odds ratio (95 % confidence interval) = 5.49 (1.54–19.54)].

The HCV-antibody positive individuals also had lower quality of life as documented by more fatigue, poorer concentration, less activity, and decreased levels of energy (all p-values < 0.05) (Table 2). The four weeks follow-up HRQOL questionnaire showed no significant changes (all $p > 0.1$) from the baseline values in individuals who tested positive for HCV (Table 4).

Discussion

This is the largest HCV screening program in the baby boomers who presented to a specialty gastroenterology practices for clinical care. The data suggest that the prevalence of HCV antibody positivity in this particular study setting (subjects visiting GE practices who have not previously been identified) is relatively low (0.5 %) as compared to the reported HCV AB positive rate in the general population at 4.1 % for males and 1.6 % for females [48]. It is important to note that, in addition to a bias introduced solely by the fact of patients being seen

Table 3 Additional socio-demographic information and link to care for HCV Ab + patients (N = 10)

	N (%) or mean ± std.dev.
Confirmed HCV ab+	10 (100.0 %)
HCV RNA-positive [a]	4 (44.4 %)
ALT, IU/mL	32.8 ± 35.4
AST, IU/mL	25.2 ± 21.7
History of:	
Past or current IV drug use	4 (40.0 %)
Blood transfusions before 1992	1 (10.0 %)
Long-term hemodialysis	0 (0.0 %)
Incarceration	1 (10.0 %)
Being born to HCV-infected mother	0 (0.0 %)
Intranasal drug use	2 (20.0 %)
Unregulated tattoo or other percutaneous exposure	4 (40.0 %)
Counseled about:	
Acetaminophen use	9 (90.0 %)
Alcohol consumption	10 (100.0 %)
Hepatitis A and B vaccination	9 (90.0 %)
Linked to care	9 (90.0 %)
Completed follow-up questionnaire	6 (60 %)

[a]one HCV ab + patient refused to give blood sample

in tertiary care centers in a small sample of localities, our study excluded individuals who had already been diagnosed with HCV or had been screened for HCV previously due to meeting certain high risk criteria. Therefore, the prevalence rate reported in this study is likely substantially lower than one that could have been obtained in a community-based screening setting, and neither does it reflect the true HCV prevalence in the GE practices (due to exclusion of those with an existing diagnosis of HCV).

Our study also indicates that about half of the individuals who were HCV antibody positive were viremic. In this HCV cohort, risk factors reported were similar to those previously known for HCV viremic patients [1–4]. Furthermore, African Americans tended to have a higher prevalence of HCV which is also consistent with previous reports. Additionally, those testing HCV positive had more depression independently associated with their HCV positivity status. All HCV positive individuals were linked to follow-up care through scheduled appointments. This is a significant finding as this part of the screening, diagnosis, and treatment continuum has been a challenge in other settings such as emergency rooms [2].

These data are similar to those reported by Sears et al. from a single GE practice for baby boomers undergoing colonoscopy. In fact, in that study, only one of 376

subjects (0.27 %) was HCV RNA positive, a rate almost identical to our HCV viremic individuals (0.2 %) [3]. There are a number of potential explanations for the relatively low prevalence of HCV in GE practices. The most important explanation may be related to the type of patients who are seen in GE practices – they are most likely insured with the majority (72 %) being Caucasians.

The low prevalence of HCV in this special population as compared to a community-based approach is of special importance as specialty practices may not be the best places to screen for HCV but may provide the best avenue for follow-up care once identified. For instance, Galbraith et al. reported screening of baby boomers in an emergency room. These authors reported an 11.1 % positive HCV antibody rate with 68 % being viremic. On the other hand, only 54 % of HCV viremic patients were able to be contacted and 38 % were able to be scheduled for follow-up appointments indicating a significant drop-off [2].

In addition to high prevalence of HCV in the baby boomers seen in the emergency department, the prevalence rates are also high for baby boomers screened in the hospital setting. In a study by Turner et al., the prevalence of newly diagnosed HCV in hospitalized baby boomers was 8 % [4]. Finally, in a study reported by Morano et al., baby boomers were screened either by point of care (POC) HCV antibody testing or traditional serologic testing in the setting of a mobile medical clinic. The reported prevalence of HCV positivity in this cohort was 6.2 %. Individuals who underwent POC testing were much more likely (93.8 %) than traditional serologic testing (18.2 %) to be linked to care [5]. In a recent modeling study from 15 countries worldwide, investigators found that diagnosing and treating a small proportion of patients with high efficacy drugs can have a significant effect on the reduction of the HCV disease burden within the countries studied [49]. At the same time, the authors caution that the best scenario would be to have increased diagnosis and treatment with high efficacy treatments to have the best results. Others, though, argue that the model used was not a dynamic model and thus may not capture any new infection or reinfections so may overestimate the true impact of the use of high efficacy drugs [50].

These findings not only assist healthcare workers in identifying better areas for the identification of HCV but may assist healthcare workers in providing a better method to link screening with follow-up care. Link to care is important to deliver the highly effective antiviral treatment to patients with HCV. Our data suggest high rates of linking to care for patients who are HCV-positive to a GE clinic. Nevertheless, given the small sample size, the generalizability of this data must be interpreted with caution. Furthermore, if a GE clinic is

Table 4 Follow-up HRQL questionnaire in HCV Ab + patients (N = 6)

Question text	Range [a]	Instrument, item (domain)	baseline	4 week f/u
How much have you been tired or fatigued during the last 2 weeks?	1–7	CLDQ-HCV, Q1 (AE)	4.00 ± 1.26	4.50 ± 1.64
How much difficulty have you had with bending, lifting, or stooping in the last 2 weeks?	1–7	CLDQ-HCV, Q4 (AE)	5.17 ± 1.83	5.33 ± 1.37
How often during the last 2 weeks have you felt a decreased level of energy?	1–7	CLDQ-HCV, Q7 (AE)	4.00 ± 1.55	4.50 ± 1.64
How often during the last 2 weeks have you felt depressed?	1–7	CLDQ-HCV, Q16 (EM)	5.17 ± 1.94	5.00 ± 1.55
How much of the time during the last 2 weeks have you had problems concentrating?	1–7	CLDQ-HCV, Q18 (AE)	5.17 ± 1.17	5.50 ± 1.05
The following questions are about activities you might do during a typical day. Does your health now limit you in these activities? If so, how much?				
Vigorous activities, such as running, lifting heavy objects, participating in strenuous sports	1–3	SF-36, PF01 (PF)	2.17 ± 0.98	2.00 ± 0.89
Moderate activities, such as moving a table, pushing a vacuum cleaner, bowling, or playing golf	1–3	SF-36, PF02 (PF)	2.33 ± 1.03	2.33 ± 0.82
Lifting or carrying groceries	1–3	SF-36, PF03 (PF)	2.50 ± 0.84	2.33 ± 0.82
Climbing several flights of stairs	1–3	SF-36, PF04 (PF)	2.33 ± 0.82	2.17 ± 0.98
Climbing one flight of stairs	1–3	SF-36, PF05 (PF)	2.33 ± 1.03	2.17 ± 0.98
Bending, kneeling, or stooping	1–3	SF-36, PF06 (PF)	2.50 ± 0.84	2.00 ± 0.89
Walking more than a mile	1–3	SF-36, PF07 (PF)	2.17 ± 0.75	2.17 ± 0.98
Walking several hundred yards	1–3	SF-36, PF08 (PF)	2.00 ± 0.89	2.33 ± 0.82
Walking one hundred yards	1–3	SF-36, PF09 (PF)	2.00 ± 1.10	2.33 ± 0.82
Bathing or dressing yourself	1–3	SF-36, PF10 (PF)	2.67 ± 0.82	2.67 ± 0.82
Please indicate how true each statement has been for you during the past 7 days.				
I feel fatigued	4–0	FACIT-F HI7 (FS)	2.00 ± 1.10	1.33 ± 1.51
I feel tired	4–0	FACIT-F An2 (FS)	2.00 ± 1.41	1.50 ± 1.38
I have trouble starting things because I am tired	4–0	FACIT-F An3 (FS)	1.33 ± 1.37	1.33 ± 1.21
I have energy	0–4	FACIT-F An5 (FS)	2.00 ± 0.63	1.67 ± 0.52
I need help doing my usual activities	4–0	FACIT-F An14 (FS)	0.50 ± 0.55	1.00 ± 0.89
Average score	0–100	Generic	63.1 ± 29.9	63.4 ± 27.9

[a] the range is from the worst to the best health status

not available another suggested method is the use of Innovative Mobile Clinics equipped with POC testing for HCV that use established pathways [5]. Using mobile clinics allow for HCV-positive patients to be immediately linked to care.

In this study, we also assessed the quality of life in all patients at baseline before they knew their HCV infection status as there are previous data which suggest that knowledge about HCV diagnosis can impair HRQL [51]. We have found that at baseline patients who were HCV AB+ had more impairment of their HRQL having more complaints of fatigue, poorer concentration, less activity, and decreased levels of energy as compared to those who were HCV AB-. This is consistent with previous data which have demonstrated that HCV-infected patients suffer from HRQL impairment possibly due to the potential effects of the virus crossing the blood-brain barrier and affecting the brain chemistry directly [52–54]. In our study, for the patients who were HCV AB+, a follow-up survey was administered 4 weeks after their initial diagnosis, and there were no statistically significant change in their reported HRQL indicating that knowing the status of being HCV AB+ did not influence their HRQL. However, the small sample size of our study may have contributed to our inability to detect this difference in the HRQOL scores.

One of the limitation of this study was the study population referred to a GE practice indicating access to insurance coverage for consultative services and colonoscopy. This could potentially introduce a bias by excluding uninsured individuals who are known to have high prevalence of HCV (30). Another limitation of our study was our focus on "the age cohort" as the risk factor for HCV. Although this was done to determine the prevalence of HCV solely based on the age-based risk factor, other risks were not included.

Conclusions

In summary, our data show that the outcome of screening and then linkage to care for the baby boomers found to be HCV-positive is feasible but may depend on the setting. In this study, GE practices appeared to have a low prevalence of HCV, but the linkage to care occurred universally. Therefore, a strategy to maximize both the yield of HCV screening and linkage to care with appropriate providers will be critical for identifying and successfully treating patients infected with HCV.

Competing interests

ZMY is a consultant to Abbvie, Gilead, BMS and GSK. Other authors have no competing interest.

Authors' contributions

ZMY-Primary investigator, research design, oversight, writing and editing the manuscript. LLLaL- Principal Investigator, subject enrollment and editing the manuscript. JJS- Principal Investigator, subject enrollment and editing the manuscript. FM- Principal Investigator, subject enrollment and editing the manuscript. VA- Principal Investigator, subject enrollment and editing the manuscript. NR- Principal Investigator, subject enrollment and editing the manuscript. LP-Research design, oversight, writing and editing the manuscript. IL- Research design, monitoring and editing the manuscript. FN-Database Management, writing and editing the manuscript. SH-Data design and review. AR-Data design and database development. All authors read and approved the final manuscript.

Funding source

Chronic Liver Disease Foundation (CLDF), Clark, NJ.

Disclosures

MS, LDP, IL, SH, FN, AR, LL, JS, FM, VA and NR – Nothing to Disclose. ZYM – Consulting: Gilead, BMS, Abbvie, GSK.

Author details

[1]Center for Liver Diseases, Inova Fairfax Hospital, Falls Church, VA, USA. [2]Center for Outcomes Research in Liver Diseases, Washington, DC, USA. [3]Digestive Disease Associates, Wyomissing, PA, USA. [4]AGA Clinical Research Associates, LLC, Egg Harbor Township, NJ, USA. [5]GastroHealth, Miami, FL, USA. [6]Central Bucks Specialists, Gastroenterology, Doylestown, PA, USA. [7]Digestive Diseases Associates, Catonsville, MD, USA. [8]Cantara Clinical Solutions, LLC, Morristown, NJ, USA. [9]Betty and Guy Beatty Center for Integrated Research, Claude Moore Health Education and Research Building, 3300 Gallows Road, Falls Church, VA 22042, USA.

References

1. Younossi ZM, Kanwal F, Saab S, Brown KA, El-Serag HB, Kim WR, Ahmed A, Kugelmas M, Gordon SC. The impact of hepatitis C burden: an evidence-based approach. Aliment Pharmacol Ther. 2014;39(5):518–31.
2. Galbraith JW, Franco RA, Donnelly JP, Rodgers JB, Morgan JM, Viles AF, Overton ET, Saag MS, Wang HE. Unrecognized chronic hepatitis C virus infection among baby boomers in the emergency department. Hepatology. 2015;61(3):776–82. doi:10.1002/hep.27410. Epub 2015 Jan 28.
3. Sears DM, Cohen DC, Ackerman K, Ma JE, Song J. Birth cohort screening for chronic hepatitis during colonoscopy appointments. Am J Gastroenterol. 2013;108(6):981–9. doi:10.1038/ajg.2013.50. Epub 2013 Mar 19.
4. Turner BJ, Taylor BS, Hanson, Perez ME, Hernandez L, Villarreal R, Veerapaneni P, Fiebelkorn K. Implementing hospital-based baby boomer

5. hepatitis c virus screening and linkage to care: Strategies, results, and costs. J Hosp Med. 2015 May 29. doi: 10.1002/jhm.2376. [Epub ahead of print].
5. Morano JP, Zelenev A, Lombard A, Marcus R, Gibson BA, Altice FL. Strategies for hepatitis C testing and linkage to care for vulnerable populations: point-of-care and standard HCV testing in a mobile medical clinic. Community Health. 2014;39(5):922–34. doi:10.1007/s10900-014-9932-9.
6. Rosenthal E, Cacoub P. Extrahepatic manifestations in chronic hepatitis C virus carriers. Lupus. 2015;24(4-5):469–82. doi:10.1177/0961203314556140.
7. Younossi ZM, Singer ME, Mir HM, Henry L, Hunt S. Impact of interferon free regimens on clinical and cost outcomes for chronic hepatitis C genotype 1 patients. J Hepatol. 2014;60(3):530–7. doi:10.1016/j.jhep.2013.11.009. Epub 2013 Nov 19.
8. Coretti S, Romano F, Orlando V, Codella P, Prete S, Di Brino E, Ruggeri M. Economic evaluation of screening programs for hepatitis C virus infection: evidence from literature. Risk Manag Healthc Policy. 2015;8:45–54. doi:10.2147/RMHP.S56911.eCollection2015.
9. Estes C, Abdel-Kareem M, Abdel-Razek W, Abdel-Sameea E, Abuzeid M, Gomaa A, Osman W, Razavi H, Zaghla H, Waked I. Economic burden of hepatitis C in Egypt: the future impact of highly effective therapies.Aliment Pharmacol Ther. 2015 Jul 22. doi: 10.1111/apt.13316. [Epub ahead of print].
10. John-Baptiste AA, Tomlinson G, Hsu PC, Krajden M, Heathcote EJ, Laporte A, Yoshida EM, Anderson FH, Krahn MD. Sustained responders have better quality of life and productivity compared with treatment failures long after antiviral therapy for hepatitis C. Am J Gastroenterol. 2009;104(10):2439–48. doi:10.1038/ajg.2009.346. Epub 2009 Jun 30.
11. North CS, Hong BA, Adewuyi SA, Pollio DE, Jain MK, Devereaux R, Quartey NA, Ashitey S, Lee WM, Lisker-Melman M. Hepatitis C treatment and SVR: the gap between clinical trials and real-world treatment aspirations. Gen Hosp Psychiatry. 2013;35(2):122–8. doi:10.1016/j.genhosppsych.2012.11.002. Epub 2012 Dec 6.
12. Younossi ZM, Stepanova M, Sulkowski M, Naggie S, Hunt SH. All Oral Therapy With Sofosbuvir Plus Ribavirin For the Treatment of Chronic Hepatitis C in Patients Co-infected With HIV (PHOTON-1 and PHOTON 2): The Impact on Patient-Reported Outcomes. J Infect Dis. 2015;212(3):367–77. doi:10.1093/infdis/jiv005. Epub 2015 Jan 12.
13. Bonkovsky HL, Snow KK, Malet PF, Back-Madruga C, Fontana RJ, Sterling RK, Kulig CC, Di Bisceglie AM, Morgan TR, Dienstag JL, Ghany MG, Gretch DR, HALT-C Trial Group. Health-related quality of life in patients with chronic hepatitis C and advanced fibrosis. J Hepatol. 2007;46(3):420–31. Epub 2006 Nov 27.
14. Fazel Y, Lam B, Golabi P, Younossi Z. Safety analysis of sofosbuvir and ledipasvir for treating hepatitis C. Expert Opin Drug Saf. 2015;14(8):1317–26. doi:10.1517/14740338.2015.1053868. Epub 2015 Jun 4.
15. Lawitz E, Mangia A, Wyles D, Rodriguez-Torres M, Hassanein T, Gordon SC, Schultz M, Davis MN, Kayali Z, Reddy KR, Jacobson IM, Kowdley KV, Nyberg L, Subramanian GM, Hyland RH, Arterburn S, Jiang D, McNally J, Brainard D, Symonds WT, McHutchison JG, Sheikh AM, Younossi Z, Gane EJ. Sofosbuvir for previously untreated chronic hepatitis C infection. N Engl J Med. 2013;368(20):1878–87. doi:10.1056/NEJMoa1214853. Epub 2013 Apr 23.
16. Poordad F, Lawitz E, Kowdley KV, Cohen DE, Podsadecki T, Siggelkow S, Heckaman M, Larsen L, Menon R, Koev G, Tripathi R, Pilot-Matias T, Bernstein B. Exploratory study of oral combination antiviral therapy for hepatitis C. N Engl J Med. 2013;368(1):45–53. doi:10.1056/NEJMoa1208809.
17. Jacobson IM, Gordon SC, Kowdley KV, Yoshida EM, Rodriguez-Torres M, Sulkowski MS, Shiffman ML, Lawitz E, Everson G, Bennett M, Schiff E, Al-Assi MT, Subramanian GM, An D, Lin M, McNally J, Brainard D, Symonds WT, McHutchison JG, Patel K, Feld J, Pianko S, Nelson DR, POSITRON Study, FUSION Study. Sofosbuvir for hepatitis C genotype 2 or 3 in patients without treatment options. N Engl J Med. 2013;368(20):1867–77. doi:10.1056/NEJMoa1214854. Epub 2013 Apr 23.
18. Afdhal N, Zeuzem S, Kwo P, Chojkier M, Gitlin N, Puoti M, Romero-Gomez M, Zarski JP, Agarwal K, Buggisch P, Foster GR, Bräu N, Buti M, Jacobson IM, Subramanian GM, Ding X, Mo H, Yang JC, Pang PS, Symonds WT, McHutchison JG, Muir AJ, Mangia A, Marcellin P, ION-1 Investigators. Ledipasvir and sofosbuvir for untreated HCV genotype 1 infection. N Engl J Med. 2014;370(20):1889–98. doi:10.1056/NEJMoa1402454. Epub 2014 Apr 11.
19. Afdhal N, Reddy KR, Nelson DR, Lawitz E, Gordon SC, Schiff E, Nahass R, Ghalib R, Gitlin N, Herring R, Lalezari J, Younes ZH, Pockros PJ, Di Bisceglie AM, Arora S, Subramanian GM, Zhu Y, Dvory-Sobol H, Yang JC, Pang PS, Symonds WT, McHutchison JG, Muir AJ, Sulkowski M, Kwo P, ION-2 Investigators. Ledipasvir and sofosbuvir for previously treated HCV genotype 1 infection. N Engl J Med. 2014;370(16):1483–93. doi:10.1056/NEJMoa1316366. Epub 2014 Apr 11.

20. Zeuzem S, Dusheiko GM, Salupere R, Mangia A, Flisiak R, Hyland RH, Illeperuma A, Svarovskaia E, Brainard DM, Symonds WT, Subramanian GM, McHutchison JG, Weiland O, Reesink HW, Ferenci P, Hézode C, Esteban R, VALENCE Investigators. Sofosbuvir and ribavirin in HCV genotypes 2 and 3. N Engl J Med. 2014;370(21):1993–2001. doi:10.1056/NEJMoa1316145. Epub 2014 May 4.

21. Kowdley KV, Gordon SC, Reddy KR, Rossaro L, Bernstein DE, Lawitz E, Shiffman ML, Schiff E, Ghalib R, Ryan M, Rustgi V, Chojkier M, Herring R, Di Bisceglie AM, Pockros PJ, Subramanian GM, An D, Svarovskaia E, Hyland RH, Pang PS, Symonds WT, McHutchison JG, Muir AJ, Pound D, Fried MW, ION-3 Investigators. Ledipasvir and sofosbuvir for 8 or 12 weeks for chronic HCV without cirrhosis. N Engl J Med. 2014;370(20):1879–88. doi:10.1056/NEJMoa1402355. Epub 2014 Apr 10.

22. Dalgard O, Bjøro K, Ring-Larsen H, Bjornsson E, Holberg-Petersen M, Skovlund E, Reichard O, Myrvang B, Sundelöf B, Ritland S, Hellum K, Frydén A, Florholmen J, Verbaan H, North-C Group. Pegylated interferon alfa and ribavirin for 14 versus 24 weeks in patients with hepatitis C virus genotype 2 or 3 and rapid virological response. Hepatology. 2008;47(1):35–42.

23. Press release- http://www.prnewswire.com/news-releases/abbvie-completes-largest-phase-iii-program-of-an-all-oral-interferon-free-therapy-for-the-treatment-of-hepatitis-c-genotype-1-242911871.html Last accessed on 30 July 2015.

24. Nachega JB, Parienti J, Olalekan J, Uthman A, Gross R, Dowdy DW, Sax DE, Gallant JE, Mugavero MJ, Mills EJ, Giordano TP. Lower Pill Burden and Once-Daily Antiretroviral Treatment Regimens for HIV Infection: A Meta-Analysis of Randomized Controlled Trials. Clin Infect Dis. 2014;58(9):1297–307.

25. Kowdley KV, Lawitz E, Poordad F, et al. Safety and efficacy of interferon-free regimens of ABT-450/r, ABT-267, ABT-333 ± ribavirin in patients with chronic HCV GT1 infection: results from the Aviator study. Poster presented at the 48th Annual Meeting of the European Association for the Study of the Liver; April 24-28, 2013; Amsterdam, The Netherlands.

26. Baran RW, Xie W, Liu Y, Cohen DE, Gooch K. Health related quality of Life (HRQoL), health state, function and wellbeing of chronic HCV patients treated with interferon-free, oral DAA regimens: patient reported outcome (PRO) results from the Aviator study. Poster presented at: 64th Annual Meeting of the American Association for the Study of Liver Disease: Nov 1-5 2013; Washington, DC. P 1113.

27. Press release: OLYSIO™ (simeprevir) Receives FDA Approval for Combination Treatment of Chronic Hepatitis C. Obtained from the world wide web at http://www.jnj.com/news/all/OLYSIO-simeprevir-Receives-FDA-Approval-for-Combination-Treatment-of-Chronic-Hepatitis-C. Last accessed on 30 July 2015.

28. Scott J, Rosa K, Fu M, Cerri K, Peeters M, Beumont M, Zeuzem S, Evon DM, Gilles L. Fatigue during treatment for hepatitis C virus: results of self-reported fatigue severity in two Phase IIb studies of simeprevir treatment in patients with hepatitis C virus genotype 1 infection. BMC Infect Dis. 2014;14(1):465. doi:10.1186/1471-2334-14-465.

29. Jacobson IM, Dore GJ, Foster GR, Fried MW, Radu M, Rafalsky VV, Moroz L, Craxi A, Peeters M, Lenz O, Ouwerkerk-Mahadevan S, De La Rosa G, Kalmeijer R, Scott J, Sinha R, Beumont-Mauviel M. Simeprevir with pegylated interferon alfa 2a plus ribavirin in treatment-naive patients with chronic hepatitis C virus genotype 1 infection (QUEST-1): a phase 3, randomised, double-blind, placebo-controlled trial. Lancet. 2014;384(9941):403–13. doi:10.1016/S0140-6736(14)60494-3. Epub 2014 Jun 4.

30. Stepanova M, Younossi ZM. Interferon-Free Regimens for Chronic Hepatitis C: Barriers Due to Treatment Candidacy and Insurance Coverage. Dig Dis Sci. 2015 May 19. doi: 10.1007/s10620-015-3709-6.

31. McGowan CE, Fried MW. Barriers to hepatitis C treatment. Liver Int. 2012;32 Suppl 1:151–6. doi:10.1111/j.1478-3231.2011.02706.x.

32. Gundlapalli AV, Nelson RE, Haroldsen C, Carter ME, LaFleur J. Correlates of Initiation of Treatment for Chronic Hepatitis C Infection in United States Veterans, 2004-2009. PLoS One. 2015;10(7), e0132056. doi:10.1371/journal.pone.0132056.eCollection2015.

33. Appleby J. VA, California Panels Urge Costly Hepatitis C Drugs For Sickest Patients. April 17,2014. Obtained from the world wide web at http://www.kaiserhealthnews.org/Stories/2014/April/17/hepatitis-c-sovaldi-panels-urge-approval.aspx. Last accessed on Jul 30, 2015.

34. Stepanova M, Kanwal F, El-Serag H, Younossi ZM. Insurance Status and Treatment Candidacy of Hepatitis C Patients: Analysis of Population-based Data from the United States. Hepatology. 2011;53(3):737–45.

35. Cohn J, Roberts T, Amorosa V, Lemoine M, Hill A. Simplified diagnostic monitoring for hepatitis C, in the new era of direct-acting antiviral treatment. Curr Opin HIV AIDS. 2015 Jul 17. [Epub ahead of print]

36. U.S. Department Of Health And Human Services/Centers for Disease Control and Prevention (CDC). Recommendations for Prevention and Control of Hepatitis C Virus (HCV) Infection and HCV-Related Chronic Disease. MMWR, Oct 16, 1998. Last accessed on 30 July 2015 at http://www.cdc.gov/mmwr/PDF/rr/rr4719.PDF.

37. Younossi ZM, Stepanova M, Afendy M, Lam BP, Mishra A. Knowledge about infection is the only predictor of treatment in patients with chronic hepatitis C. J Viral Hepat. 2013;20(8):550–5.

38. U.S. Department Of Health And Human Services/Centers for Disease Control and Prevention (CDC). HEPATITIS C: Why Baby Boomers Should Get Tested. Available at: http://www.cdc.gov/knowmorehepatitis/Media/PDFs/FactSheet-Boomers.pdf. Last accessed at 30 July 2015.

39. Galbraith JW, Donnelly JP, Franco RA, Overton ET, Rodgers JB, Wang HE. National estimates of healthcare utilization by individuals with hepatitis C virus infection in the United States. Clin Infect Dis. 2014;59(6):755–64. doi:10.1093/cid/ciu427. Epub 2014 Jun 9.

40. Razavi H, Elkhoury AC, Elbasha E, Estes C, Pasini K, Poynard T, Kumar R. Chronic hepatitis C virus (HCV) disease burden and cost in the United States. Hepatology. 2013;57(6):2164–70. doi:10.1002/hep.26218. Epub 2013 May 6.

41. Smith B, Morgan R, Beckett G, Falk-Yetter Y, Holtzman D, Teo C, et al. Recommendations for the identification of chronic hepatitis C virus infection among persons born during 1945-1965. MMWR Recomm Rep. 2012;61(RR-4);1–32.

42. Moyer VA. Screening for Hepatitis C Virus Infection in Adults: U.S. Preventive Services Task Force Recommendation Statement Ann Intern Med. 2013; 159(5):349–58.

43. Ware JE, Kosinski M. Interpreting SF-36 summary health measures: a response. Qual Life Res. 2001;10(5):405–13. discussion 415-20.

44. Younossi ZM, Guyatt G, Kiwi M, Boparai N, King D. Development of a disease specific questionnaire to measure health related quality of life in patients with chronic liver disease. Gut. 1999;45(2):295–300.

45. Younossi ZM, Stepanova M, Henry L. Performance and Validation of Chronic Liver Disease Questionnaire-Hepatitis C Version (CLDQ-HCV) in Clinical Trials of Patients with Chronic Hepatitis C. Value in Health 2016 (In Press).

46. Webster K, Odom L, Peterman A, et al. The Functional Assessment of Chronic Illness Therapy (FACIT) measurement system: Validation of version 4 of the core questionnaire. Qual Life Res. 1999;8(7):604.

47. Reilly MC, Zbrozek AS, Dukes EM. The validity and reproducibility of a work productivity and activity impairment instrument. Pharmaco Economics. 1993;4:353–65.

48. Chou R, Clark E, Helfand.Screening for Hepatitis C Virus Infection- Systematic Evidence Reviews, No. 24. http://www.ncbi.nlm.nih.gov/books/NBK43249/.

49. Wedemeyer H, Duberg AS, Buti M, Rosenberg WM, Frankova S, Esmat G, Örmeci N, et al. Strategies to manage hepatitis C virus (HCV) disease burden. J Viral Hepat. 2014;21 Suppl 1:60–89. 10.1111/jvh.12249.

50. Razavi H, Bruggmann P, Wedemeyer H, Dore G. Response to letter to the editor: Strategies to reduce HCV disease burden and HCV transmission need different models, as what works for end-stage liver disease may not work for HCV prevalence: a comment on the results presented in JVH Special Issue. J Viral Hepat. 2014;21(12):e169–70. doi: 10.1111/jvh.12339. Epub 2014 Sep 29.

51. Rodger AJ, Jolley D, Thompson SC, Lanigan A, Crofts N. The impact of diagnosis of hepatitis C virus on quality of life. Hepatology. 1999; 30(5):1299–301.

52. Loria A, Doyle K, Weinstein AA, Winter P, Escheik C, Price J, Wang L, Birerdinc A, Baranova A, Gerber L, Younossi ZM. Multiple Factors Predict Physical Performance in People with Chronic Liver Disease. Am J Phys Med Rehabil. 2014 Jan 6. [Epub ahead of print]

53. Kallman J, O'Neil MM, Larive B, Boparai N, Calabrese L, Younossi ZM. Fatigue and health-related quality of life (HRQOL) in chronic hepatitis C virus infection. Dig Dis Sci. 2007;52(10):2531–9. Epub 2007 Apr 4.

54. Boscarino JA1, Lu M, Moorman AC, Gordon SC, Rupp LB, Spradling PR, Teshale EH, Schmidt MA, Vijayadeva V, Holmberg SD. Predictors of poor mental and physical health status among patients with chronic hepatitis C infection: The chronic hepatitis cohort study (CHeCS). Hepatology. 2014 Sep 9. doi: 10.1002/hep.27422. [Epub ahead of print].

23

Epilepsy as a risk factor for hepatic encephalopathy in patients with cirrhosis

Peter Jepsen[1,2]* iD, Jakob Christensen[3], Karin Weissenborn[4], Hugh Watson[5] and Hendrik Vilstrup[1]

Abstract

Background: Epilepsy is associated with an increased mortality among cirrhosis patients, but the reasons are unknown. We aimed to determine whether epilepsy is a risk factor for developing hepatic encephalopathy (HE), which is a strong predictor of mortality.

Methods: We used data from three randomized 1-year trials of satavaptan in cirrhosis patients with ascites. With Cox regression, we compared the hazard rates of HE grade 1–4 between those cirrhosis patients who did or did not have epilepsy. We adjusted for confounding by gender, age, cirrhosis etiology, diabetes, history of HE, Model for Endstage Liver Disease (MELD) score, serum sodium, albumin, lactulose use, rifaximin use, and benzodiazepine/barbiturate sedation. In a supplementary analysis we examined the association between epilepsy and the hazard rate of HE grade 2–4.

Results: Of the 1120 cirrhosis patients with ascites, 21 (1.9 %) were diagnosed with epilepsy. These patients had better liver function at inclusion than the patients without epilepsy (median MELD score 7.9 vs. 11.4), and only one died during the trials. Nevertheless, seven patients with epilepsy had an HE episode during the follow-up, and the adjusted hazard ratio of HE grade 1–4 for patients with epilepsy vs. controls was 2.12 (95 % CI 0.99–4.55). The corresponding hazard ratio of HE grade 2–4 was 3.83 (95 % CI 1.65–8.87).

Conclusions: Our findings suggest that epilepsy is associated with an increased risk of HE in patients with cirrhosis.

Keywords: End-stage liver disease, Neurology, Seizures, Liver failure, Prognosis

Background

We have previously shown that patients with liver cirrhosis who have been given a diagnosis of epilepsy have a higher mortality than other patients with cirrhosis [1]. Unfortunately, we could not determine the reasons for that association, and no one else has studied it. However, sporadic case reports have described that hepatic encephalopathy (HE) may manifest as status epilepticus [2, 3], and since HE is a very strong predictor of mortality in cirrhosis patients [4], we thought that epilepsy might increase the risk of HE in cirrhosis patients.

Epilepsy has a prevalence of about 3 % among Danish cirrhosis patients [1], and these patients have a 1-year HE risk around 15 % [4]. Therefore it is necessary to have a large cohort of cirrhosis patients to obtain meaningful estimates of the association between epilepsy and HE risk. We had access to the complete original dataset from three large randomized controlled trials of satavaptan treatment of ascites in nearly 1200 patients with cirrhosis who were followed for 1 year, and these data presented a unique opportunity to study epilepsy as a risk factor for HE. Satavaptan had no effect on the development of HE [5].

Given this background, the aim of this study was to examine the effect of epilepsy on HE risk in patients with cirrhosis. Understanding the risk of HE in patients with epilepsy may add to our understanding of the pathogenesis of HE and improve our management of cirrhosis patients who have epilepsy.

* Correspondence: pj@clin.au.dk
[1]Department of Hepatology and Gastroenterology, Aarhus University Hospital, Nørrebrogade 44, DK-8000 Aarhus, Denmark
[2]Department of Clinical Epidemiology, Aarhus University Hospital, Aarhus, Denmark
Full list of author information is available at the end of the article

Methods

Between July 2006 and December 2008 three multinational randomized controlled trials were conducted to examine whether satavaptan was efficacious in treating ascites in cirrhosis patients [6]. The three trials included patients with differing severity of ascites, but were otherwise similar and included 1,198 patients in total. Patients with a functioning transjugular intrahepatic portosystemic shunt were excluded from the trials, as were patients with variceal bleeding or spontaneous bacterial peritonitis in the 10 days before randomization. Other reasons for exclusion were: serum creatinine >151 μmol/L, serum potassium ≥5.0 mmol/L, serum sodium >143 mmol/L (because satavaptan may increase the serum sodium concentration), serum bilirubin >150 μmol/L, INR >3.0, platelets <30,000/mm^3, neutrophils <1,000/mm^3, hepatocellular carcinoma exceeding the Milan criteria, use of a potent modifier of the cytochrome P450 3A pathway, or use of drugs that increase the risk of Q-T interval prolongation [6]. We excluded 78 patients who were encephalopathic at the time of randomization (because they were not at risk of developing HE), leaving 1120 patients for inclusion (Fig. 1). Patients with a history of HE before randomization were included in the analyses.

Study design

The planned treatment duration in the trials was 52 weeks, but the second and third trials were stopped early due to a poor risk-benefit ratio [6]. In all three trials, some patients discontinued the study medication prematurely, primarily due to adverse events [6]. Irrespective of the reason for discontinuation, all patients were followed for one additional week to assess drug safety. For the analysis presented here, we stopped follow-up on the date of the last drug safety assessment, i.e. 1 week after study completion or premature discontinuation.

Data collection

Data on epilepsy, seizures, and use of antiepileptic drugs were collected at the time of randomization. The case report forms described why patients used antiepileptic drugs, but contained no details about their type of epilepsy or seizures. In our primary analysis, we categorized patients as having or not having epilepsy on the basis of epilepsy diagnoses recorded at randomization. Due to concern that epilepsy diagnoses were incorrect, we conducted a secondary analysis in which our neurologist coauthors (JC and KW) used all the available information to re-categorize patients as follows: patients with definite epilepsy (all 8 patients with a recorded diagnosis of epilepsy who were using antiepileptic drugs), patients with unspecified seizures (12 of 13 patients with a recorded diagnosis of epilepsy who were not using antiepileptic drugs; 1 of 13 patients was re-categorized as a control), patients who used antiepileptic drugs for neuropathy or other indications, and controls. We defined antiepileptic drugs by the ATC-code N03A*. Of the 12 patients with unspecified seizures, three had a history of HE before inclusion. We did not have the data to determine whether these patients' HE episodes were related to the seizures.

During the follow-up, patients were seen every 4 weeks in their hepatology departments, and at those visits all current medications including their indications and dosages were recorded, and blood tests were taken. All HE episodes and other clinical events were recorded during the follow-up as part of the safety assessment. Every

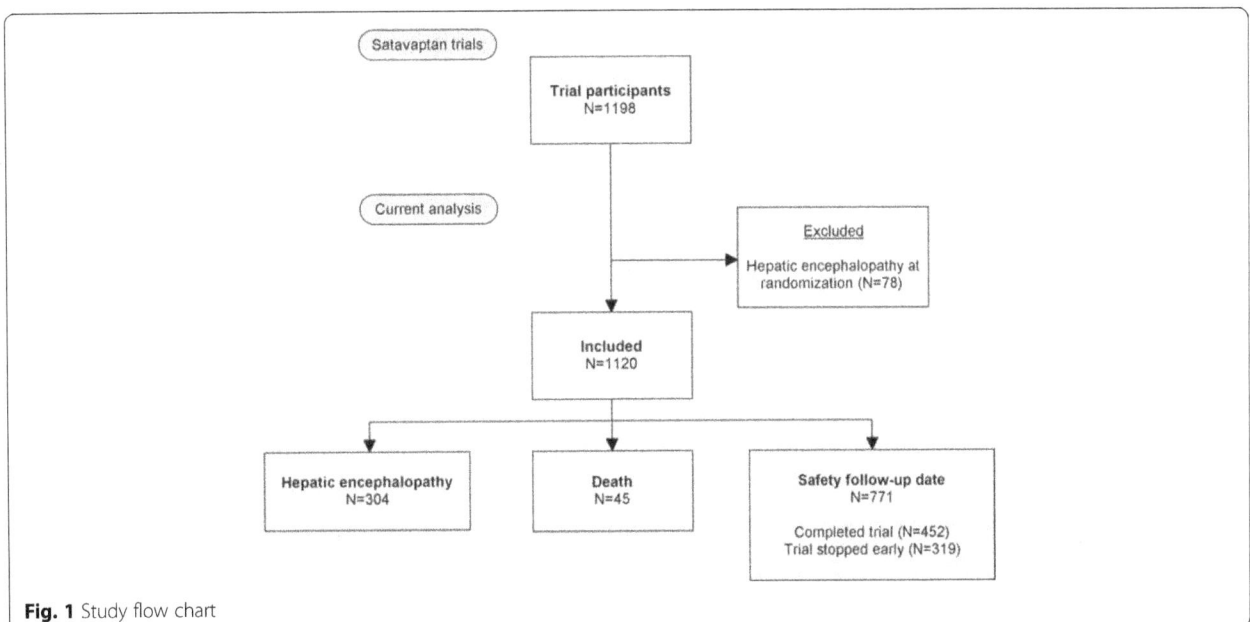

Fig. 1 Study flow chart

four-week visit also included a formal examination for signs and symptoms of HE by an experienced clinician, and at the same time the clinician took a history of HE episodes since the previous visit. There was no psychometric testing for minimal HE. For every HE episode clinicians recorded the severity according to the West Haven criteria [7], the dates of onset and resolution, and likely precipitants.

Statistical analysis

For the present analysis, follow-up began at randomization and continued until the first occurrence of one of the following: onset of an HE episode (grade 1, 2, 3, or 4), death, or the safety follow-up date following study completion or premature discontinuation of the study treatment (Fig. 1). We used the chi-square test (for categorical variables) and the Mann-Whitney test (for continuous variables) to compute the p-value of the hypothesis that baseline characteristics were identical between cirrhosis patients with or without epilepsy. We used Cox proportional hazards regression to examine the association between patient category and HE hazard rate. We adjusted for confounding by patient gender, age, cirrhosis etiology (alcohol only [reference], chronic hepatitis C only, or other etiology), diabetes, history of HE before randomization, Model for Endstage Liver Disease (MELD) score, serum sodium, serum albumin, lactulose use, rifaximin use, and benzodiazepine/barbiturate sedation. This last variable was defined by the ATC codes N05BA, N05CA, N05CB, N05CD, and N05CF. Benzodiazepines and barbiturates counted as antiepileptic drugs if they were given for epilepsy (in which case they had the ATC code N03AA or N03AE), and as sedatives if they were given

for anxiety or as sedation. Age, MELD score, biochemistry, and diuretics were included as continuous, linear variables, and all confounders were included as time-dependent variables. In addition, we repeated the Cox regression analysis within the stratum of patients with cirrhosis due to alcoholism.

Sensitivity analysis

The clinical diagnosis of the low grades of HE may be uncertain so we repeated our analyses with overt HE as the outcome, i.e. HE grades 2, 3, or 4 [8]. We also repeated our analyses excluding patients who had experienced one or more HE episodes before randomization. This exclusion reduced the possibility that we included patients who had minimal HE, but it also reduced the number of patients in the study.

Results

We included 1120 cirrhosis patients, 21 (1.9 %) of whom had a recorded diagnosis of epilepsy. During the total follow-up time of 622.2 person-years, 304 cirrhosis patients had an HE episode, and 45 died without having developed HE. The 21 cirrhosis patients who had epilepsy had less severe cirrhosis, as judged by their MELD scores (Table 1), and only one of them died during the trials. This patient died after his first HE episode, i.e. after follow-up ended in our current analysis of the trial data. Despite their favorable MELD scores, seven of the 21 cirrhosis patients with epilepsy had an HE episode during the follow-up. The HE incidence rate was 0.67 episodes per person-year for the 21 cirrhosis patients with epilepsy (seven episodes during 10.5 person-years,

Table 1 Characteristics of the study cohort at the beginning of follow-up

	Epilepsy	Not epilepsy	p-value
Number of patients	21	1099	
Men (%)	18 (86 %)	760 (69 %)	0.10
Age (median, IQR)	54 (45–59)	57 (50–64)	0.04
Cirrhosis etiology			0.22
Alcohol alone (%)	16 (76 %)	634 (58 %)	
Hepatitis C alone (%)	1 (5 %)	147 (13 %)	
Other (%)	4 (19 %)	318 (29 %)	
Diabetes (%)	4 (19 %)	256 (23 %)	0.65
History of HE before randomization (%)	4 (19 %)	251 (23 %)	0.68
MELD score (median, IQR)	7.9 (4.6–11.3)	11.4 (8.1–14.4)	0.02
Sodium, mmol/L (median, IQR)	136 (133–138)	137 (134–139)	0.34
Albumin, g/L (median, IQR)	33 (29–37)	33 (29–37)	0.68
Lactulose, any dose (%)	14 (19 %)	330 (30 %)	0.28
Rifaximin, any dose (%)	0 (0 %)	27 (2 %)	0.45
Benzodiazepine/barbiturates, any dose (%)	2 (10 %)	95 (9 %)	0.89

IQR interquartile range, 25th percentile to 75th percentile

median 0.42 years of follow-up per patient) compared with 0.49 episodes per person-year for the 1099 cirrhosis patients without epilepsy (297 episodes during 611.7 person-years, median 0.58 years of follow-up per patient). After confounder adjustment, the rate of HE for patients with epilepsy vs. controls was more than doubled (adjusted HR = 2.12, 95 % CI 0.99–4.55), but the association was not statistically significant (Table 2). Among the 650 patients with alcoholic cirrhosis, the corresponding confounder-adjusted HR was 2.44 (95 % CI 0.96–6.17).

When we re-categorized patients, eight patients (0.7 %) had definite epilepsy; 12 (1.1 %) had a history of seizures but did not currently use antiepileptic drugs; 16 (1.4 %) used antiepileptic drugs for non-epilepsy indications, primarily neuropathic pain; and the remaining 1084 (96.8 %) were controls. Thus, one patient with a recorded diagnosis of epilepsy was re-categorized as a control after neurologists reviewed the available data. The eight patients with definite epilepsy used very different drug regimens: two used topiramate, one used phenytoin + gabapentin (and developed HE), one used phenytoin + valproate, one used gabapentin (and developed HE), one used carbamazepine, one used oxcarbazepine (and developed HE), and one used phenobarbital. In this analysis with four patient categories the hazard ratio estimates had wider confidence intervals because the patient groups were smaller, but the point estimate for 'definite epilepsy' vs. controls (adjusted HR = 2.49, 95 % CI 0.78–7.90) was essentially the same as the estimate for 'epilepsy' vs. controls in the primary analysis (Table 3). Also the patients we classified as having unspecified seizures and those who used antiepileptic drugs

Table 2 Confounder-adjusted effect of a recorded diagnosis of epilepsy on the hazard rate of HE episodes grade 1, 2, 3, or 4

	Adjusted hazard ratio
Epilepsy (as recorded)	2.12 (0.99–4.55)
Male vs. female	1.07 (0.83–1.39)
Age, per 10-year increase	1.17 (1.04–1.32)
Cirrhosis etiology	
Alcohol alone (%)	1 (reference)
Hepatitis C alone (%)	1.64 (1.18–2.28)
Other (%)	1.35 (1.03–1.76)
Diabetes	1.41 (1.09–1.82)
History of HE before randomization	1.72 (1.34–2.20)
MELD score, per point	1.09 (1.07–1.11)
Sodium, per 5 mmol/L increase	0.64 (0.58–0.71)
Albumin, per 5 g/L increase	0.78 (0.70–0.87)
Lactulose, any dose vs. none	1.79 (1.41–2.28)
Rifaximin, any dose vs. none	0.59 (0.32–1.10)
Benzodiazepines/barbiturates, any dose vs. none	1.22 (0.85–1.74)

Table 3 Confounder-adjusted effects of definite epilepsy, unspecified seizures, and use of antiepileptic drugs for non-epilepsy indications on the hazard rate of HE episodes grade 1, 2, 3, or 4

	Adjusted hazard ratio
Patient category (after re-categorization)	
Definite epilepsy	2.49 (0.78–7.90)
Unspecified seizures	1.50 (0.47–4.76)
Antiepileptic drugs for non-epilepsy indications	1.52 (0.74–3.12)
Controls	1 (reference)
Male vs. female	1.08 (0.83–1.40)
Age, per 10-year increase	1.17 (1.03–1.32)
Cirrhosis etiology	
Alcohol alone (%)	1 (reference)
Hepatitis C alone (%)	1.65 (1.19–2.30)
Other (%)	1.35 (1.03–1.76)
Diabetes	1.38 (1.06–1.78)
History of HE before randomization	1.70 (1.33–2.18)
MELD score, per point	1.09 (1.07–1.11)
Sodium, per 5 mmol/L increase	0.63 (0.57–0.70)
Albumin, per 5 g/L increase	0.78 (0.70–0.87)
Lactulose, any dose vs. none	1.80 (1.41–2.29)
Rifaximin, any dose vs. none	0.59 (0.32–1.11)
Benzodiazepines/barbiturates, any dose vs. none	1.23 (0.86–1.76)

for non-epilepsy indications had higher HE rates than the controls, but their HE rates were not as high as the HE rate among patients with definite epilepsy (Table 3).

Sensitivity analysis

There were 151 overt HE episodes during the follow-up, including six among the 21 cirrhosis patients with a recorded diagnosis of epilepsy. These 21 patients' adjusted hazard ratio of overt HE vs. controls was 3.83 (95 % CI 1.65–8.87). When we re-categorized patients, the adjusted hazard ratio for patients with definite epilepsy vs. controls was 3.60 (95 % CI 0.86–15.06). It was 2.99 (95 % CI 0.92–9.75) for patients with unspecified seizures vs. controls, and 1.20 (95 % CI 0.38–3.86) for patients who used antiepileptic drugs for non-epilepsy indications vs. controls.

Finally, when we excluded the 255 patients with an HE episode before randomization the association between epilepsy and HE strengthened. The adjusted hazard ratio was 4.78 (95 % CI 1.92–11.88) for epilepsy patients vs. controls. After re-categorization it was 6.12 (95 % CI 1.47–25.44) for patients with definite epilepsy vs. controls, 2.97 (95 % CI 0.71–12.44) for patients with unspecified seizures vs. controls, and 2.76 (95 % CI

1.11–6.86) for patients who used antiepileptic drugs for non-epilepsy indications vs. controls.

Discussion

This study was based on an unparalleled dataset with detailed clinical data on more than 1100 cirrhosis patients. We examined the association between epilepsy and HE and found similar hazard ratio estimates whether we defined epilepsy per the recorded diagnoses, or we used all available information to identify patients with definite epilepsy. Moreover, the association strengthened when we considered only episodes of overt HE, or when we excluded patients with HE episodes before inclusion. Therefore, this study provides evidence that epilepsy is a risk factor for developing HE, despite the small number of patients with epilepsy.

Our motivation for this study was to understand why epilepsy was associated with a 1.31-fold increased mortality among patients with cirrhosis [1]. We could not confirm that association in these trial data because the 21 patients with epilepsy had so well-preserved liver function that only one of them died during the 1-year follow-up in the trials. Nevertheless, epilepsy's association with HE development in the trial data suggests that epilepsy might also have been a risk factor for mortality if patients had been followed for longer than 1 year. It is evident that this study is limited by the small number of patients with epilepsy and the short duration of follow-up, but a stronger dataset will not emerge in the foreseeable future.

The cirrhosis-related data for these analyses were rigorously defined, but the data regarding epilepsy were not. Epilepsy diagnoses were recorded by the hepatologists caring for the patients, and we had no information that explained why patients with epilepsy were not receiving antiepileptic treatment—were they uncompliant with recommended antiepileptic treatment, or did they in fact not have epilepsy? That uncertainty led us to recategorize patients and define a patient group with definite epilepsy. It is a crucial finding that the hazard ratio estimates were similar for the larger 'epilepsy' and the smaller 'definite epilepsy' group (2.12 and 2.49, respectively). It is obvious that the confidence interval was wider for the smaller group, but the fact that the *estimates* were similar supports the conclusion that epilepsy is indeed a risk factor for developing HE.

It is likely that some of those with a recorded diagnosis of epilepsy who did not receive antiepileptic treatment (those we categorized as having 'unspecified seizures') did in fact have epilepsy. That possibility might explain why this group of patients had an increased HE risk. The effect of antiepileptic drugs for non-epilepsy indications was ambiguous, and we are concerned that the HE episodes might be related to the *indication* for the antiepileptic drug rather than to the drug itself. For example, some of the cirrhosis patients without epilepsy who used antiepileptic drugs suffered from diabetes or alcoholism, both of which are risk factors for neuropathy, the prevailing indication for some antiepileptic drugs. Diabetes itself is a risk factor for HE [9], and alcoholism can cause symptoms and signs that might be mistaken for HE [7]. Although we controlled for both conditions in our analysis, these patients could have *worse* diabetes or *worse* alcoholism than other patients, in which case residual confounding would cause us to overestimate the effect of antiepileptic drugs. That concern, coupled with the imprecise hazard ratio estimate, means that we do not claim that antiepileptic drugs cause HE, although the sedative properties of some antiepileptic drugs could potentially increase the risk of HE.

It is conceivable that some events perceived as HE episodes were in fact non-convulsive status epilepticus, which may resemble grade 4 HE [2, 3]. However, only one patient with epilepsy had a grade 4 HE episode, and that episode had an identified precipitant (electrolyte disturbance) and occurred in a patient who had previously had HE. We are not concerned by the risk of mistaking grade 1 HE episodes for post-ictal disorientation because our sensitivity analysis showed that epilepsy was an even stronger risk factor for *overt* HE, which is considered a more reliable clinical diagnosis [8].

Our data on the association between epilepsy and HE are merely observational and do not clarify any pathogenetic aspect of HE beyond the obvious disturbed function of the central nervous system [10]. It remains very intriguing that a condition with overshoot of excitatory neurotransmission increases the risk of developing a condition characterized by neuroinhibition [11, 12]. Our findings are probably best viewed in light of the concept of the 'frail brain' [13], whereby the cirrhosis patient's brain responds with HE to *anything* that affects neurotransmission, but the links between epilepsy, antiepileptic drugs, and HE risk clearly deserve further investigation.

Conclusions

In these data from three worldwide randomized trials in cirrhosis patients with ascites, epilepsy seemed to cause an increased risk of HE. This finding may help us understand the pathogenesis of HE and improve our clinical management of patients with cirrhosis and epilepsy.

Abbreviations
HE, hepatic encephalopathy; MELD, model for endstage liver disease

Acknowledgements
Not applicable.

Funding
Peter Jepsen received funding from the Danish Council for Independent
Research under the Danish Agency for Science, Technology and Innovation
(10-081838/FSS).

Authors' contributions
PJ and HV conceived and designed the study, and PJ, JC, KW, HW, and HV
contributed to the analysis and interpretation of the data. PJ drafted the
manuscript, and PJ, JC, KW, HW, and HV revised it critically for important
intellectual content. PJ, JC, KW, HW, and HV have approved the version to be
published.

Authors' information
Not applicable.

Competing interests
The authors declare that they have no competing interest.

Consent for publication
Not applicable.

Author details
[1]Department of Hepatology and Gastroenterology, Aarhus University
Hospital, Nørrebrogade 44, DK-8000 Aarhus, Denmark. [2]Department of
Clinical Epidemiology, Aarhus University Hospital, Aarhus, Denmark.
[3]Department of Neurology, Aarhus University Hospital, Aarhus, Denmark.
[4]Department of Neurology, Hannover Medical School, Hannover, Germany.
[5]Sanofi Aventis R&D, Paris, France.

References
1. Jepsen P, Vilstrup H, Lash TL. Development and validation of a comorbidity
    scoring system for patients with cirrhosis. Gastroenterology. 2014;146:147–56.
2. Eleftheriadis N, Fourla E, Eleftheriadis D, Karlovasitou A. Status epilepticus as a
    manifestation of hepatic encephalopathy. Acta Neurol Scand. 2003;107:142–4.
3. Delanty N, French JA, Labar DR, Pedley TA, Rowan AJ. Status epilepticus
    arising de novo in hospitalized patients: an analysis of 41 patients. Seizure.
    2001;10:116–9.
4. Jepsen P, Ott P, Andersen PK, Sørensen HT, Vilstrup H. The clinical course of
    alcoholic liver cirrhosis: a Danish population-based cohort study.
    Hepatology. 2010;51:1675–82.
5. Watson H, Jepsen P, Wong F, Gines P, Cordoba J, Vilstrup H. Satavaptan
    treatment for ascites in patients with cirrhosis: a meta-analysis of effect on
    hepatic encephalopathy development. Metab Brain Dis. 2013;28:301–5.
6. Wong F, Watson H, Gerbes A, Vilstrup H, Badalamenti S, Bernardi M, Gines P.
    Satavaptan for the management of ascites in cirrhosis: efficacy and safety
    across the spectrum of ascites severity. Gut. 2012;61:108–16.
7. Vilstrup H, Amodio P, Bajaj J, Cordoba J, Ferenci P, Mullen KD, Weissenborn
    K, Wong P. Hepatic encephalopathy in chronic liver disease: 2014 practice
    guideline by the American Association for the study of liver diseases and
    the European Association for the study of the liver. Hepatology. 2014;60:
    715–35.
8. Bajaj JS, Wade JB, Sanyal AJ. Spectrum of neurocognitive impairment in
    cirrhosis: implications for the assessment of hepatic encephalopathy.
    Hepatology. 2009;50:2014–21.
9. Jepsen P, Watson H, Andersen PK, Vilstrup H. Diabetes as a risk factor for
    hepatic encephalopathy in cirrhosis patients. J Hepatol. 2015;63:1133–8.
10. Ott P, Vilstrup H. Cerebral effects of ammonia in liver disease: current
    hypotheses. Metab Brain Dis. 2014;29:901–11.
11. van der Rijt CC, Schalm SW, de Groot GH, de Vlieger M. Objective
    measurement of hepatic encephalopathy by means of automated EEG
    analysis. Electroencephalogr Clin Neurophysiol. 1984;57:423–6.
12. Moshe SL, Perucca E, Ryvlin P, Tomson T. Epilepsy: new advances. Lancet.
    2015;385:884–98.
13. Malmstrom TK, Morley JE. The frail brain. J Am Med Dir Assoc. 2013;14:453–5.

24

Effect of coexisting diabetes mellitus and chronic kidney disease on mortality of cirrhotic patients with esophageal variceal bleeding

Chia-Chi Lung[1,2*], Zhi-Hong Jian[1], Jing-Yang Huang[1] and Oswald Ndi Nfor[1]

Abstract

Background: Esophageal variceal bleeding (EVB) is a serious and common complication of cirrhosis. Diabetes mellitus (DM) and chronic kidney disease (CKD) increase mortality in patients with cirrhosis. However, whether coexisting DM and CKD increase mortality in cirrhotic patients with EVB remains unclear.

Methods: We enrolled cirrhotic patients hospitalized with the first presentation of EVB from 2005 through 2010 using Longitudinal Health Insurance Database 2005. The hazard ratios (HRs) of 42-day and one-year EVB mortality were calculated using Cox regression model.

Results: We identified 888 patients hospitalized with the first presentation of EVB. Among the cirrhotic patients with EVB, all-cause mortality at 42-day and one-year were 21.3 and 45.0 %, respectively. The respective HRs for the 42-day and one-year mortality were 1.80 (95 % confidence interval [CI], 1.10–2.97) and 1.52 (95 % CI, 1.06–2.17) for patients with CKD and 0.79 (95 % CI, 0.57–1.10) and 0.88 (95 % CI, 0.71–1.09) for patients with DM. Specifically, coexisting CKD and DM increased the 42-day and one-year mortality with respective HRs of 1.99 (95%CI, 1.03–3.84) and 1.84 (95%CI, 1.14–2.98) compared with those without CKD and DM. The HRs for 42-day and 1-year mortality in female patients with DM and CKD were 4.03 (95%CI, 1.40–11.59) and 2.84 (95%CI, 1.31–6.14) respectively, and were 2.93 (95%CI, 1.14–7.57) and 2.42 (95%CI, 1.28–4.57) in male patients with DM and CKD.

Conclusion: We identified that coexisting DM and CKD increased risk of mortality at 42 days and 1 year following EVB.

Keywords: Chronic kidney disease, Cirrhosis, Diabetes mellitus, Esophageal variceal bleeding

Background

Bleeding from esophageal varices is a life-threatening condition with an annual mortality of 57 %. Nearly half these deaths occur within 6 weeks from the initial episode of bleeding [1]. Various factors have been proposed as predictors of outcome of variceal bleeding, some of which include age, gender, stage of cirrhosis, etiology, and associated conditions like renal failure and diabetes mellitus (DM) [2–5].

Renal function is a critical prognostic factor in cirrhotic patients with esophageal variceal bleeding (EVB) [6, 7]. Patients with chronic kidney disease (CKD) have many long-term complications, such as increased immunocompromised status [8], as well as an increased risk of metabolic disorders [9], and cardiovascular events [10]. Physiological mechanisms contributing to an increased bleeding tendency included uremic platelet dysfunction, use of antiplatelet agents, and anticoagulants [11, 12]. In addition, usage of aspirin is associated with the occurrence of EVB in cirrhotic patients [13].

The Verona Diabetes Study, a population-based study with 7,148 patients with DM, showed an increased risk of mortality from chronic liver disease and cirrhosis compared with the general population [14]. Insulin resistance,

* Correspondence: dinoljc@csmu.edu.tw
[1]Department of Public Health and Institute of Public Health, Chung Shan Medical University, Taichung City, Taiwan
[2]Department of Family and Community Medicine, Chung Shan Medical University Hospital, Taichung City, Taiwan

a characteristic feature of DM, has been proven to be a predictor of portal hypertension [15] and the development of esophageal varices [16]. In a hospital-based study with 146 patients with cirrhosis, DM significantly correlated with gastroesophageal variceal bleeding [2].

The presence of metabolic syndrome and the number of metabolic syndrome components have been associated with higher prevalence of CKD [9]. CKD is one of the most common long-term complications of DM [17]. The prevalence of DM and CKD in Taiwan has been reported as 7,570 and 892 per 100,000 population, respectively [18, 19]. How DM and/or CKD per se, is/are independent mortality risk factors, and how they further increase the risk of mortality is still unclear. This study aimed to investigate DM and CKD on mortality of cirrhotic patients with first presentation of EVB.

Methods

Data source

This retrospective cohort study used data from the Longitudinal Health Insurance Database 2005 (LHID2005), which is a subset of the National Health Insurance Research Database (NHIRD). The LHID2005 database was derived by the Bureau of National Health Insurance, Ministry of Health and Welfare of Taiwan and maintained by the National Health Research Institutes so as to make it accessible for research purposes. The LHID2005 is broadly used in academic studies [20–23]. LHID2005 contains all the original claims data of one million out of 23 million National Health Insurance enrollees, randomly sampled from the year 2005 registry for beneficiaries of the NHIRD. There was no significant difference in the age and sex distribution between patients in the LHID2005 and the original NHIRD [24]. The use of the data was reviewed and granted by the National Health Research Institutes. The source data was encrypted and the data extracted was anonymous. This study was approved by the Institutional Review Board of the Chung-Shan Medical University Hospital, Taiwan.

Patient identification

This retrospective study included cirrhotic patients who were hospitalized with a first presentation of EVB between 2005 and 2010. Subjects with incomplete information, such as sex and registry data were excluded. EVB was confirmed by the International Classification of Diseases, Ninth Revision, Clinical Modification (ICD-9-CM) code (ICD-9-CM code 456.0 and 456.20) and esophageal variceal ligation or sclerotherapy.

Variables of exposure

To reduce bias, the diagnoses of comorbidities were confirmed by more than two outpatient visits or one admission in 1 year. Comorbidities were defined using the following ICD-9-CM codes: DM (250), CKD (585 and 586), hepatitis B virus (HBV) infection (070.2, 070.3, and V02.61), hepatitis C virus (HCV) infection (070.41, 070.44, 070.51, 070.54, 070.7, and V02.62), alcohol-related disorders (291, 303, 305.00–305.03, and 571.0–571.3), hepatocellular carcinoma (HCC) (155.0 and 155.2), ascites (789.5 or ICD-9 Volume 3 procedure code 54.91), hepatic encephalopathy (572.2), spontaneous bacterial peritonitis (SBP) (567.2, 567.8, or 567.9, excluding the procedure codes for the abdominal surgery), chronic obstructive pulmonary disease (COPD) (490, 491, 492, 494, and 496), asthma (493), pulmonary tuberculosis (TB) (010 - 012), acute coronary syndrome (410–414)), cerebrovascular accident (430–438), and bacterial infections. The bacterial infections during hospitalization included pneumonia (ICD-9-CM 481–487, excluding 484), liver abscess (ICD-9-CM 572.0), empyema (ICD-9-CM 510), cellulitis (ICD-9-CM 681 and 682), necrotizing fasciitis (ICD-9-CM 728.86), central nervous system infection (ICD-9-CM 324 and 320), sepsis (ICD-9-CM 038 and 790.7), infective endocarditis (ICD-9-CM 421), urinary tract infection (ICD-9-CM 590.1, 595.0, 595.9, and 599.0), biliary tract infection (ICD-9-CM 574.00, 574.01, 574.30, 574.31, 574.60, 574.61, 574.80, 574.81, 575.0, and 576.1), septic arthritis (ICD-9-CM 711), and perianal abscess (ICD-9-CM 566).

Statistical analysis

All analyses were made using SAS 9.3 software (SAS Institute, Cary, NC). Chi square test was used to exam the differences in sociodemographic characteristics and comorbidities. Multivariate Cox proportional hazards regression was performed to determine mortality for independent variables, such as sex, age, low income, urbanization, comorbidities, etiology, and complications of cirrhosis. Furthermore, in order to evaluate the effect of coexisting DM and CKD on all-cause mortality, 4 separate models were conducted: 42-day mortality of all patients (Model 1), 42-day mortality stratified by gender (Model 2), 1-year mortality of all patients (Model 3), and 1-year mortality stratified by gender (Model 4). All comparisons with a p-value < 0.05 were considered statistically significant.

Results

The demographic characteristics and comorbidities of cirrhotic patients with EVB are listed in Table 1. The 42-day and 1-year EVB mortalities were 21.3 and 45.0 %, respectively. HBV, CKD, HCC, and hospitalization due to ascites, hepatic encephalopathy, and SBP were more common in non-survivors. The possible etiologies of CKD were as follows: diabetes alone, 3 cases (4.6 %), diabetes + hypertension, 8 (12.3 %), diabetes + hypertension + coronary artery disease, 2 (3.1 %), diabetes + hypertension + hyperlipidemia, 2 (3.1 %), diabetes + hypertension +

Table 1 Characteristics of cirrhotic patients with first esophageal variceal bleeding and mortality, Taiwan, 2005–2010

	42-day mortality			One-year mortality		
	Survivors (n = 699) (%)	Death (n = 189) (%)	p-value	Survivors (n = 488) (%)	Death (n = 400) (%)	p-value
Year of first diagnosis of EVB						
2005 (n = 167)	132 (18.9)	35 (18.5)	0.909	84 (17.2)	83 (20.8)	0.585
2006 (n = 151)	122 (17.4)	29 (15.3)	0.808	84 (17.2)	67 (16.8)	0.864
2007 (n = 142)	101 (14.4)	41 (21.7)	0.170	72 (14.8)	70 (17.5)	0.686
2008 (n = 134)	102 (14.6)	32 (16.9)	0.769	79 (16.2)	55 (13.7)	0.729
2009 (n = 146)	120 (17.2)	26 (13.8)	0.648	83 (17.0)	63 (15.7)	0.864
2010 (n = 148)	122 (17.5)	26 (13.8)	0.615	86 (17.6)	62 (15.5)	0.793
Sex						
Female (n = 243)	202 (28.9)	41 (21.7)	0.049	151 (30.9)	92 (23.0)	0.008
Age at the first diagnosis of EVB						
< 50 (n = 261)	212 (30.3)	49 (25.9)	0.433	165 (33.8)	96 (24.0)	0.002
50–69 (n = 437)	335 (47.9)	102 (54.0)	0.302	230 (47.1)	207 (51.8)	0.171
≥70 (n = 190)	152 (21.8)	38 (20.1)	0.626	93 (19.1)	97 (24.2)	0.061
Complication of cirrhosis						
HCC (n = 359)	247 (35.3)	112 (59.3)	<0.001	127 (26.0)	232 (58.0)	<0.001
Infection during hospitalization (n = 58)	40 (5.7)	18 (9.5)	0.061	26 (5.3)	32 (8.0)	0.109
Previous episodes of decompensation required hospitalization within 1 year before EVB						
Ascites						
0 (n = 711)	577 (82.6)	134 (70.9)	<0.001	417 (85.4)	294 (73.5)	<0.001
1 (n = 114)	82 (11.7)	32 (16.9)	0.058	52 (10.7)	62 (15.5)	0.038
≥ 2 (n = 63)	40 (5.7)	23 (12.2)	0.002	19 (3.9)	44 (11.0)	<0.001
Hepatic encephalopathy						
0 (n = 789)	628 (89.9)	161 (85.2)	0.247	447 (91.6)	342 (85.4)	0.026
1 (n = 60)	47 (6.7)	13 (6.9)	0.940	31 (6.4)	29 (7.3)	0.724
≥ 2 (n = 39)	24 (3.4)	15 (7.9)	0.041	10 (2.0)	29 (7.3)	0.001
SBP						
0 (n = 846)	670 (95.9)	176 (93.1)	0.329	477 (97.8)	369 (92.3)	<0.001
1 (n = 35)	28 (4.0)	7 (3.7)	0.850	10 (2.0)	25 (6.2)	0.003
≥ 2 (n = 7)	1 (0.1)	6 (3.2)	<0.001	1 (0.2)	6 (1.5)	0.028
Etiology of cirrhosis						
HBV (n = 340)	250 (35.8)	90 (47.6)	0.003	168 (34.4)	172 (43.0)	0.009
HCV (n = 306)	248 (35.5)	58 (30.7)	0.219	168 (34.4)	138 (34.5)	0.982
Alcoholism (n = 382)	313 (44.8)	69 (36.5)	0.042	236 (48.4)	146 (36.5)	<0.001
Comorbidities						
DM (n = 332)	270 (38.6)	62 (32.8)	0.142	187 (38.3)	145 (36.3)	0.526
CKD (n = 65)	43 (6.2)	22 (11.6)	0.010	23 (4.7)	42 (10.5)	0.001
COPD (n = 216)	174 (24.9)	42 (22.2)	0.448	124 (25.4)	92 (23.0)	0.405
Asthma (n = 87)	69 (9.9)	18 (9.5)	0.887	49 (10.0)	38 (9.5)	0.787
TB (n = 28)	24 (3.4)	4 (2.1)	0.358	18 (3.7)	10 (2.5)	0.313
Previous episode of acute coronary syndrome (n = 184)	145 (20.7)	39 (20.6)	0.974	96 (19.7)	88 (22.0)	0.395
Previous episode of cerebrovascular accident (n = 102)	73 (10.4)	29 (15.3)	0.061	45 (9.2)	57 (14.3)	0.019

Table 1 Characteristics of cirrhotic patients with first esophageal variceal bleeding and mortality, Taiwan, 2005–2010 *(Continued)*

Low income						
Yes (n = 24)	20 (2.9)	4 (2.1)	0.575	7 (1.4)	17 (4.3)	0.010
Urbanization						
Urban (n = 438)	339 (48.5)	99 (52.4)	0.357	246 (50.4)	192 (48.0)	0.475
Normal (n = 316)	243 (34.8)	73 (38.6)	0.357	160 (32.8)	156 (39.0)	0.120
Rural (n = 134)	117 (16.7)	17 (9.0)	0.030	82 (16.8)	52 (13.0)	0.214

CKD chronic kidney disease, *COPD* chronic obstructive pulmonary disease, *DM* diabetes mellitus, *EVB* esophageal variceal bleeding, *HBV* hepatitis B virus, *HCC* hepatocellular carcinoma, *HCV* hepatitis C virus, *SBP* spontaneous bacterial peritonitis, *TB* pulmonary tuberculosis

coronary artery disease + hyperlipidemia, 5 (7.7 %), diabetes + other etiologies, 4 (6.1 %), and etiologies other than diabetes, 41 (63.1 %). For CKD patients with or without DM, the 42-day mortalities were 41.7 % (10/24) and 29.3 % (12/41), and the 1-year mortality were 79.2 % (19/24) and 56.1 % (23/41), respectively (data not shown).

Table 2 shows the HRs for 42-day and 1-year mortality. At 42 days following EVB, the risk of mortality was high in patients with CKD (hazard ratio [HR], 1.80; 95 % confidence interval [CI], 1.10–2.97), HCC (HR, 2.13; 95 % CI, 1.54–2.95), and previous hospitalization due to ascites and SBP. Similarly, at 1 year following EVB, risk of mortality was also high in men (HR,1.54; 95 % CI, 1.19–2.00), CKD (HR,1.52; 95 % CI, 1.06–2.17), HCC (HR, 2.48; 95%CI, 1.99–3.10), infections during hospitalization (HR:1.50; 95 % CI, 1.03–2.18), and previous hospitalization due to ascites and SBP.

Table 3 illustrates the adjusted HRs of EVB mortality at 42 days and 1 year in patients with either DM, CKD, or both by gender. For 42-day mortality (Model 1), the HRs were 1.99 (95 % CI, 1.03–3.84) and 0.72 (95%CI, 0.50–1.02) among DM patients with or without CKD, respectively. The HR for patients with CKD was 1.25 (95 % CI, 0.62–2.52). When stratified by gender and disease combinations (Model 2), the HRs were higher in female diabetic patients with CKD (HR, 4.03; 95 % CI, 1.40–11.59) and male diabetic patients with CKD (HR, 2.93; 95 % CI, 1.14–7.57).

For 1-year mortality, the HRs were 1.84 (95 % CI, 1.14–2.98) and 0.80 (95 % CI, 0.64–1.02) in diabetic patients with or without CKD (Model 3). The HR for patients with CKD was 1.07 (95 % CI, 0.65–1.76). There was significant interaction between DM and CKD (p = 0.028). In Model 4, the HRs for male and female diabetic patients with CKD were 2.84 (95 % CI, 1.31–6.14) and 2.42 (95 % CI, 1.28–4.57), respectively.

Discussion

We found that coexistence of CKD and DM was independently associated with 42-day and 1-year mortality in both sexes. These risk factors are easy to identify following the initial EVB event and are valuable for predicting

clinical outcomes. They may also be useful for guiding the clinical management of cirrhotic patients with EVB. Identifying patients at high risk will be important for cost-effective management of EVB.

Globally, 57 % of cirrhosis is attributable to either hepatitis B (30 %) or hepatitis C (27 %) [25]. Alcohol consumption is another important cause, accounting for about 20 % of the cases. The seroprevalence of HBV and HCV was 17.3 and 4.4 % in Taiwan, respectively [26]. More than 70 % of cirrhosis and HCC were the sequelae of chronic HBV infection in 1990s [27]. Our results showed that HBV infection was higher in non-survivors and the prevalence of HBV infection in HCC was 46.2 %. When HBV infection was put into the multivariate model for analyses, there was no significant association between HBV infection and EVB mortality. The efficacy of universal immunization has been proven with substantial reductions of HBV carriage in children, adolescents and young adults since 1984 [28]. HCC in Taiwan also falls after universal hepatitis B vaccination [29]. We also showed improvement in the 42-day mortality rate over time perhaps due to treatment advances, such as variceal ligation, appropriate vasoconstrictor usage, and antiviral treatment for the underlying cirrhosis [30, 31].

Bleeding from ruptured esophageal varices is the most severe complication of cirrhosis and 6-week mortality rates have been reported to be 15–20 % [30]. The inpatient bleeding rate among cirrhotic patients has been reported as 13 % [32]. Around 30 to 60 % of cirrhotic patients suffer from DM with insulin resistance and hyperinsulinemia [33]. The presence of DM appears to be associated with failure to control esophageal variceal bleeding and re-bleeding [34]. Hyperglycemia induces splanchnic hyperemia, increases portal pressure and azygos vein blood flow, and may increase the risk of variceal bleeding [35, 36]. However, in this study, DM individually failed to show significant association with 42-day and 1-year mortality.

In an analysis involving 2,592 cirrhotic patients hospitalized with SBP in 2004, the respective HRs for 30-day and 1-year mortality were 1.37 (95%CI, 0.85–2.21) and 1.37 (95%CI, 1.01–1.84) in patients with CKD [37]. Increased long-term mortality rates of SBP in cirrhotic

Table 2 Estimation of hazard ratios of mortality in patients with esophageal variceal bleeding between 2005 and 2010 using cox proportional model

	42-day mortality			One-year mortality		
	HR	95 % C.I.	p-value	HR	95 % C.I.	p-value
Sex (reference: Female)						
Male	1.37	0.93–2.02	0.109	1.54	1.19–2.00	0.001
Age at the first diagnosis of EVB (reference: <50)						
50–69	0.93	0.63–1.38	0.721	1.03	0.77–1.38	0.831
≥ 70	0.77	0.45–1.34	0.361	1.24	0.85–1.81	0.269
Comorbidities						
DM	0.79	0.57–1.10	0.163	0.88	0.71–1.09	0.241
CKD	1.80	1.10–2.97	0.021	1.52	1.06–2.17	0.023
COPD	0.88	0.59–1.31	0.533	0.85	0.65–1.12	0.251
Asthma	1.19	0.70–2.00	0.526	1.08	0.75–1.55	0.699
TB	0.68	0.27–1.88	0.460	0.65	0.34–1.24	0.191
Previous episode of acute coronary syndrome	1.01	0.68–1.51	0.954	1.04	0.79–1.36	0.779
Previous episode of cerebrovascular accident	1.54	0.99–2.38	0.054	1.21	0.89–1.65	0.214
Etiology of cirrhosis						
HBV	1.13	0.82–1.54	0.465	1.07	0.86–1.33	0.559
HCV	0.81	0.57–1.14	0.224	0.86	0.68–1.09	0.217
Alcoholism	0.76	0.52–1.11	0.157	0.74	0.57–0.97	0.031
Complication of cirrhosis						
HCC	2.13	1.54–2.95	<0.001	2.48	1.99–3.10	<0.001
Infection during hospitalization	1.65	0.99–2.75	0.055	1.50	1.03–2.18	0.035
Previous episodes of decompensation required hospitalization within 1 year before EVB						
Ascites (reference: 0)						
1	1.66	1.10–2.52	0.017	1.60	1.18–2.18	0.003
≥ 2	1.77	1.04–3.02	0.036	1.73	1.18–2.55	0.005
Hepatic encephalopathy (reference: 0)						
1	0.98	0.54–1.79	0.949	1.09	0.72–1.67	0.680
≥ 2	1.09	0.59–1.99	0.793	1.28	0.82–1.99	0.271
SBP (reference: 0)						
1	0.63	0.28–1.41	0.258	1.20	0.76–1.92	0.435
≥ 2	3.42	1.38–8.50	0.008	2.93	1.24–6.93	0.015
Low income	0.70	0.25–1.99	0.503	1.63	0.95–2.79	0.078
Urbanization (reference: Urban)						
Sub-urban	1.02	0.75–1.39	0.891	1.09	0.87–1.35	0.455
Rural	0.58	0.34–0.98	0.043	0.84	0.61–1.15	0.270

CI confidence interval, *CKD* chronic kidney disease, *COPD* chronic obstructive pulmonary disease, *DM* diabetes mellitus, *EVB* esophageal variceal bleeding, *HBV* hepatitis B virus, *HCC* hepatocellular carcinoma, *HCV* hepatitis C virus, *HR* hazard ratio, *SBP* spontaneous bacterial peritonitis, *TB* pulmonary tuberculosis

patients may be attributed to the impaired immune functions caused by CKD [38]. Hung et al. evaluated 4,932 cirrhotic patients with hepatic encephalopathy and showed that the adjusted HR of 3-year mortality for CKD was 1.93 (95 % CI, 1.55–2.40) compared with those with normal renal function [39]. However, patients with end-stage renal disease (ESRD) receiving hemodialysis had better 3 year survival rate (HR, 0.66; 95 % CI, 0.46–0.94) than those with CKD. This implied that CKD may be associated with poor clearance of circulatory neurotoxic substances that increases the susceptibility to mortality in cirrhotic patients with hepatic encephalopathy. Hung et al. evaluated 6,740 cirrhotic patients who were hospitalized with EVB in 2007 and showed that

Table 3 Adjusted Risk for 42-Day and One-Year Mortality Stratified by DM, Chronic Kidney Diseases, and Sex

	42-day mortality						One-year mortality					
	Model 1[a]			Model 2[b]			Model 3[a]			Model 4[b]		
	HR	95 % CI	P value	HR	95 % CI	P value	HR	95 % CI	P value	HR	95 % CI	P value
All patients												
Non-DM & CKD	Ref.						Ref.					
Only DM	0.72	0.50–1.02	0.062				0.80	0.64–1.02	0.066			
Only CKD	1.25	0.62–2.52	0.541				1.07	0.65–1.76	0.801			
DM + CKD	1.99	1.03–3.84	0.042				1.84	1.14–2.98	0.012			
P for DM × CKD interaction	0.100						0.028					
Women												
Non-DM & CKD				Ref.						Ref.		
Only DM				1.11	0.56–2.21	0.772				0.77	0.49–1.21	0.260
Only CKD				3.40	0.75–15.48	0.113				1.30	0.39–4.28	0.672
DM + CKD				4.03	1.40–11.59	0.010				2.84	1.31–6.14	0.008
Men												
Non-DM & CKD				2.00	1.14–3.52	0.016				1.61	1.13–2.29	0.009
Only DM				1.25	0.67–2.32	0.487				1.32	0.90–1.92	0.154
Only CKD				2.02	0.83–4.94	0.123				1.64	0.90–2.98	0.108
DM + CKD				2.93	1.14–7.57	0.026				2.42	1.28–4.57	0.007
P for gender × diseases interaction				0.920						0.559		

CI confidence interval, *CKD* chronic kidney disease, *DM* diabetes mellitus, *HR* hazard ratio, *Ref* reference
[a]Adjusted for sex, age, comorbidities, etiology of cirrhosis, complications of cirrhosis, low income and urbanization
[b]Adjusted for age, comorbidities, etiology of cirrhosis, complications of cirrhosis, low income and urbanization

ESRD was associated with 1-year mortality (HR,1.50; 95 % CI, 1.18–1.91), but not a risk factor for 42-day mortality (HR,1.19; 95 % CI, 0.79–1.78) [5]. They implicated that the ESRD-related platelet dysfunction contributed higher EVB and mortality. In our study, we identified that CKD was independent prognostic factor for both 42-day and one-year mortality in cirrhotic patients with first presentation of EVB.

Coexisting DM and CKD are important prognostic factors in cirrhotic patients regardless of the causes of liver diseases. CKD and DM have many long-term complications such as increased immunocompromised status, as well as increased risk of metabolic disorders and cardiovascular events [40–42]. DM increases portal blood flow secondary to fluctuating blood sugar levels leading to an increase in portal pressure [35, 43]. There is increased bleeding tendency due to uremic platelet dysfunction, use of antiplatelet agents, and anticoagulants [11, 12]. In addition, usage of aspirin increases the occurrence of EVB in cirrhotic patients [13]. These complications could indicate why the 42-day and 1-year overall mortality was higher among the coexisting DM and CKD than DM or CKD individuals. A gender-stratified comparative analysis indicated that coexisting DM and CKD exhibited mortality risk in both genders.

In a cohort study with patients with chronic hepatitis C (CHC), patients with new-onset diabetes subsequently were found to have an increased risk of developing cirrhosis, or decompensation in those with established cirrhosis [44]. Persico et al. retrospectively evaluated 852 consecutive patients (726 CHC and 126 chronic hepatitis B) who had undergone liver biopsy [45]. Liver fibrosis (odds ratio [OR], 4.70; 95%CI, 2.75–8.03) was independent risk factors for the presence of significant steatosis (>30 %) in patient with CHC. Camma et al. analyzed 104 patients with CHC cirrhosis (Child-Pugh class A) receiving upper gastrointestinal endoscopy [16]. They found a high homeostasis model assessment score (OR, 1.37; 95 % CI, 1.01–1.86) as an independent predictor of the presence of esophageal varices. Cirrhosis, per se, independently by the viral etiology, may be associated with the development of insulin resistance and diabetes.

Although HCV and HBV infection were not associated with increased risk of mortality, they have been reported to be associated with renal diseases. HCV is also associated with extra-hepatic diseases, including various types of glomerulonephritis, even in the absence of cirrhosis [46]. A high baseline HCV viral load was an independent predictor of CKD [47]. Soma et al. indicated that HCV infection leads to a rapid decline in the renal function of patients with diabetic nephropathy [48]. HBV-related renal injury is associated with the deposition of immune complexes of HBV antigens and host antibodies [49]. Untreated chronic HBV infection is also associated with increased risk of CKD [50].

Hepatic steatosis or fatty liver is characterized by lipid accumulation within the cytoplasm of hepatocytes, and includes a spectrum of liver disease from a benign simple steatosis, steatohepatitis, to fibrosis [51]. In Taiwan, the prevalence of non-alcoholic fatty liver disease (NAFLD) is about 11.5 % [52], and the rates are higher in subgroups, from 66.4 % in healthy taxi drivers [53] to 80 % in obese individuals enrolled in weight reduction programs [54]. In a cross-sectional community study that included 11.4 % (372/3,260) individuals with elevated alanine aminotransferase (ALT), NAFLD was the most common cause of ALT elevation with a prevalence of 33.6 %, and followed by HBV (28.5 %), unexplained cause (21.8 %), HCV (13.2 %), both HBV and HCV (2.2 %), and excess alcohol consumption (0.8 %) [55]. Approximately 1 % of patients with NAFLD develop cirrhosis [56], where as in non-alcoholic steatohepatitis (NASH), the estimated figure is up to 20 % [57]. However, NAFLD was not available in the NHIRD.

Our data included all EVB patients hospitalized in a variety of hospitals in Taiwan; hence, selection bias was minimized. There were some significant limitations to this study. First, the basic laboratory data (e.g. prothrombin times, bilirubin, creatinine, and albumin levels) were not available. For the severity of cirrhosis, Child-Pugh or Model of End-Stage Liver Disease (MELD) scores could not be calculated using the ICD-9 coding in the database. We put previous episodes of decompensation that required hospitalization, such as asictes, hepatic encephalopathy, and SBP into multiple variable analyses. This information could obviate the important limitation of not having laboratory data to calculate the MELD score. Second, the exact cases of NAFLD-related cirrhosis were not available. Data on NAFLD-related cirrhosis are limited and only one case report has been reported in Taiwan [58]. Third, the diagnoses of EVB and other comorbidities were based on ICD-9 codes, and misclassification could be possible. We included cirrhotic patients who were hospitalized with first presentation of EVB and received esophageal variceal ligation or sclerotherapy to minimize ascertainment bias.

Conclusions

This study provides evidence that coexistence of CKD and DM has a higher impact on 42-day and one-year mortality than DM or CKD individually.

Abbreviations
ALT: alanine aminotransferase; CHC: chronic hepatitis C; CI: confidence interval; CKD: chronic kidney disease; COPD: chronic obstructive pulmonary disease; DM: diabetes mellitus; ESRD: end-stage renal disease;

EVB: esophageal variceal bleeding; HBV: hepatitis B virus; HCC: hepatocellular carcinoma; HCV: hepatitis C virus; HR: hazard ratio; ICD-9-CM: International Classification of Diseases, Ninth Revision, Clinical Modification; LHID2005: Longitudinal Health Insurance Database 2005; MELD: Model of End-Stage Liver Disease; NAFLD: non-alcoholic fatty liver disease; NASH: non-alcoholic steatohepatitis; NHIRD: National Health Insurance Research Database; OR: odds ratio; SBP: spontaneous bacterial peritonitis; TB: pulmonary tuberculosis.

Competing interests
The authors declare that they have no competing interests.

Authors' contributions
The study was designed by CCL, ZHJ and JYH. JYH carried out data analysis, and CCL, ZHJ and ONN wrote the paper. All the authors had access to the data. All authors read and approved the final manuscript as submitted.

Acknowledgments
The authors acknowledge the National Health Research Institute of Taiwan for providing the NHIRD. The descriptions or conclusions herein do not represent the viewpoint of the Bureau.

References
1. D'Amico G, Garcia-Tsao G, Pagliaro L. Natural history and prognostic indicators of survival in cirrhosis: a systematic review of 118 studies. J Hepatol. 2006;44:217–31.
2. Yang CH, Chiu YC, Chen CH, Chen CH, Tsai MC, Chuah SK, et al. Diabetes mellitus is associated with gastroesophageal variceal bleeding in cirrhotic patients. Kaohsiung J Med Sci. 2014;30:515–20.
3. Augustin S, Muntaner L, Altamirano JT, Gonzalez A, Saperas E, Dot J, et al. Predicting early mortality after acute variceal hemorrhage based on classification and regression tree analysis. Clin Gastroenterol Hepatol. 2009;7:1347–54.
4. Kwon SY, Kim SS, Kwon OS, Kwon KA, Chung MG, Park DK, et al. Prognostic significance of glycaemic control in patients with HBV and HCV-related cirrhosis and diabetes mellitus. Diabet Med. 2005;22:1530–5.
5. Hung TH, Tseng CW, Tseng KC, Hsieh YH, Tsai CC, Tsai CC. Is end stage renal disease a risk factor for the mortality of cirrhotic patients with esophageal variceal bleeding? Hepatogastroenterol. 2014;61:1871–5.
6. del Olmo JA, Pena A, Serra MA, Wassel AH, Benages A, Rodrigo JM. Predictors of morbidity and mortality after the first episode of upper gastrointestinal bleeding in liver cirrhosis. J Hepatol. 2000;32:19–24.
7. Cardenas A, Gines P, Uriz J, Bessa X, Salmeron JM, Mas A, et al. Renal failure after upper gastrointestinal bleeding in cirrhosis: incidence, clinical course, predictive factors, and short-term prognosis. Hepatology. 2001;34:671–6.
8. Pesanti EL. Immunologic defects and vaccination in patients with chronic renal failure. Infect Dis Clin North Am. 2001;15(3):813–32.
9. Kurata M, Tsuboi A, Takeuchi M, Fukuo K, Kazumi T. Association of Metabolic Syndrome with Chronic Kidney Disease in Elderly Japanese Women: Comparison by Estimation of Glomerular Filtration Rate from Creatinine, Cystatin C, and Both. Metab Syndr Relat Disord. 2015; [Epub ahead of print]
10. Holzmann MJ, Carlsson AC, Hammar N, Ivert T, Walldius G, Jungner I, et al. Chronic kidney disease and 10-year risk of cardiovascular death. Eur J Prev Cardiol. 2015; [Epub ahead of print]
11. Escolar G, Diaz-Ricart M, Cases A. Uremic platelet dysfunction: past and present. Curr Hematol Rep. 2005;4:359–67.
12. Kringen MK, Narum S, Lygren I, Seljeflot I, Sandset PM, Troseid AM, et al. Reduced platelet function and role of drugs in acute gastrointestinal bleeding. Basic Clin Pharmacol Toxicol. 2011;108:194–201.
13. De Ledinghen V, Heresbach D, Fourdan O, Bernard P, Liebaert-Bories MP, Nousbaum JB, et al. Anti-inflammatory drugs and variceal bleeding: a case-control study. Gut. 1999;44:270–3.
14. Trombetta M, Spiazzi G, Zoppini G, Muggeo M. Review article: type 2 diabetes and chronic liver disease in the Verona diabetes study. Aliment Pharmacol Ther. 2005;22 Suppl 2:24–7.
15. Francque S, Verrijken A, Mertens I, Hubens G, Van Marck E, Pelckmans P, et al. Visceral adiposity and insulin resistance are independent predictors of the presence of non-cirrhotic NAFLD-related portal hypertension. Int J Obes. 2011;35:270–8.

16. Camma C, Petta S, Di Marco V, Bronte F, Ciminnisi S, Licata G, et al. Insulin resistance is a risk factor for esophageal varices in hepatitis C virus cirrhosis. Hepatology. 2009;49:195–203.

17. Collins AJ, Foley RN, Chavers B, Gilbertson D, Herzog C, Johansen K, et al. United states renal data system 2011 annual data report: atlas of chronic kidney disease & end-stage renal disease in the United States. Am J Kidney Dis. 2012;59(1 Suppl 1):A7, e1–420.

18. Cheng JS, Tsai WC, Lin CL, Chen L, Lang HC, Hsieh HM, et al. Trend and factors associated with healthcare use and costs in type 2 diabetes mellitus: a decade experience of a universal health insurance program. Med Care. 2015;53:116–24.

19. Chan TC, Fan I, Liu MS, Su MD, Chiang PH. Addressing health disparities in chronic kidney disease. Int J Environ Res Public Health. 2014;11:12848–65.

20. Kuo RN, Lai MS. Comparison of Rx-defined morbidity groups and diagnosis-based risk adjusters for predicting healthcare costs in Taiwan. BMC Health Serv Res. 2010;10:126.

21. Liao YH, Lin CC, Li TC, Lin JG. Utilization pattern of traditional Chinese medicine for liver cancer patients in Taiwan. BMC Complement Altern Med. 2012;12:146.

22. Liu ME, Tsai SJ, Chang WC, Hsu CH, Lu T, Hung KS, et al. Population-based 5-year follow-up study in Taiwan of dementia and risk of stroke. PLoS One. 2013;8:e61771.

23. Lee YT, Nfor ON, Tantoh DM, Huang JY, Ku WY, Hsu SY, et al. Herpes zoster as a predictor of HIV infection in Taiwan: a population-based study. PLoS One. 2015;10:e0142254.

24. National Health Insurance Research Database, Taiwan. http://nhird.nhri.org.tw/en/Data_Subsets.html. Accessed 31 Oct 2015.

25. Perz JF, Armstrong GL, Farrington LA, Hutin YJ, Bell BP. The contributions of hepatitis B virus and hepatitis C virus infections to cirrhosis and primary liver cancer worldwide. J Hepatol. 2006;45(4):529–38.

26. Chen CH, Yang PM, Huang GT, Lee HS, Sung JL, Sheu JC. Estimation of seroprevalence of hepatitis B virus and hepatitis C virus in Taiwan from a large-scale survey of free hepatitis screening participants. J Formos Med Assoc. 2007;106:148–55.

27. Tsai JF, Chang WY, Jeng JE, Ho MS, Lin ZY, Tsai JH. Hepatitis B and C virus infection as risk factors for liver cirrhosis and cirrhotic hepatocellular carcinoma: a case-control study. Liver. 1994;14:98–102.

28. Kao JH. Hepatitis B, vaccination and prevention of hepatocellular carcinoma. Best Pract Res Clin Gastroenterol. 2015;29:907–17.

29. Mayor S. Liver cancer in Taiwan falls after universal hepatitis B vaccination. BMJ. 1997;315:7.

30. Fortune B, Garcia-Tsao G. Current management strategies for acute esophageal variceal hemorrhage. Curr Hepatol Rep. 2014;13:35–42.

31. Chang TT, Liaw YF, Wu SS, Schiff E, Han KH, Lai CL, et al. Long-term entecavir therapy results in the reversal of fibrosis/cirrhosis and continued histological improvement in patients with chronic hepatitis B. Hepatology. 2010;52:886–3.

32. Carbonell N, Pauwels A, Serfaty L, Fourdan O, Levy VG, Poupon R. Improved survival after variceal bleeding in patients with cirrhosis over the past two decades. Hepatology. 2004;40:652–9.

33. Garcia-Compean D, Jaquez-Quintana JO, Maldonado-Garza H. Hepatogenous diabetes. Current views of an ancient problem. Ann Hepatol. 2009;8:13–20.

34. Majid S, Azam Z, Shah HA, Salih M, Hamid S, Abid S, et al. Factors determining the clinical outcome of acute variceal bleed in cirrhotic patients. Indian J Gastroenterol. 2009;28:93–5.

35. Pugliese D, Lee SS, Koshy A, Cerini R, Ozier Y, Lebrec D. Systemic and splanchnic hemodynamic effects of intravenous hypertonic glucose in patients with cirrhosis. Hepatology. 1988;8:643–6.

36. Jeon HK, Kim MY, Baik SK, Park HJ, Choi H, Park SY, et al. Hepatogenous diabetes in cirrhosis is related to portal pressure and variceal hemorrhage. Dig Dis Sci. 2013;58:3335–41.

37. Hung TH, Tsai CC, Hsieh YH, Tsai CC, Tseng CW, Tsai JJ. Effect of renal impairment on mortality of patients with cirrhosis and spontaneous bacterial peritonitis. Clin Gastroenterol Hepatol. 2012;10:677–81.

38. Verkade MA, van Druningen CJ, Vaessen LM, Hesselink DA, Weimar W, Betjes MG. Functional impairment of monocyte-derived dendritic cells in patients with severe chronic kidney disease. Nephrol Dial Transplant. 2007;22:128–38.

39. Hung TH, Tseng CW, Tseng KC, Hsieh YH, Tsai CC, Tsai CC. Effect of renal function impairment on the mortality of cirrhotic patients with hepatic

encephalopathy: a population-based 3-year follow-up study. Medicine. 2014;93:e79.

40. Saito I. Epidemiological evidence of type 2 diabetes mellitus, metabolic syndrome, and cardiovascular disease in Japan. Circ J. 2012;76:1066–73.

41. Koh GC, Peacock SJ, van der Poll T, Wiersinga WJ. The impact of diabetes on the pathogenesis of sepsis. Eur J Clin Microbiol Infect Dis. 2012;31:379–88.

42. Kato S, Chmielewski M, Honda H, Pecoits-Filho R, Matsuo S, Yuzawa Y, et al. Aspects of immune dysfunction in end-stage renal disease. Clin J Am Soc Nephrol. 2008;3:1526–33.

43. Moreau R, Chagneau C, Heller J, Chevenne D, Langlet P, Deltenre P, et al. Hemodynamic, metabolic and hormonal responses to oral glibenclamide in patients with cirrhosis receiving glucose. Scand J Gastroenterol. 2001;36:303–8.

44. Huang YW, Yang SS, Fu SC, Wang TC, Hsu CK, Chen DS, et al. Increased risk of cirrhosis and its decompensation in chronic hepatitis C patients with new-onset diabetes: a nationwide cohort study. Hepatology. 2014;60:807–14.

45. Persico M, Masarone M, La Mura V, Persico E, Moschella F, Svelto M, et al. Clinical expression of insulin resistance in hepatitis C and B virus-related chronic hepatitis: differences and similarities. World J Gastroenterol. 2009;15:462–6.

46. Arase Y, Ikeda K, Murashima N, Chayama K, Tsubota A, Koida I, et al. Glomerulonephritis in autopsy cases with hepatitis C virus infection. Intern Med. 1998;37:836–40.

47. Satapathy SK, Lingisetty CS, Williams S. Higher prevalence of chronic kidney disease and shorter renal survival in patients with chronic hepatitis C virus infection. Hepatol Int. 2012;6:369–78.

48. Soma J, Saito T, Taguma Y, Chiba S, Sato H, Sugimura K, et al. High prevalence and adverse effect of hepatitis C virus infection in type II diabetic-related nephropathy. J Am Soc Nephrol. 2000;11:690–9.

49. Bhimma R, Coovadia HM. Hepatitis B virus-associated nephropathy. Am J Nephrol. 2004;24:198–211.

50. Chen YC, Su YC, Li CY, Hung SK. 13-year nationwide cohort study of chronic kidney disease risk among treatment-naive patients with chronic hepatitis B in Taiwan. BMC Nephrol. 2015;16:110.

51. Serfaty L, Lemoine M. Definition and natural history of metabolic steatosis: clinical aspects of NAFLD, NASH and cirrhosis. Diabetes Metab. 2008;34:634–7.

52. Chen CH, Huang MH, Yang JC, Nien CK, Yang CC, Yeh YH, et al. Prevalence and risk factors of nonalcoholic fatty liver disease in an adult population of taiwan: metabolic significance of nonalcoholic fatty liver disease in nonobese adults. J Clin Gastroenterol. 2006;40:745–52.

53. Tung TH, Chang TH, Chiu WH, Lin TH, Shih HC, Chang MH, et al. Clinical correlation of nonalcoholic fatty liver disease in a Chinese taxi drivers population in Taiwan: Experience at a teaching hospital. BMC Res Notes. 2011;4:315.

54. Hsiao TJ, Chen JC, Wang JD. Insulin resistance and ferritin as major determinants of nonalcoholic fatty liver disease in apparently healthy obese patients. Int J Obes Relat Metab Disord. 2004;28:167–72.

55. Chen CH, Huang MH, Yang JC, Nien CK, Yang CC, Yeh YH, et al. Prevalence and etiology of elevated serum alanine aminotransferase level in an adult population in Taiwan. J Gastroenterol Hepatol. 2007;22:1482–9.

56. Dam-Larsen S, Franzmann M, Andersen IB, Christoffersen P, Jensen LB, Sorensen TI, et al. Long term prognosis of fatty liver: risk of chronic liver disease and death. Gut. 2004;53:750–5.

57. McCullough AJ. The clinical features, diagnosis and natural history of nonalcoholic fatty liver disease. Clin Liver Dis. 2004;8:521–33.

58. Tang CP, Huang YS, Tsay SH, Chang FY, Lee SD. Nonalcoholic fatty liver disease manifesting esophageal variceal bleeding. J Chin Med Assoc. 2006;69:175–8.

Permissions

The contributors of this book come from diverse backgrounds, making this book a truly international effort. This book will bring forth new frontiers with its revolutionizing research information and detailed analysis of the nascent developments around the world.

We would like to thank all the contributing authors for lending their expertise to make the book truly unique. They have played a crucial role in the development of this book. Without their invaluable contributions this book wouldn't have been possible. They have made vital efforts to compile up to date information on the varied aspects of this subject to make this book a valuable addition to the collection of many professionals and students.

This book was conceptualized with the vision of imparting up-to-date information and advanced data in this field. To ensure the same, a matchless editorial board was set up. Every individual on the board went through rigorous rounds of assessment to prove their worth. After which they invested a large part of their time researching and compiling the most relevant data for our readers.

The editorial board has been involved in producing this book since its inception. They have spent rigorous hours researching and exploring the diverse topics which have resulted in the successful publishing of this book. They have passed on their knowledge of decades through this book. To expedite this challenging task, the publisher supported the team at every step. A small team of assistant editors was also appointed to further simplify the editing procedure and attain best results for the readers.

Apart from the editorial board, the designing team has also invested a significant amount of their time in understanding the subject and creating the most relevant covers. They scrutinized every image to scout for the most suitable representation of the subject and create an appropriate cover for the book.

The publishing team has been an ardent support to the editorial, designing and production team. Their endless efforts to recruit the best for this project, has resulted in the accomplishment of this book. They are a veteran in the field of academics and their pool of knowledge is as vast as their experience in printing. Their expertise and guidance has proved useful at every step. Their uncompromising quality standards have made this book an exceptional effort. Their encouragement from time to time has been an inspiration for everyone.

The publisher and the editorial board hope that this book will prove to be a valuable piece of knowledge for researchers, students, practitioners and scholars across the globe.

List of Contributors

Wenhui Qiao
Department of General Surgery, First Hospital of Lanzhou University, Lanzhou, China

Feng Yu
Department of Hepatobiliary Surgery, No.101 Hospital of CPLA, Wuxi, China

Lupeng Wu, Bin Li and Yanming Zhou
Department of Hepato-Biliary-Pancreato-Vascular Surgery, First affiliated Hospital of Xiamen University, Xiamen, China

Folasade P. May
Division of Digestive Diseases, Department of Medicine, David Geffen School of Medicine at UCLA, 650 Charles E. Young Drive; Suite A2-125, Los Angeles, CA 90095-6900, USA
Department of Health Policy and Management, UCLA Fielding School of Public Health, Los Angeles, CA, USA

Vineet S. Rolston
Department of Medicine, Cedars-Sinai Medical Center, Los Angeles, CA, USA

Elliot B. Tapper
Division of Gastroenterology, Beth Israel Deaconess Medical Center, Harvard Medical School, Boston, MA, USA

Ashwini Lakshmanan
Department of Pediatrics, Center for Fetal and Neonatal Medicine, Children's Hospital Los Angeles, Keck School of Medicine, University of Southern California, Los Angeles, CA, USA

Sammy Saab
Division of Digestive Diseases, Department of Medicine, David Geffen School of Medicine at UCLA, 650 Charles E. Young Drive; Suite A2-125, Los Angeles, CA 90095-6900, USA
Department of Surgery, David Geffen School of Medicine at UCLA, Los Angeles, CA, USA

Vinay Sundaram
Division of Gastroenterology and Hepatology and Comprehensive Transplant Center, Cedars-Sinai Medical Center, Los Angeles, CA, USA

Hyun Ju Min, Ja Yun Choi, Hyun Chin Cho, Hong Jun Kim and Chang Yoon Ha
Department of Internal Medicine, Gyeongsang National University School of Medicine and Gyeongsang National University Hospital, 15, Jinju-daero 816 beon-gil, Jinju, Gyeongnam 52727, Republic of Korea

Tae Hyo Kim and Ok-Jae Lee
Department of Internal Medicine, Gyeongsang National University School of Medicine and Gyeongsang National University Hospital, 15, Jinju-daero 816 beon-gil, Jinju, Gyeongnam 52727, Republic of Korea
Institute of Health Sciences, Gyeongsang National University, Jinju, Republic of Korea

Hyun Jin Kim
Department of Internal Medicine, Gyeongsang National University School of Medicine and Gyeongsang National University Hospital, 15, Jinju-daero 816 beon-gil, Jinju, Gyeongnam 52727, Republic of Korea
Institute of Health Sciences, Gyeongsang National University, Jinju, Republic of Korea
Department of Internal Medicine, Gyeongsang National University School of Medicine and Gyeongsang National University Changwon Hospital, Jinju, Republic of Korea

Jin Hyun Kim
Biomedical Research Institute, Gyeongsang National University Hospital, Jinju, Republic of Korea

Sang Soo Lee, Jin Joo Kim and Jae Min Lee
Department of Internal Medicine, Gyeongsang National University School of Medicine and Gyeongsang National University Hospital, 15, Jinju-daero 816 beon-gil, Jinju, Gyeongnam 52727, Republic of Korea
Department of Internal Medicine, Gyeongsang National University School of Medicine and Gyeongsang National University Changwon Hospital, Jinju, Republic of Korea

Norio Akuta, Yusuke Kawamura, Fumitaka Suzuki, Satoshi Saitoh, Yasuji Arase, Shunichiro Fujiyama, Hitomi Sezaki, Tetsuya Hosaka, Masahiro Kobayashi, Yoshiyuki Suzuki, Kenji Ikeda and Hiromitsu Kumada
Department of Hepatology, Toranomon Hospital and Okinaka Memorial Institute for Medical Research, 2-2-2 Toranomon, Minato-ku, Tokyo 105-0001, Japan

Mariko Kobayashi
Liver Research Laboratory, Toranomon Hospital, Tokyo, Japan

Jian Kang, Yinhua Zhang, Deqiang Ma, Changzheng Ke and Yue Chen
Department of Infectious Diseases, Taihe Hospital, Hubei University of Medicine, Shiyan, China

Ping Liu
Department of Infectious Diseases, Taihe Hospital, Hubei University of Medicine, Shiyan, China
Department of Infectious Diseases, Renmin Hospital of Wuhan University, Zhangzhidong Road. 99, 430060 Wuhan, China

Zhongji Meng
Department of Infectious Diseases, Taihe Hospital, Hubei University of Medicine, Shiyan, China
Institute of Biomedicine, Taihe Hospital, Hubei University of Medicine, Shiyan, China

Zhiqiang Wei
Institute of Biomedicine, Taihe Hospital, Hubei University of Medicine, Shiyan, China

Yonghong Zhang
Institute of Wudang Chinese Medicine, Taihe Hospital, Hubei University of Medicine, Shiyan, China

Jie Luo
Department of Neurology, Taihe Hospital, Hubei University of Medicine, South Renmin Road. 32, 442000 Shiyan, Hubei, China

Zuojiong Gong
Department of Infectious Diseases, Renmin Hospital of Wuhan University, Zhangzhidong Road. 99, 430060 Wuhan, China

Hella Wobser and Agnetha Gunesch
Department of Internal Medicine and Gastroenterology, University Hospital of Regensburg, Regensburg 93042, Germany

Frank Klebl
Department of Internal Medicine and Gastroenterology, University Hospital of Regensburg, Regensburg 93042, Germany
Praxiszentrum Alte Mälzerei, Regensburg, Germany

Bensong Duan and Jiangfeng Hu
Department of Gastroenterology, Tongji Hospital, Tongji University School of Medicine, Shanghai, China

Tongyangzi Zhang
Department of Respiration, Tongji Hospital, Tongji University School of Medicine, Shanghai, China

Xu Luo, Yi Zhou and Liang Zhu
Department of Gastroenterology, Changzheng Hospital, Second Military Medical University, Shanghai, China.

Shun Liu
Department of Epidemiology, School of Public Health, Guangxi Medical University, Nanning, Guangxi, China

Cheng Wu
Digestive Endoscopic Center, Department of Gastroenterology, South Building General Hospital of PLA, Beijing, China.

Wenxiang Liu and Chao Chen
Department of Gastroenterology, First Affiliated Hospital of Chinese PLA General Hospital, Beijing, China

Hengjun Gao
National Engineering Center for Biochip at Shanghai, Shanghai, China
Department of Gastroenterology, Institute of Digestive Diseases, Tongji University School of Medicine, Shanghai, China

Catherine Atkin, Philip Earwaker, Pankaj Punia and Yuk Ting Ma
The Cancer Centre, University Hospitals Birmingham NHS Foundation Trust
Edgbaston, Birmingham B15 2TH, UK

Arvind Pallan
Department of Radiology, University Hospitals Birmingham NHS Foundation Trust, Edgbaston, Birmingham B15 2TH, UK

Shishir Shetty
The Liver Unit, University Hospitals Birmingham NHS Foundation Trust, Edgbaston, Birmingham B15 2TH, UK

Jia-Qi Li, Jing-Yu Gong, Mei-Hong Zhang and Wei-Sha Luan
Department of Pediatrics, Jinshan Hospital of Fudan University, Shanghai
201508, China

Yi-Ling Qiu, Li-Min Dou, Yi Lu and Jian-She Wang
The Center for Pediatric Liver Diseases, Children's Hospital of Fudan University, Shanghai 201102, China

A. S. Knisely
Institut für Pathologie, Medizinische Universität Graz, Auenbruggerplatz 25, A-8036 Graz, Austria

Jun Zhang, Jia Fan, Chongming Zhou and Yanyu Qi
Department of Oncology, The third people's hospital of Chengdu, Chengdu 610031, China

Yasushi Honda, Takaomi Kessoku, Takashi Kobayashi, Takayuki Kato, Yuji Ogawa, Wataru Tomeno, Kento Imajo, Koji Fujita, Masato Yoneda, Satoru Saito and Atsushi Nakajima
Department of Gastroenterology and Hepatology, Yokohama City University Graduate School of Medicine, Yokohama, Japan

Yoshio Sumida
Division of Hepatology and Pancreatology, Department of Internal Medicine, Aichi Medical University, Aichi, Japan

Koshi Kataoka, Masataka Taguri and Takeharu Yamanaka
Department of Biostatistics, Yokohama City University Graduate School of Medicine, Yokohama, Japan

Yuya Seko and Yoshito Itoh
Department of Gastroenterology and Hepatology, Kyoto Prefectural University of Medicine, Kyoto, Japan

Saiyu Tanaka
Center for Digestive and Liver Diseases, Nara City Hospital, Nara, Japan

Masafumi Ono
Department of Gastroenterology and Hepatology, Kochi Medical School, Kochi, Japan

Satoshi Oeda and Yuichiro Eguchi
Liver Center, Saga University Hospital, Saga, Japan

Wataru Aoi
Division of Applied Life Sciences, Graduate School of Life and Environmental Sciences, Kyoto Prefectural University, Kyoto, Japan

Kenji Sato
Division of Applied Biosciences, Graduate School of Agriculture, Kyoto University, Kyoto, Japan

Shunichiro Fujiyama, Satoshi Saitoh, Yusuke Kawamura, Hitomi Sezaki, Tetsuya Hosaka, Norio Akuta, Masahiro Kobayashi, Yoshiyuki Suzuki, Fumitaka Suzuki, Yasuji Arase, Kenji Ikeda and Hiromitsu Kumada
Department of Hepatology, Toranomon Hospital, Toranomon 2-2-2, Minato-ku, Tokyo 105-8470, Japan

Siriwardana Rohan Chaminda, Thilakarathne Suchintha, Gunathilake Mahen Bhagya and Liyanage Chandika Anuruddha Habarakada
Department of surgery, Faculty of Medicine, University of Kelaniya Sri Lanka, Kelaniya, Sri Lanka

Niriella Madunil Anuk and De Silva Hithadurage Janaka
Department of medicine, Faculty of Medicine, University of Kelaniya Sri Lanka, Kelaniya, Sri Lanka

Dassanayake Anuradha Supun
Department of pharmacology, Faculty of Medicine, University of Kelaniya Sri Lanka, Kelaniya, Sri Lanka

Shreena Shakya, Anjeela Bhetwal, Puspa Raj Khanal, Roshan Pandit and Jyotsna Shakya
Department of Laboratory Medicine, Manmohan Memorial Institute of Health Sciences, Kathmandu, Nepal

Bashu Dev Pardhe
Department of Laboratory Medicine, Manmohan
Memorial Institute of Health Sciences, Kathmandu,
Nepal
Department of Health Science, National Open
College, Sanepa, Lalitpur, Nepal

Jennifer Mathias
Department of Health Science, National Open
College, Sanepa, Lalitpur, Nepal

Hari Om Joshi
Department of Radiology, Bhaktapur District
Hospital, Bhaktapur, Nepal

Sujan Babu Marahatta
Department of Public Health, Manmohan Memorial
Institute of Health Sciences, Kathmandu, Nepal

Lin Li and Wenzhuo Zhao
Department of Gastroenterology, Tangdu Hospital,
Military Medical University of PLA Airforce (Fourth
Military Medical University), 1 Xinsi Road, Xi'an
710038, China

Mengmeng Wang
Department of Drug and Equipment, Aeromedicine
Identification and Training Centre of Air Force,
Lintong District, Xi'an, China

Jie Hu and Enxin Wang
Department of Liver Disease and Digestive
Interventional Radiology, Xijing
Hospital of Digestive Diseases, Military Medical
University of PLA Airforce
(Fourth Military Medical University), Xi'an, China

Yan Zhao
Department of Gastroenterology, First Affiliated
Hospital of Xi'an Jiaotong University, 277 West
Yanta Road, Xi'an 710061, China

Lei Liu
Department of Gastroenterology, Tangdu Hospital,
Military Medical University of PLA Airforce (Fourth
Military Medical University), 1 Xinsi Road, Xi'an
710038, China
Cell Engineering Research Center and Department
of Cell Biology, State Key Laboratory of Cancer
Biology, Military Medical University of PLA
Airforce), Xi'an, China

Yan Wang, Ya Li and Feng Xu
Department of Gastroenterology, The First
Affiliated Hospital of Zhengzhou University, 1
Jianshe Donglu, Zhengzhou 450052, Henan, China

Dan Qiao
Department of Zhengzhou Center for Disease
Control and Prevention, Zhengzhou, China

Huiyong Wu and Jianjun Han
Department of Intervention, Shandong Tumor
Hospital Affiliated to Shandong University, Jinan
250117, China

Wei Zhao
Department of Radiotherapy, Shandong Tumor
Hospital Affiliated to Shandong University, Jinan
250117, China

Jianbo Zhang
Department of pathology, Shandong Tumor
Hospital Affiliated to Shandong University, Jinan
250117, China

Shuguang Liu
Department of Thoracic Oncology Surgery,
Shandong Tumor Hospital Affiliated to Shandong
University, No. 440, Jiyan Road, Jinan 250117, China

Jian Yang, Bin Yan, Lihong Yang and Jie Zheng
Clinical Research Center, the First Affiliated
Hospital, Xi'an Jiaotong University, Xi'an 710061,
People's Republic of China

Huimin Li, Yajuan Fan and Xiancang Ma
Department of Psychiatry, the First Affiliated
Hospital, Xi'an Jiaotong University, No.277 Yanta
West Road, Yanta District, Xi'an 710061, People's
Republic of China

Feng Zhu
Center for Translational Medicine, the First
Affiliated Hospital, Xi'an Jiaotong
University, Xi'an 710061, People's Republic of
China

**Jing-Hua Li, Ning Zhu, Ying-Bin Min, Xiang-
Zhou Shi, Yun-You Duan and Yi-Lin Yang**
Department of Ultrasound Diagnosis, Tangdu
Hospital, Fourth Military Medical University, Xi'an
710038, Shaanxi Province, China

Kun-Ming Chan, Chun-Yi Tsai, Chun-Nan Yeh, Ta-Sen Yeh, Wei-Chen Lee, Yi-Yin Jan and Miin-Fu Chen
Department of General Surgery, Chang Gung Memorial Hospital at Linkou, Chang Gung University College of Medicine, 5 Fu-Hsing Street, Kwei-Shan District, Taoyuan City 33305, Taiwan

Chuan-Mo Lee, Tsung-Hui Hu, Sheng-Nan Lu, Jing-Houng Wang, Chao-Hung Hung, Chien-Hung Chen and Yi-Hao Yen
Division of Hepatogastroenterology, Department of Internal Medicine, Kaohsiung Chang Gung Memorial Hospital, 123 Ta Pei Road, Niao Sung Dist. 833, Kaohsiung City, Taiwan
School of Medicine, College of Medicine, Chang Gung University, Taoyuan, Taiwan

Zobair M. Younossi
Center for Liver Diseases, Inova Fairfax Hospital, Falls Church, VA, USA
Center for Outcomes Research in Liver Diseases, Washington, DC, USA
Betty and Guy Beatty Center for Integrated Research, Claude Moore Health Education and Research Building, 3300 Gallows Road, Falls Church, VA 22042, USA

Fatema Nader, Sharon Hunt, Andrei Racila and Maria Stepanova
Center for Outcomes Research in Liver Diseases, Washington, DC, USA

Louis L. LaLuna
Digestive Disease Associates, Wyomissing, PA, USA

John J. Santoro
AGA Clinical Research Associates, LLC, Egg Harbor Township, NJ, USA

Flavia Mendes
GastroHealth, Miami, FL, USA

Victor Araya
Central Bucks Specialists, Gastroenterology, Doylestown, PA, USA

Natarajan Ravendhran
Digestive Diseases Associates, Catonsville, MD, USA

Lisa Pedicone and Idania Lio
Cantara Clinical Solutions, LLC, Morristown, NJ, USA

Hendrik Vilstrup
Department of Hepatology and Gastroenterology, Aarhus University Hospital, Nørrebrogade 44, DK-8000 Aarhus, Denmark

Peter Jepsen
Department of Hepatology and Gastroenterology, Aarhus University Hospital, Nørrebrogade 44, DK-8000 Aarhus, Denmark
Department of Clinical Epidemiology, Aarhus University Hospital, Aarhus, Denmark

Jakob Christensen
Department of Neurology, Aarhus University Hospital, Aarhus, Denmark

Karin Weissenborn
Department of Neurology, Hannover Medical School, Hannover, Germany

Hugh Watson
Sanofi Aventis R&D, Paris, France

Zhi-Hong Jian, Jing-Yang Huang and Oswald Ndi Nfor
Department of Public Health and Institute of Public Health, Chung Shan
Medical University, Taichung City, Taiwan

Chia-Chi Lung
Department of Public Health and Institute of Public Health, Chung Shan Medical University, Taichung City, Taiwan
Department of Family and Community Medicine, Chung Shan Medical University Hospital, Taichung City, Taiwan

Index

www.ingramcontent.com/pod-product-compliance
Lightning Source LLC
Chambersburg PA
CBHW082013190326
41458CB00010B/3176